MENTAL HEALTH INFORMATICS

Mental Health Informatics

Ardis Hanson, PhD, ML3
COLLEGE OF BEHAVIORAL & COMMUNITY SCIENCES
UNIVERSITY OF SOUTH FLORIDA
TAMPA, FL

Bruce Lubotsky Levin, DrPH, MPH
GRADUATE STUDIES IN BEHAVIORAL HEALTH PROGRAM
DEPARTMENT OF COMMUNITY & FAMILY HEALTH
COLLEGE OF PUBLIC HEALTH AND
DEPARTMENT OF CHILD & FAMILY STUDIES
COLLEGE OF BEHAVIORAL & COMMUNITY SCIENCES
UNIVERSITY OF SOUTH FLORIDA
TAMPA, FL

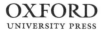

OXFORD
UNIVERSITY PRESS

OXFORD
UNIVERSITY PRESS

Oxford University Press is a department of the University of Oxford.
It furthers the University's objective of excellence in research, scholarship,
and education by publishing worldwide.

Oxford   New York
Auckland   Cape Town   Dar es Salaam   Hong Kong   Karachi
Kuala Lumpur   Madrid   Melbourne   Mexico City   Nairobi
New Delhi   Shanghai   Taipei   Toronto

With offices in
Argentina   Austria   Brazil   Chile   Czech Republic   France   Greece
Guatemala   Hungary   Italy   Japan   Poland   Portugal   Singapore
South Korea   Switzerland   Thailand   Turkey   Ukraine   Vietnam

Oxford is a registered trademark of Oxford University Press in the UK and certain other
countries.

Published by Oxford University Press, Inc.
198 Madison Avenue, New York, NY 10016
www.oup.com

Library of Congress Cataloging-in-Publication Data
Hanson, Ardis.
   Mental health informatics / Ardis Hanson, Bruce Lubotsky Levin.
   p.; cm.
   Includes bibliographical references and index.
   ISBN 978–0–19–518302–3 (hardcover: alk. paper)
I. Levin, Bruce Lubotsky.   II. Title.
[DNLM: 1. Medical Informatics.   2. Mental Health Services. WM 26.5]
LC Classification not assigned
610.28'5—dc23
2012010956

Ardis Hanson and Dr. Bruce Lubotsky Levin report no biomedical financial
interests or potential conflicts of interest.

9 8 7 6 5 4 3 2 1
Printed in the United States of America
on acid-free paper

Contents

Preface

INFORMATICS IS THE creative use of information and technologies in support of patient care, education, and research. Informatics deals with resources, devices, applications, and formalized methods for optimizing the storage, retrieval, and management of information for clinical problem solving and decision making.

More specifically, health informatics is an interdisciplinary field based upon literature in the computer and information sciences, the cognitive and decision sciences, the health sciences (including public health and epidemiology), the medical sciences, and the telecommunication sciences. Whether we are looking at e-health, m-health, or x-health (as in the still-unknown application), health informatics continues to develop new methods and techniques to enhance health care, academic and applied services research, and education. From our perspective, informatics technology ranges from the plain old telephone service (POTS) to high bandwidth applications, from a focus on individual care to administrative analyses to systems-wide public sector care.

Mental Health Informatics examines critical issues of how computers and information technology improve the organization, financing, and delivery of mental health services and services research. It combines a discussion of the core issues in informatics (including data and standards, management information systems, adoption, legal issues, and information strategies) together with research competencies, databases, globalization of information, and implications for policy and practice in mental health.

This book evolved from our experiences in teaching a graduate-level behavioral health course in mental health informatics at the University of South Florida (USF) College of Public Health and the College of Behavioral and Community Sciences. No single text provided an adequate knowledge base for our course. Other health and mental health informatics textbooks have examined mental health from a clinical perspective or have focused primarily on database design. As we taught the class, we realized that we lacked a definitive text that would address the structural knowledge necessary to understand how health information is used in decision making, public health programming, and outcomes assessment. Even more important, we needed a book that would provide a good overview of the complexity of health services research from an information perspective as well as the perspective of the secondary and tertiary data user.

This text presents a unique public health perspective of mental health informatics. The course blends the public health, mental health, services research, and library and information sciences perspectives of mental health informatics. We examine informatics from a wider behavioral health perspective, which encompasses the areas of alcohol, drug abuse, and mental health services. The text covers public sector (local, state, and federal government agencies) and private sector practice, as well as the practice, administrative, and educational aspects of behavioral health (defined as alcohol, drug abuse, and mental disorders viewed from a public health perspective).

Mental health includes elements of many other specialty fields, including medicine, the social and behavioral health sciences, criminal justice, social work, and rehabilitation. Public mental health care may be acute or long-term care, and it emphasizes a focus on a particular at-risk population. Mental health services are offered in hospitals, general and specialty providers' offices, community mental health centers, peer-run centers, religious organizations (pastoral care), academic health centers, jails and prisons, state and local government facilities, military and Veterans Administration medical centers, and private facilities. At the same time, users of data generated by mental health services include a wide range of stakeholders, including consumers, families, providers, payers, managed care organizations, state mental health authorities, federal agencies, administrators, researchers, policy makers, advocates, and criminal justice personnel.

In 2003, the New Freedom Commission on Mental Health made a number of recommendations to fundamentally transform the delivery of mental health services in the United States. Goal 6 from the New Freedom Commission on Mental Health specifically addressed technology to improve access to and coordination of mental health care. The use of technology has two major aims. The first aim addresses advancing research in the development of evidence-based practices to treat individuals with mental and substance use disorders, with the ultimate goal of preventing mental disorders and promoting recovery among individuals with mental illnesses. The second aim is the effective use of technology to maximize diffusion, early adoption, and effective implementation of efficacious and effective practices and to improve service provision and service utilization.

Technology is also relevant to workforce development issues in assuring that current and future practitioners have access to and utilize evidence-based services. In addition, technology is a critical component in developing the knowledge base in mental and substance use disorders, particularly in the areas of disparities, trauma, acute care, and long-term consequences of medications. Finally, integrated information technology (e.g., electronic health records) and communications infrastructure (e.g., telehealth networks) require substantial investments, but are critical to the effective delivery of mental health services.

Informatics also builds upon and links numerous other national initiatives, starting with the electronic health record (EHR). With the implementation of the EHR come new data standards that have changed in terms of what is measured, what is counted, what is assessed, and what the outcomes are to establish the quality and effectiveness of mental health services.

Tied closely to the EHR is the national health information infrastructure (NHII). Numerous governmental and nongovernmental organizations are involved in the development of the NHII within the United States, setting standards related to the architecture, content, storage, security, confidentiality, exchange, functionality, and communication of health and mental health information. Communication of health and mental health information addresses record formats, such as the continuity of care record (CCR) standard that is a longitudinal record of all of a patient's treatment trajectories, and the standardization of existing clinical vocabularies and messaging standards into an interoperable federal health data system.

The emergence of translational research in public health has pushed informatics to an even more prominent role in health and mental health services research as it seeks to integrate health information technology, electronic medical record systems, clinical trial management systems, clinical research informatics, statistical analyses, and data mining.

Telecommunication and information technology, including the Internet, holds enormous potential for transforming mental health services delivery systems in America. Central to the application of information science and technology to promote mental health and prevent mental disorders in at-risk populations is the establishment of an infrastructure to develop comprehensive integrated health surveillance and information systems that bridge programmatic boundaries within communities. Thus, there remains great potential for mental health informatics to play an important role in the integration of a variety of data (e.g., census, surveillance, and hospital) if more emphasis is placed upon updating national efforts to collect more current mental health and substance abuse data.

Mental Health Informatics offers an examination of contemporary issues that focuses on the innovative use of computers and information technology in support of patient care, education, and mental health services research and delivery. Fourteen chapters are divided into four main parts: (I) Introduction; (II) Standards and Implementation; (III) Competencies and Strategies; and (IV) Globalization and the Future.

Part I covers basic concepts, definitions, and the history of mental health informatics. It has been our experience that students had an understanding of either mental health or technology but not an integrative perspective of how informatics is used in mental health services, research, or policy.

Building upon the overview, Part II of the book provides an account of the development of a national electronic health record, the issues involved in developing data sets for a variety of uses within mental health organizations, current standards development, and the implications and future of the electronic health record in mental health. With a focus on decision making, operations management, cognitive support, and usability, we also discuss comparative effectiveness research, patient portals, and report cards as key components in mental health management information systems. Part II also explores the issues involved in the adoption and implementation of mental health information technology, including the nature of teamwork in health and mental health, as well as legal and ethical issues involved in the use of informatics in the provision of care.

The intensive computational and technology skill sets necessary to work with data today require additional approaches to literacy. With that in mind, Part III focuses on the research competencies that are needed to move research to practice, preparing researchers to work in increasingly data-intensive information and computing environments. Understanding how competencies are framed across knowledge, skills, and attitudes allows us to work from and across macro-, meso-, and micro-levels of how information and processes intersect. We also examine how data establishes future research priorities and explore information-seeking strategies.

In Part IV, we step outside the United States and review international aspects of telemental health, including the creation of globally accepted measures and standards, issues in tracking health care services, and operational reforms in developing and emerging nations. We conclude the book by examining the challenges faced by public health and mental health providers, educators, and researchers. We present emergent trends, upcoming legislation, and new ways of conceptualizing the intersection of mental health services research, public health practice, and informatics.

Although it is impossible to examine all of the relevant issues in mental health informatics in a single volume, this text underscores the importance of establishing a public health framework for the study of mental health informatics. We hope that our public health approach provides a useful starting point for future research and policy making in the area of mental health informatics.

The text has been designed for a variety of audiences, including: (1) graduate students and post-doctoral fellows in the public health, behavioral health, and information science fields; (2) professionals currently managing mental health programs and information systems in hospitals, managed care organizations, mental health clinics, and community mental health centers; and (3) policy makers and professionals in mental health services delivery within local, regional, state, and national levels of government.

Throughout the preparation of this text, several individuals at Oxford University Press provided encouragement and continued support. We are grateful to Craig Panner and Kathryn Winder for their valuable suggestions and advice, and to the Press's staff for copyediting and design supports. In addition, special thanks to Ms. Meghan Haggard and Ms. Melissa Tirotti at USF for their valuable support in the final preparation of this text. Finally, we would like to dedicate this book to our families for their love, generous understanding, and unwavering encouragement in our efforts to write and complete this text.

Ardis Hanson
Bruce Lubotsky Levin
Tampa, Florida

Part 1   Introduction

> [Public health is] the science and art of preventing disease, prolonging life, and promoting
> health and efficiency through organized community effort for the sanitation of the
> environment, the control of communicable infections, the organization of medical and
> nursing services for the early diagnosis and prevention of disease, the education of the
> individual in personal health and the development of the social machinery to assure
> everyone a standard of living adequate for the maintenance or improvement of health.
>
> CHARLES-EDWARD AMORY WINSLOW, 1920, pp. 6–7

1   Informatics and Public Health

Introduction

Informatics is a field that focuses on the creative use of computers, information systems, and other information technology in support of education, research, and applications for improving the overall quality of life. It is found in all disciplines and deals with resources, devices, and formalized methods for optimizing the storage, retrieval, and management of information for problem solving and decision making. More specifically, health informatics is an interdisciplinary field, based upon literature in computer and information sciences, the cognitive and decision sciences, the health sciences (including public health and epidemiology), medical sciences, and telecommunication sciences. Researchers in health informatics have discovered new methods and techniques to enhance health care, academic and applied services research, and education through the application of information technology.

The emergence of health informatics can be attributed to three major factors: (1) the rapid evolution of technology; (2) the growth of information management; and (3) the continued development of decision support systems. The changes in computing and communications technology are now read, viewed, or heard daily in the media. For example, e-business is presented as a high-profile commodity via daily advertisements. It is apparent that traditional paper-based methods for handling daily communication, patient information, and biomedical knowledge have become unmanageable and expensive, particularly with the continued demand for technology within managed health care. Finally, it is important to realize that other information databases are as important to current health and mental health management decision making as the traditional clinical and research databases.

Telecommunication also plays an increasingly important and prominent role within the health care field, where the most remarkable opportunities, along with associated challenges and obstacles, have emerged in relation to telecommunication initiatives. For example, telecommunication or "telehealth" strategies continue to broaden access to health and mental health care, health education, and health services delivery for at-risk populations in America. The development of computer-based patient records, personal health information systems, and unified electronic claims systems utilize various electronic communication technologies to streamline and centralize databases (Levin & Hanson, 2011).

For the purposes of this text, health informatics will be viewed from both public health and behavioral health perspectives. Behavioral health encompasses primarily the areas of alcohol, drug abuse, and mental health services, all specialty areas within public health. Nevertheless, throughout this text, the terms *mental health* and *behavioral health* will be used interchangeably. In addition, this text will primarily cover the public sector (local, state, and federal government agencies) and private sector practice, as well as the administrative, services delivery, and educational aspects of behavioral health informatics.

Telemedicine, Telehealth, and Health Informatics

Telemedicine "began" in the 1950s as physicians who were geographically remote from their patients rendered treatment or provided consultations over the telephone and/or through wire services. Today, although the principles are largely the same, the technology and milieu of contemporary telemedicine are vastly different. In the age of high-speed data lines, advanced data compression technologies, the privatization of federal technologies, and the computerization of patient medical records, clinical outcomes, and physician practices, telemedicine promises to be the next milestone in health care advances.

Telehealth has been described as the use of communications and information technology to deliver a variety of health care services, information, and education to participants who are not able to be at the same place to receive these services (Field, 2002). This helps to improve access to health care and helps to overcome the geographic, transportation infrastructure, and socioeconomic barriers to treatment in a timely fashion. Telehealth may include clinical consultation, continuing professional education, health promotion, and health and mental health care management and administration. Telehealth technologies initially included videoconferencing, telephones, computers, the Internet, e-mail, fax, radio, and television. More recently, technologies are increasingly being introduced and utilized in health care, through a variety of social media, including blogs, texting, Twitter, wikis, digital portfolios, and portals. In addition, programs deliver health care using a combination of audio graphic, store-and-forward, and telemetry technologies (the automatic transmission and measurement of data from remote sources by wire, radio, or wireless technologies).

Health informatics covers a very wide range of applications for delivering services and for applied services research, all dedicated to the improvement of patient care and public health. Health informatics continues to incorporate rapidly changing information environments and continues to encounter emerging public health issues, some created by the advent of new technological opportunities, while others emerge through the application of technology to complex public health problems. For example, applications range from electronic patient records to national health databases in the establishment of clinical guidelines and clinical (referral) pathways to care. The key component of health informatics is the process of converting data to accessible and usable information that enables improvements in the quality, value, and effectiveness of health and mental health services.

Electronic information systems are revolutionizing health care practice, health research, and health education. Efficient management of information improves patient satisfaction and creates the development of new aspects of clinical practice, as well as creating new opportunities for implementing health education initiatives. Many health care professionals realize that they are in need of additional skills and knowledge in finding and using information, and in assessing health information systems.

The proliferation of interest in health informatics has centered on the technical and sociological aspects of the medium. It is only recently, however, that legal and regulatory issues have been discussed. In fact, the potential for mass availability of telemedicine and telehealth information and services will likely depend upon how the legal and regulatory issues are resolved. The rapid development and growth of health information and communication technologies provide a wealth of opportunities to create new approaches for the delivery of health, mental health, and substance use services. Accordingly, mental health informatics is the systematic application of health information and computer science and technology to mental health practice and applied services research.

The remainder of this chapter will present some basic concepts in public health so that readers will understand the public health approach to informatics. The next chapter will address basic topics in mental health services delivery from a public health or population perspective.

Public Health

INTRODUCTION

Historically, in academic research and in the academy, it is common to examine problems from a (single) discipline-specific perspective. The advantage of this discipline-specific perspective includes a comprehensive literature base with theoretical frameworks that help guide future research and teaching in that discipline. The disadvantage of examining problems from a single perspective lies in the loss of potential contributions from other related disciplines in examining issues or problems that might draw contributions from a multidisciplinary perspective.

Unlike academics, where knowledge-based areas are traditionally organized by discipline-oriented departments, the field of health care has historically utilized a multidisciplinary team approach to services delivery, where improving health and clinical outcomes involves the utilization of evidence-based practices, with multidisciplinary health care teams providing services to patients. This was particularly true with the advent of prepaid health plans in early twentieth-century America.

The field of public health, by definition, utilizes a multidisciplinary approach to examining health and mental health problems in at-risk populations. It draws heavily from the areas of biostatistics and epidemiology, environmental and occupational health, health policy and management, and community and family health to address health issues and problems from a population perspective.

While most definitions of public health include advancing a healthy lifestyle for communities through the promotion of health and the prevention of disease, one particular definition of public health was suggested in the early twentieth century by Charles-Edward Amory Winslow, a pioneer in public health practice in America:

> [Public health is] the science and art of preventing disease, prolonging life, and promoting health and efficiency through organized community effort for the sanitation of the environment, the control of communicable infections, the organization of medical and nursing services for the early diagnosis and prevention of disease, the education of the individual in personal health and the development of the social machinery to assure everyone a standard of living adequate for the maintenance or improvement of health. (Winslow, 1920, pp. 6–7)

Toward the end of the twentieth century, the Institute of Medicine's (IOM) Committee for the Study of the Future of Public Health (IOM Committee) published *The Future of Public Health*, which examined public health programs and the coordination of services across U.S. government agencies and within state and local health departments. The Committee defined the *substance* of public health as "organized community efforts aimed at the prevention of disease and promotion of health" (Institute of Medicine, 1988, p. 41) and defined the *mission* of public health as "the fulfillment of society's interest in assuring conditions in which people can be healthy" (Institute of Medicine, 1988, p. 40).

The IOM Committee also identified three core functions of public health: (1) assessment; (2) policy development; and (3) assurance (of providing necessary public health services in the community). Subsequently, the U.S Public Health Service convened the Public Health Functions Steering Committee (1994), a national work group chaired by the Surgeon General, which developed 10 essential public health services needed to carry out the basic public health core functions in a community:

1. Monitor health status to identify community health problems;
2. Diagnose and investigate identified health problems and health hazards in the community;
3. Inform, educate, and empower people about health issues;
4. Mobilize community partnerships to identify and solve health problems;
5. Develop policies and plans that support individual and community health efforts;
6. Enforce laws and regulations that protect health and ensure safety;
7. Link people to needed personal health services and assure the provision of health care;
8. Assure a competent public health and personal health care workforce;

9. Assess effectiveness, accessibility, and quality of personal and population-based health; and
10. Research for new insights and innovative solutions to health problems.

Thus, while there are a variety of definitions and functions of public health, common elements include a population-based, multidisciplinary approach that emphasizes health promotion and disease prevention, even at an international level (World Health Organization, 2012). Furthermore, a public health approach involves both formal activities undertaken within government, combined with efforts by private and voluntary organizations and individuals, working together to focus on maintaining the health of populations. This public health framework of problem solving includes (1) problem identification (utilizing epidemiologic surveillance); (2) identifying risks and protective factors; (3) development, implementation, and evaluation of interventions; and (4) monitoring implementation in relation to the impact on policy and cost-effectiveness. It also requires the determination if a disease is preventable or not preventable, controllable or not controllable, as well as its priority compared to other incidences of disease outbreak.

The remainder of this chapter will examine selected topics in public health. Where possible, the public health topics included below will contain a brief discussion of how that area is related to the field of informatics.

EPIDEMIOLOGY

Epidemiology, a fundamental science of public health, is the study of the factors that determine the frequency and distribution of disease in (human) populations. In medicine, physicians focus on individual patients; in public health, on the other hand, epidemiologists focus at a population level, that is, on a community or a specific population at risk for selected diseases. Thus, in public health, the community replaces the individual patient as the primary focus of concern (i.e., the "unit of analysis"). The objective is to evaluate the health of a defined community, including those members who would benefit from, but often do not seek, health care services. In epidemiology, disease does not occur in random fashion and may have multiple causal factors. Factors whose presence is associated with an increased likelihood that disease will develop at a later time are called risk factors.

Epidemiologic studies may be applied to all diseases, conditions, and health-related events. *Endemic occurrence* is defined as the habitual presence of a disease or infectious agent within a geographic area, or the usual prevalence of a given disease within such an area. The term is used in contrast with *epidemic*, or the occurrence in a community (or region) of a group of illnesses of similar nature, clearly in excess of normal expectancy. An epidemic includes any kind of disease, exists whenever the number of cases exceeds what is expected on the basis of past experience for a given population, has no specific geographic limitations, and may encompass any time period.

Two common terms used in the measurement of disease frequency in epidemiologic studies are *incidence* and *prevalence*. Incidence rates are designed to provide a measure of the rate at which people without a disease develop the disease during a specified period of time, that is, the number of new cases of a disease in a population during a specified interval of time (e.g., the number of new cases of schizophrenia per 100,000 persons in one year). The population in which the incidence is measured is restricted to those who are susceptible to getting the disease during the observation time period. This restricted population generally is called the *at-risk population* because they are at risk for contracting the disease. Incidence allows researchers to study the impact of harmful exposures or preventive interventions on the occurrence of disease because it does not depend upon the length of disease course or its fatality.

Prevalence rate measures the number of people in a population who have a disease (i.e., the existing cases) in the total population at a particular time (point prevalence), or during a stated period of time (period prevalence). Thus, incidence reveals the rate at which new illness occurs, whereas prevalence measures the "residual" of such illness, the amount existing at a given point in time in a community. Prevalence depends upon two factors: how many people have become ill in the past, and the duration of their illnesses.

SURVEILLANCE

Surveillance is the ongoing systematic collection, analysis, and interpretation of health incidence data. Comprising population- and/or individual-based data, surveillance data monitors the incidence of disease to establish patterns of progression. Surveillance helps us to predict, observe, and minimize the harm caused by chronic and acute illnesses, such as outbreaks, epidemics, and pandemics. It also increases our knowledge of the factors that may contribute to the diagnosis and treatment of disorders. A key part of modern disease surveillance is case reporting. Examples of mental health surveillance data are the Centers for Disease Control and Prevention's (CDC) Behavioral Risk Factor Surveillance System (BRFSS) and the Substance Abuse and Mental Health Services Administration's (SAMHSA) National Survey on Drug Use and Health (NSDUH).

PREVENTION

Primary, secondary, and tertiary prevention provide the foundation for the public health model of prevention and form the underlying principles for avoiding and controlling public health problems. However, in the case of mental health, these concepts are more difficult to apply. The causes of many mental disorders are not fully understood, due to the complexity of the etiology of mental disorders, the lack of knowledge on disease triggers, and the lack of complete understanding of disease emergence, progression, and subsidence from a physiological perspective. Hence, the avoidance of the occurrence of an illness, which is true primary prevention, often eludes researchers and practitioners in the field of mental health. Although great progress has been made in the genetics of diseases such as early onset Alzheimer's disease, we are still very distant from a basic knowledge of the genetic predispositions of many mental disorders. Even though there has been a great deal of "social engineering" attempted to prevent the occurrence of mental disorders, there is little evidence that these efforts have been successful (Levin, Hanson, & Hennessy, 2004; Levin, Hanson, Coe, & Kuppin, 2000).

Secondary prevention is the avoidance of disease recurrences or exacerbations post–disease diagnosis. This has been a more achievable goal in mental health. With early identification and intervention, it is possible to stabilize many mood disorders, allowing individuals to lead productive, relatively unimpaired lives (Levin, Hanson, & Hennessy, 2004). Early intervention in other diagnostic groups of mental disorders has varying chances of success (Bird et al., 2010). However, considering the magnitude of the disabilities, particularly from a developmental perspective, such intervention is justifiable. To show the efficacy of secondary prevention, high-quality program evaluation is critical.

Finally, tertiary prevention is the reduction of disability and the utilization of rehabilitation. A substantial portion of mental health services for individuals with serious mental disorders is categorized as tertiary prevention. The mental health field can document considerable success through a number of program initiatives, including community support programs, positive assertive community treatment, psychosocial rehabilitation, and systems of integrated services delivery (U.S. Department of Health and Human Services, 1999). When we examine the direct and indirect costs of the suffering and the care of individuals with mental illnesses and their families, mental health professionals readily justify costs. However, the funding of public mental health programs is a political process, and it is critical to clearly demonstrate the cost-benefits of mental health treatment to the public, as well as to state and federal lawmakers. Effective data collection and analyses, including cost, efficacy, and outcomes, are key to defending these programs in terms of cost-effectiveness and long-term successful outcomes for persons with serious mental illnesses.

EVIDENCE-BASED PRACTICE

Clinical guidelines are those guidelines developed to assist in "best practice" treatment initiatives in order to be useful in diagnosis and treatment. These guidelines are often the foundation of evidence-based practices (EBP). EBPs are those research practices that have undergone and passed rigorous scientific and clinical practice review.

Evidence-based practice in behavioral health, for example, is an emerging field. There are a number of organizations and agencies that are authoritative sources for clinical guidelines, best practices, and EBP in the behavioral health field, including the National Registry of Evidence-Based Programs and Practices (http://www.nrepp.samhsa.gov/), the Cochrane Collaboration (http://www.cochrane.org/), and Blueprints for Violence Prevention: Center for the Study and Prevention of Violence (http://www.colorado.edu/cspv/blueprints/index.html). Data from EBP provide new ways of thinking about services delivery and what works best for whom, helping to reframe clinical treatment as well as services delivery frameworks. This allows more systemic and innovative approaches to translating research to clinical practice and clinical practice to research.

MANAGED CARE

Managed care is an evolving array of health care review and service coordination mechanisms that ultimately attempts to control (i.e., reduce) health services utilization and costs, to improve efficiency and services coordination, to increase access to preventive services, and to improve the quality of health care (Frank & McGuire, 2004). Managed care organizations (MCOs) are constantly evolving entities of various organizational structures and arrangements. A managed health care plan (MHCP) may be one or more products or entities that integrate financing and management with the delivery of health care services to an enrolled population. An MHCP may employ or contract with an organized provider network that delivers services and that (as a network or individual provider) either shares financial risk or incorporates various incentives to deliver high-quality and cost-effective services. Most MHCPs use information systems capable of monitoring and evaluating utilization and cost patterns of their enrolled population.

COMMUNITY MENTAL HEALTH

The history of caring for individuals with mental illnesses is crucial in understanding the development of public health services, particularly the role of deinstitutionalization, which led to the development of the community mental health system in America (Deutsch, 1946; Regier et al., 1978; Drake et al., 2003). Table 1.1 briefly summarizes the prevailing eras for how individuals with mental illnesses were treated in America.

Community mental health services are the treatment of persons with mental illnesses in a community-based setting rather than in a hospital or psychiatric hospital environment.

TABLE 1.1

Eras of Mental Health

Era	Time	Advocates	Location	Theoretical framework
Age of Restraint	1773–1836		Home or wilderness	Containment
Moral Treatment	1836–1862	Pinel, Tuke, Rush, Dix	Asylum	Humane, restorative treatment
Custodial Care	1862–1900		Asylum	Personal and public safety
Mental Hygiene	1900–1955	Beers, Meyer, Deutsch	Mental hospital or clinic	Prevention, early intervention, promotion
Community Mental Health	1955–1977	Felix, Anthony, Chamberlin,	Community mental health center	Deinstitutionalization, community (re) integration
Systems Delivery	1977–1981	Carter, Hatfield, Lefley, Anthony, Deegan	Local communities (CASSP, PAMII)	Social welfare concern
Managed Care	1974–1990	Frank, McGuire, Pardes	Local communities	Community support, recovery
Behavioral Health	1990–Present	Rubinow,	Local communities	Decade of the brain, disease management, prevention

Ten elements were determined to be essential to ensure successful outcomes for persons with mental illnesses in the community. These included (1) a responsible case management team; (2) residential care; (3) emergency care; (4) Medicare care; (5) halfway houses; (6) supervised (supported) apartments; (7) outpatient therapy; (8) vocational training and opportunities; (9) social and recreational opportunities; and (10) family and network attention (Turner & Tenhoor, 1978).

Today, community mental health services provide a variety of mental health services, from traditional mental health treatment programs to vocational programs and rehabilitation counseling. A variety of additional programs are provided, including supported housing, employment, and education; partial hospitalization; local primary care medical services; clubhouses and peer-run services; and self-help groups for mental health. The significance of community mental health services is to provide the necessary services and supports so that persons with mental illnesses can remain integrated in their local communities and can be productive as well as functioning members of society.

PHYSICAL HISTORY

A physical history is the patient's treatment history, defined as whether he or she had ever received treatment prior to the current episode of care, and, if so, where. A history often is in the form of an interview and may include physical examinations, basic patient demographics, medications, allergies, and the presenting problem(s) or complaint(s) that brought the patient to the practitioner. In addition, the practitioner usually takes a family history, developmental history (including stresses and transitions), and a social history (education, occupational history, religion, etc.), which also documents linguistic and cultural issues that may be relevant in determining treatment. The service history is an essential part of the evaluative process, not just of the patient's current state but also in determining effectiveness of treatment and short- and long-term patient outcomes. Traditionally, this data may be kept in paper files, but increasingly these data are now part of the electronic health record.

LEVEL OF FUNCTIONING

Severity and level of functioning measures an individual's level of everyday functioning and comparison with pre-morbid (before onset of diseases) functioning (Murray & Lopez, 1996). Relevant aspects of daily living include daily living skills, social and recreational skills, financial skills, vocational skills, interpersonal skills, and parental skills. The point of measuring level of functioning is to assess how much the illness has affected the person and to use that information in designing appropriate levels of psychosocial treatment.

PROGRAM EVALUATION

Effective program evaluation is a systematic way to improve and account for public health services delivery and programmatic improvement. Program evaluation addresses how effectively decision making and administrative functions are performed, services are delivered, and whether outcomes meet quality, patient, and service goals, as well as accountability guidelines. Quality assessment tools include system performance indicators, report cards, and consumer outcome measures, all of which use guideline fidelity measures (standards). They comprise domains that are issues, categories, or topics of interest. Indicators are measurable activities, events, characteristics, or items that represent a domain. Measures are the instruments used to assess, evaluate, and measure an indicator.

In public health evaluation, the following questions are asked:

- What will be evaluated? (i.e., what is the program and in what context does it exist?)
- What aspects of the program will be considered when judging program performance?
- What standards (i.e., type or level of performance) must be reached for the program to be considered successful?
- What evidence will be used to indicate how the program has performed?
- What conclusions regarding program performance are justified by comparing the available evidence to the selected standards?; and
- How will the lessons learned from the inquiry be used to improve public health effectiveness? (Milstein & Wetterhall, 1999).

The data collected to effectively answer these questions come from a variety of sources (including census data, surveillance data, and needs assessments) and from numerous data sources at local, state, regional, and national levels. The synthesis of data and information required to determine the effectiveness of programs, including patient outcomes, requires an understanding of public health systems and informatics.

IMPLICATIONS FOR MENTAL HEALTH INFORMATICS

This chapter was designed to give readers a basic understanding of public health and how the field views the world through an informatics perspective. For those with a basic understanding of public health, part of this chapter may seem like a review of basic principles. However, for those who are looking at the dual areas of public health and informatics for the first time, this overview is necessary.

The next chapter will briefly highlight some basic areas of mental health and mental disorders, viewed from a public health perspective. This will be followed by an overview of informatics in mental health services delivery.

References

Bird, V., Premkumar, P., Kendall, T., Whittington, C., Mitchell, J., & Kuipers, E. (2010). Early intervention services, cognitive-behavioural therapy and family intervention in early psychosis: Systematic review. *British Journal of Psychiatry, 197*(5), 350–356.

Field, M. (2002). *Telemedicine: A guide to assessing telecommunications in health care.* Washington, DC: National Academy Press. Retrieved from www.nap.edu/books/0309055318/html/index.html.

Frank, R. G., & McGuire, T. G. (2004). Insuring mental health care in the age of managed care. In B. L. Levin & J. Petrila (Eds.), *Mental health services: A public health perspective* (pp. 15–41). New York: Oxford University Press.

Deutsch, A. (1946). *The mentally ill in America: A history of their care and treatment from colonial times*. New York: Columbia University Press.

Drake, R. E., Green, A. I., Mueser, K. T., et al. (2003). The history of community mental health treatment and rehabilitation for persons with severe mental illness. *Community Mental Health Journal, 39*(5), 427–440.

Institute of Medicine Committee for the Study of the Future of Public Health. (1988). *The future of public health*. Washington, DC: National Academy Press. Retrieved from http://www.nap.cdu/catalog.php?record_id=1091.

Levin, B. L. & Hanson, A. (2011). Mental health informatics. In N. Cummings & W. T. O'Donohue (Eds.), *Understanding the behavioral healthcare crisis: The promise of integrated care and diagnostic reform* (pp. 59–82). New York: Routledge.

Levin B. L., Hanson, A., Coe, R., & Kuppin, S. A. (2000). *Mental health parity: National and state perspectives 2000*. Tampa: University of South Florida, the Louis de la Parte Florida Mental Health Institute.

Levin, B. L., Hanson, A., & Hennessy K. D. (2004). Overview of prevention, integration, and parity. In B. L. Levin, J. Petrila, & K. D., Hennessy (Eds.), *Mental health services: A public health perspective*, 2nd ed. (pp. 3–14). New York: Oxford University Press.

Milstein, R. L., & Wetterhall, S. F. (1999). Framework for program evaluation in public health, *MMWR: Recommendations & Reports, 48*(RR11), 1–40. Retrieved from http://www.cdc.gov/mmwr/preview/mmwrhtml/rr4811a1.htm.

Murray, C. J., & Lopez, A. D. (1996). *The global burden of disease: A comprehensive assessment of mortality and disability from diseases, injuries, and risk factors in 1990 and projected to 2020*. Cambridge, MA: Harvard University Press.

Public Health Functions Steering Committee. (1994). *Public health in America statement*. Washington, DC: U.S. Department of Health & Human Services. Retrieved from http://www.health.gov/phfunctions/public.htm.

Regier, D. A., Goldberg, I. D., & Taube, C. A. (1978). The de facto U. S. mental health services system: A public health perspective. *Archives of General Psychiatry, 35*, 685–693.

Turner, J. C., & TenHoor, W. J. (1978). The NIMH Community Support Program: Pilot approach to a needed social reform. *Schizophrenia Bulletin, 4*, 319–349.

U.S. Department of Health and Human Services. (1999). *Mental health: A report of the Surgeon General*. Rockville, MD: Substance Abuse and Mental Health Services Administration, National Institute of Mental Health.

Winslow, C.-E.A. (1920). The untilled field of public health. *Modern Medicine, 2*, 1–9.

World Health Organization. (2012). *The public health approach*. Geneva. Retrieved from http://www.who.int/violenceprevention/approach/public_health/en/index.html.

The neuroscience of mental health—a term that encompasses studies extending from molecular events to psychological, behavioral, and societal phenomena—has emerged as one of the most exciting arenas of scientific activity and human inquiry.

DAVID SATCHER, former U.S. surgeon general, in USDHHS, 1999

2 Mental Health

Introduction

In addition to the definition, substance, mission, and functions of public health noted in the previous chapter in this volume, public health may also be viewed within the larger context of health. The World Health Organization defines health as "a state of complete physical, mental, and social well-being and not merely the absence of disease or infirmity" (World Health Organization, 2006). Accordingly, mental health may be conceptualized as an integral part of the overall health of individuals and populations, although different cultures and ethnicities may vary in their definitions of what constitutes "mental health" and "mental illness."

Mental health spans both private and public services. It also includes elements of many other specialty fields, including medicine, social and behavioral sciences, social work, and rehabilitation. Public mental health care may be acute or long-term care. It usually emphasizes a focus on a particular at-risk population. Mental health services are offered in hospitals, general and specialty providers' offices, community mental health centers, peer-run centers, religious organizations (pastoral care), academic health centers, jails and prisons, state and local government facilities, and private facilities. At the same time, users of data generated by mental health services include a wide range of stakeholders, including consumers, families, providers, payers, managed care organizations, state mental health authorities, federal agencies, administrators, researchers, policy makers, advocates, and criminal justice personnel.

This chapter will present an overview of mental health services from a public health perspective. It will also briefly discuss selected topics in mental health services as background information for the next chapter on informatics and mental health.

The Burden of Mental Disorders

Mental disorders are common worldwide and comprise some of the most significant and complex problems in public health. Individuals who suffer from mental disorders endure social isolation and experience a poor quality of life as well as have increased mortality when compared to persons without mental disorders. In addition, mental disorders contribute to significant economic and social costs (both direct and indirect costs) to society (World Health Organization, 2005).

EPIDEMIOLOGY

An estimated 450 million people throughout the world suffer from mental disorders, including alcohol and drug use disorders. Approximately 20% of these individuals will develop one or more mental disorders in their lifetime. Globally, depression, alcohol and drug use disorders, bipolar disorders, schizophrenia, Alzheimer and other dementias, and panic disorder are among the 20 leading causes of disability and premature death worldwide (Mathers, Boerma, and Fat, 2008). In addition, over 154 million people globally suffer from depression, 25 million people suffer from schizophrenia, 91 million people are affected by alcohol use disorders, and 15 million people have drug use disorders (World Health Organization, 2002). About one-half of mental disorders begin before individuals reach the age of 14 years (World Health Organization, 2005). Individuals with mental disorders are more at risk for medical illnesses, for communicable and non-communicable diseases, and for injury (World Health Organization, 2001).

Mental disorders in the United States are also significant public health problems. Approximately 20% of adults 18 years or older suffer from a mental disorder, and of these individuals, nearly 20% also have suffered from a substance use or dependence disorder. Further, nearly 9% of the U.S. population 12 years and older suffer from a substance use disorder (Substance Abuse and Mental Health Services Administration, 2010a, 2010b).

EXPENDITURES

Mental illnesses also have serious consequences for worker performance, absenteeism, accidents, and overall productivity in the workplace (Harnois and Gabriel, 2000). The significance of the substantial burden of mental disorders on individuals, worker productivity, and society is underscored by expenditures for mental health and substance use services. In 1986, expenditures for mental health and substance abuse treatment in the United States were $42 billion. By 2003, expenditures had increased to $121 billion, and expenditures for mental health and substance abuse treatment are projected to reach $239 billion by 2014 (Levit, Kassed, Coffey, et al., 2008). While private financing of services has increased, public financing is still considered the major funding source for mental health and substance abuse services in the United States.

The previous paragraph uses the most current data available, from the year 2003, for national health care expenditures for mental health and substance abuse treatment. However, data for national health care expenditures for all health services are available for the year 2009 (National Health Care Expenditure Fact Sheet, 2012). Thus, the collection of national information for mental health and substance abuse expenditures, as well as other data in the mental health field, is seriously behind data collection for all health services.

Selected Issues in Mental Health

SERVICE SYSTEMS DELIVERY

Through the 1950s, state-run mental hospitals were the primary location for providing care to people with serious mental disorders in the United States. As de-institutionalization occurred, the publicly financed mental health system evolved from state-run hospital settings to a variety of specialty (sector) services within a number of different organizational settings, largely independent from public health systems. The Institute of Medicine (IOM) Committee for the Study of the Future of Public Health emphasized this fragmented (or de facto) mental health delivery system (Regier, Goldberg, Taube, 1978; Regier et al., 1993) as well as the lack of integration between public health and mental health services. Ultimately, the IOM Committee called for the integration of future public health initiatives with mental health initiatives, particularly in the areas of disease prevention and health promotion (Institute of Medicine, 1988).

The de facto mental health system in the United States is not an organized system of care. Rather, it comprises numerous health and mental health delivery systems, as well as other social, justice, and educational systems, where individuals with mental disorders are commonly found seeking assistance. These systems include both public and private sector services, each having their own agencies, funding streams, specific services, and overall mission and objectives. Collectively, these systems provide acute and long-term mental health care in homes, communities, and institutional settings, across the specialty mental health sector, the general medical/primary care sector, and the voluntary care sector. Professional licensing and accreditation organizations, managed care provider entities, insurance companies, advocacy and regulatory agencies, and health care policy-making groups potentially influence how mental health care is accessed, organized, delivered, and financed. Thus, the assessment and treatment of individuals with mental illnesses often occur in other systems whose primary missions have little to do with the identification of mental illnesses.

INSURANCE AND FINANCING

Historically, the provision of mental health services has been the responsibility of individual practitioners and hospitals in the private sector and by community mental health centers, the Veterans Administration, and city/county/state hospitals in the public sector. The passage of federal entitlement programs in the 1960s encouraged counties and states to provide mental health services outside the state and county mental health facilities. The private sector has moved toward insurance-based service delivery systems since an increasing percentage of individuals obtain their primary health and mental health insurance coverage through their place of employment. Today, funding for mental health and substance abuse services comes from a blended array of public and private sources.

The provision and financing of mental health services have remained separated rather than integrated with physical health services. This lack of integration between health and mental health services has contributed to the development of a number of dubious public health policies, including insurance providers' unequal coverage of mental health services in comparison to physical health services.

In 1996, Congress passed the Mental Health Parity Act, which made it unlawful for companies with more than 50 employees to put limits on mental health care (unless similar dollar limits apply to medical and surgical care). Although the original 1996 Act did not provide coverage for substance abuse or chemical dependency, the Mental Health Parity and Addiction Equity Act of 2008 provided parity for coverage of substance abuse and chemical dependency disorders.

In addition, the historical reliance on the public sector for long-term mental health care and on the private sector for acute mental health care has contributed to limited overall continuity of care, as well as limited sharing of information between mental health service delivery systems. Mental health services increasingly have been financed through multiple (public and private) payers as well as numerous (public and private) providers of mental health care.

MANAGED CARE

Historically in the United States, health insurance has been based upon an acute care model and has been confined to traditional medical care. Generally, it has not been defined within a long-term care treatment environment. The greatest unmet needs of individuals with severe mental illnesses have involved rehabilitation and long-term services that typically have not been covered under private health insurance policies.

The concept of "managing" health care in the United States began during the early twentieth century with the evolution of prepaid health plans and the development of the Kaiser Permanente medical care programs in California. These prepaid health plans provided health, mental health, and substance abuse services at one location for a defined population on a monthly (capitated) fee. The design of these health plans included the emphasis on prevention initiatives. However, controlling costs and service utilization of health and behavioral health services became the critical bottom line for many of these organizations.

Today, managed care dominates health and mental health coverage for individuals (Merrick & Reif, 2010). This continued growth of managed care " ... has [increasingly] blurred the distinction between organizations bearing financial risk for health care (insurers), organizations managing care (health maintenance and utilization management organizations), and organizations making clinical treatment decisions (provider groups or individual clinicians)" (Sturm, 2002, p. 362). At the same time, the rapid growth of managed care in the United States has raised concerns that reduction in health and mental health care costs may have resulted in cost shifting to public programs and/or consumers themselves.

Managed care organizations (MCOs) have rapidly expanded into the public sector. Increasingly, public mental health systems have shifted their priorities from providing mental health and substance abuse services to purchasing these services. Hence, public mental health systems often utilize a "systems of care" approach rather than primarily maintaining institutions and other more traditional services.

ENTITLEMENT PROGRAMS

The Medicare and Medicaid programs finance much of the mental health and substance use services, and the Social Security Disability Insurance (SSDI) and Supplemental Security Income (SSI) programs, which provide income support to many people with severe and persistent mental illness, are examples of social insurance programs. Social insurance programs serve two primary purposes: (1) they are a means of overcoming market failure in private markets; and (2) they serve a redistributive function in providing "safety net" resources to vulnerable populations. The Medicare program, enacted in 1965, serves both functions. Medicare Part A, which covers hospital services, was made compulsory explicitly to overcome adverse selection problems and is funded by general revenue. Nearly all people 65 and older are covered by Part A. Medicare, after a two-year waiting period, also covers those under the age of 65 who have qualified for the SSDI program (those with a disability who paid into the Social Security system for 40 or more quarters).

The Medicare Part B program, which covers office-based and other services, while not compulsory, is funded in part (25%) by Medicare beneficiaries, with the remaining 75% funded by general revenue. The premiums for the optional Medicare Part D drug benefit are similarly heavily subsidized, encouraging high rates of participation, as well. The large subsidy also has been effective in overcoming adverse selection: 90% of Medicare beneficiaries eligible for Part D prescription drug coverage have some form of coverage (Duggan, Healy, & Scott Morton, 2008).

The Medicaid program, unlike Medicare, was not designed to provide broad-based coverage for the population, but as an insurer of last resort for vulnerable populations. It provides coverage to low-income children and their parents (many with Temporary Assistance to Needy Families), low-income pregnant women, low-income elderly, and people with disabilities. Eligibility varies widely from state to state. Medicaid is an especially important source of coverage for people with mental disorders who qualify for SSI income support (many of whom do not have enough quarters of work to qualify for SSDI and, thus, Medicare). It also plays an important role in filling the gaps for Medicare, which requires significant cost-sharing and does not cover many mental health and substance abuse services. Concerns regarding the potential loss of Medicaid and Medicare coverage create strong disincentives for people with disabilities to seek work; this situation has led to a number of initiatives, such as the Ticket to Work program (Social Security Administration, 2006).

RESEARCH TO PRACTICE

There has been more than a half century of research on mental illness. The field has made great strides over the years in psychopharmacology and the integration of biological, neurological, and behavioral sciences. New medications and psychosocial interventions have provided new treatment opportunities for individuals with mental disorders, requiring new approaches in evaluating their effectiveness. Some of these new approaches have come from the evaluation of somatic health care interventions.

Evidence-based practice distinguishes research that is of direct clinical significance. Using a set of simple rules for evaluating research evidence, it provides a framework for making clinical decisions on the basis of research findings and for applying research findings to individual patients. It consists of five explicit steps: (1) the clinician constructs a specific clinical question concerning the care of a patient or group of patients; (2) the clinician finds the best evidence to answer the question; (3) the clinician evaluates the evidence for validity and usefulness; (4) the results are applied to the specific patient or group of patients; and (5) the outcome of the intervention is evaluated as to its effectiveness and efficacy (Straus & Sackett, 1998). Evidence-based practice increases accountability as well as increasing access to resources and dissemination.

There has been considerable discussion on the role of evidence-based practice in mental health. Barkham et al. (2001, 2008) suggest that practice-based evidence should help determine evidence-based practice, along with the contributions of random clinical trials and qualitative methods. Practice research networks should collaborate to collect and analyze large bodies of effectiveness data rather than efficacy data, particularly since observational or audit data may be more clinically relevant than data gathered under experimental conditions (Hennessy, 2010).

STIGMA

Historically in the United States, there has been a significant amount of literature on public attitudes toward and understanding of mental disorders. The literature has shown that attitudes toward persons with mental disorders generally have been negative (Compagni & Manderscheid, 2006; Ben-Zeev, Young, & Corrrigan, 2010; Sharac et al., 2010), even when the individuals surveyed were educated about the "facts" of mental disorders.

Over a half century later, the stigma of mental illness is still an issue in the United States. In a now-classic ethnographic study of persons with mental disorders in the community, the study participants felt that mental disorders still carried a public stigma in the dominant culture and, although persons with mental disorders desired normalcy, they still feared rejection by the "dominant" culture (Estroff, 1981).

TECHNOLOGY, RECOVERY, AND PREVENTION

The New Freedom Commission on Mental Health (2003) made a number of recommendations to fundamentally transform the delivery of mental health services in the United States. Of the five goals the Commission identified, three address technology, recovery, and prevention.

The use of technology has two major aims. The first addresses advancing research in the development of evidence-based practices to treat individuals with mental and substance use disorders, with the ultimate goal of preventing mental disorders and promoting recovery among individuals with mental illnesses. The second aim is the effective use of technology to maximize diffusion, early adoption, and effective implementation of efficacious and effective practices and to improve service provision and service utilization. Technology is also relevant to workforce development issues in assuring that current and future practitioners have access to and utilize evidence-based services. Technology is also a critical component in developing the knowledge base in mental and substance use disorders, particularly in the areas of disparities, trauma, acute care, and long-term consequences of medications. Finally, integrated information technology (e.g., electronic health records) and communications infrastructure (e.g., telehealth systems) require substantial investments, but are critical to the effective delivery of mental health services.

Mental health systems that are driven by consumer and family participation are one focus of the New Freedom Commission report. The report emphasizes the need for individualized plans for care, stakeholder participation, protection and advocacy for persons with mental disorders, and improved access and accountability for mental health services. Emphasis on applied mental health research to promote recovery and resiliency is a cornerstone of transforming mental health services.

The basic message of recovery from serious mental disorder is hope for the restoration of a meaningful life for each individual. This message of hope offers the possibility of an identity that is simultaneously *within* and *beyond* the limits of disability. According to Anthony (1993), recovery requires "the development of new meaning and purpose in one's life as one grows beyond the catastrophic effects of mental illness" (p. 11). What is critical about recovery as a process and as an outcome, however, is the personal meaning that each individual attaches to the concept.

Prevention is included in the Commission's recommendation for early mental health screening, assessment, and referral to services and with the emphasis on developing integrated mental health systems. With the dissemination, adoption, and implementation of evidence-based practices, together with an improved workforce, a fundamental transformation of the varied approaches to mental health care in the United States may be achieved.

Implications for Mental Health Informatics

Currently, the evolution of separate and distinct physical health, mental health, and substance abuse services has created fragmented de facto health and mental health care delivery systems throughout the United States, as well as within each state. Furthermore, the national collection of mental health expenditures and service utilization appear at least five years behind data collection vis-à-vis total health care expenditures and service utilization. Thus, there remains great potential for mental health informatics to play an important role in the integration of a variety of data (census, surveillance, and hospital) if more emphasis is placed upon updating national efforts to collect more current mental health and substance abuse data.

References

Anthony, W. A. (1993). Recovery from mental illness: The guiding vision of the mental health service system in the 1990s. *Psychosocial Rehabilitation Journal, 16*(4), 11–23.

Barkham, M., Margison, F., Leach, C., Lucock, M., Mellor-Clark, J., Evans, C., Benson, L., Connell, J., Audin, K., & McGrath, G. (2001). Service profiling and outcomes benchmarking using the CORE-OM: Toward practice-based evidence in the psychological therapies: Clinical outcomes in toutine evaluation-outcome measures. *Journal of Consulting & Clinical Psychology, 69*(2), 184–196.

Barkham, M., Stiles, W. B., Connell, J., Twigg, E., Leach, C., Lucock, M., Mellor-Clark, J., Bower, P., King, M., Shapiro, D. A., Hardy, G. E., Greenberg, L., & Angus, L. (2008). Effects of psychological therapies in randomized trials and practice-based studies. *British Journal of Clinical Psychology, 47*(Pt. 4), 397–415. doi:10.1348/014466508X311713.

Ben-Zeev, D., Young, M. A, & Corrigan, P. W. (2010). DSM-V and the stigma of mental illness. *Journal of Mental Health, 19*(4), 318–327.

Compagni, A., & Manderscheid, R. W. (2006). A neuroscientist-consumer alliance to transform mental health care. *Journal of Behavioral Health Services & Research, 33*(2), 265–274.

Duggan, M., Healy, P., & Scott Morton, F. (2008). Providing prescription drug coverage to the elderly: America's experiment with Medicare Part D. *Journal of Economic Perspectives, 22*(4), 69–92.

Estroff, S. E. (1981). *Making it crazy: An ethnography of psychiatric clients in an American community*. Berkeley: University of California Press.

Harnois, G., & Gabriel, P. (2000). *Mental health and work: Impact, issues, and good practices*. Geneva: World Health Organization.

Hennessy, K. D. (2010). Quality improvement. In B. L. Lubotsky, K. D. Hennessy, & J. Petrila (Eds.), *Mental health services: A public health perspective*, 3rd ed. (pp. 67–82). New York: Oxford University Press.

Institute of Medicine. (1988). Committee for the Study of the Future of Public Health, Division of Health Care Services. *The future of public health*. Washington, DC: National Academy Press.

Levit, K. R., Kassed, C. A., Coffey, R. M., Mark, T. L., McKusick, D. R., King, E., Vandivort, R., Buck, J., Ryan, K., & Stranges, E. (2008). Projections of national expenditures for mental health services and substance abuse treatment, 2004–2014 (SAMHSA Publication No. SMA 08-4326). Rockville, MD: Substance Abuse and Mental Health Services Administration.

Mathers, C., Boerma, T., & Fat, D. M. (2008). *The glodal burden of disease, 2004 update*. Geneva: World Health Organization. Retrieved from http://www.who.int/healthinfo/global_burden_disease/GBD_report_2004update_full.pdf.

Merrick, E. L., & Reif, S. (2010). Services in an era of managed care. In B. L. Lubotsky & M. A. Becker (Eds.), *A public health perspective of women's mental health* (pp. 201–227). New York: Oxford University Press.

National Health Care Expenditure Fact Sheet. Baltimore, MD: Centers for Medicare and Medicaid Services, 2012. Retrieved from https://www.cms.gov/NationalHealthExpendData/25_NHE_Fact_Sheet.asp#TopOfPage.

New Freedom Commission on Mental Health. (2003). *Achieving the promise: Transforming mental health care in America. Final Report*. DHHS Pub. No. SMA-03-3832. Rockville, MD: U.S. Department of Health and Human Services.

Regier, D., Goldberg, I., & Taube, C. (1978). The de facto U.S. mental health services system: A public health perspective. *Archives of General Psychiatry, 35*, 685–693.

Regier, D. A., Narrow, W. E., Rae, D. S., Manderscheid, R. W., Locke, B. Z., & Goodwin, F. K. (1993). The de facto US mental and addictive disorders service system. Epidemiologic Catchment Area prospective 1-year prevalence rates of disorders and services. *Archives of General Psychiatry, 50*(2), 85–94.

Sharac, J., McCrone, P., Clement, S., & Thornicroft, G. (2010). The economic impact of mental health stigma and discrimination: A systematic review. *Epidemiology and Psychiatric Science, 19*(3), 223–232.

Social Security Administration. (2006). Exemption of work activity as a basis for a continuing disability review: Final rules. *Federal Register, 71*(222), 66840–66860.

Straus, S. E., & Sackett, D. L. (1998). Using research findings in practice. *BMJ, 317*(7154), 339–342.

Sturm, R. (2002). Effect of managed care and financing on practice constraints and career satisfaction in primary care. *Journal of the American Board of Family Practice, 15*(5), 367–377.

Substance Abuse and Mental Health Services Administration. (2010a). *Results from the 2009 National Survey on Drug Use and Health: Mental Health Findings* (Office of Applied Studies, NSDUH Series H-39, HHS Publication No. SMA 10–4609). Rockville, MD: SAMHSA.

Substance Abuse and Mental Health Services Administration. (2010b). *Results from the 2009 National Survey on Drug Use and Health:* Volume I. *Summary of National Findings* (Office of Applied Studies, NSDUH Series H-38A, HHS Publication No. SMA10–4856 Findings). Rockville, MD: SAMHSA, 2010.

World Health Organization. (2001). *The world health report 2001: Mental health: New understanding, new hope.* Geneva: World Health Organization.

World Health Organization. (2002). *The world health report 2002: Reducing risks, promoting healthy life.* Geneva: World Health Organization.

World Health Organization. (2005). Preventing chronic diseases: A vital investment. *WHO global report.* Geneva: World Health Organization.

World Health Organization. (2006). *Constitution of the World Health Organization.* Geneva: World Health Organization. Retrieved from http://www.who.int/governance/eb/who_constitution_en.pdf.

Man-computer symbiosis is an expected development in cooperative interaction between men and electronic computers. It will involve very close coupling between the human and the electronic members of the partnership. The main aims are (a) to let computers facilitate formulative thinking as they now facilitate the solution of formulated problems, and (b) to enable men and computers to cooperate in making decisions and controlling complex situations without inflexible dependence on predetermined programs. In the anticipated symbiotic partnership, men will set the goals, formulate the hypotheses, determine the criteria, and perform the evaluations. Computing machines will do the routinizable work that must be done to prepare the way for insights and decisions in technical and scientific thinking.

JOSEPH CARL ROBNETT LICKLIDER, 1960

3 Informatics and Mental Health

Introduction

The emergence and evolution of technology in the provision of mental health services, research, and education are not recent developments. Although the Internet has played a major role in providing new opportunities for mental health professionals to collaborate and for their professional development, mental health informatics began in the mid-twentieth century. This chapter will cover a brief history of mental health informatics and will set the stage for the transition from telephone to fiber, including infrastructure developments crucial to today's informatics landscape, as well as legislation. Implications and future trends will also be addressed in this chapter.

The history of informatics in mental health begins with the use of early telecommunication networks, such as telephone and television, by the clinical disciplines, by state and federal initiatives, and by individual and family support and consumer initiatives. Throughout the history of informatics, the use of technology has ranged widely, from plain old telephone service (POTS) to high bandwidth applications, from a focus on individual care to administrative analyses to systems-wide public sector care. However, through all of the technology, programs, and services, the primary focus still remains on how best to improve mental health care and the quality of life for those individuals who have mental illnesses.

From a historical perspective, *computing* and *computers* are found throughout time, from the use of the abacus in China to the Pascaline in 1654 (Ball, 1960, 1908). During the 1880s, a "computer" was a person who handled or taught complex arithmetical and mathematical work (Scripture, 1891). In 1834, the modern analytic computer was invented (Babbage, 1899), the forerunner of the modern electronic digital computer, with binary algebra (Boolean) developed in 1854 (Boole, 1951, 1854). In the early 1900s, use of these analytic computers, also known as calculating machines, was urged to ensure greater accuracy with minimum expenditure of time and energy (Dunlap, 1913). Computing tables that could shorten the processing of complex data sets and numeric calculations were common (Tippett, 1927). Thanks to Vannevar Bush and colleagues, differential analyzer technology developed in the 1930s (Owens, 1986), and analog computers dominated the field of computing.

The first digital computer, Electronic Numerical Integrator and Computer (ENIAC), was built in 1944 at the University of Pennsylvania (Hartree, 1946; Moore School of Electrical Engineering, 1944). Five years later, the first-generation digital computer, Universal Automatic Computer (UNIVAC), was patented, with the ability to process numerical as well as textual data (Paul, 2003).

Emergence of Mental Health Informatics

THE 1950S

This decade ushered in significant technology as we think of it today. By 1955, IBM was known for its commercial computers (Chamberlain, 1954). The literature contains notices of the emergence of "the many different automatic and semi-automatic computing devices now available [that] may be used to handle the computations; the data are so set up they may be programmed into one of these devices. The more complicated of these computers are not ordinarily accessible, as yet, to researchers in the social sciences" (Katz, 1950, p. 110).

The literature reflected concerns over the growing use of media (radio) in airing mental health issues. Psychologists addressed the ethical consequences of radio-aired "personal advice columns" in letters to the American Psychological Association. There was concern that these "personal problems as entertainment" settings would have adverse consequences for individuals who might take such advice seriously (Snyder, 1949). Psychologists also suggested that the American Psychological Association consider creating a library of radio broadcast transcriptions that would be available to licensed professionals (Newland, 1948).

The space race, Sputnik, and Memex (Bush, 1945) were the news of the day. *Cybernetics*, or the analogies between man and machine, also captured the world's imagination (Rentchnick, 1950; Weiner, 1948). *Cybernetics*, a Greek word meaning "steersman," was seen as "embracing the entire field of control and communication theory as applied to both animals and machines" (Taylor, 1949, p. 236). Cybernetics offered the possibility of extending the precision of mathematics to human processes, clearly involving ideas of information, control, and feedback. Terms such as *feed-forward*, which describes the search activity of individuals, began entering the vocabulary in the field of cybernetics (von Foerster, Mead, & Teuber, 1953).

Concepts originating in mathematics and engineering were applied to biology and the behavioral sciences. Computerization and simulation, set theory, graph theory, net theory, automata theory, decision theory, queuing theory, game theory, and general systems theory became part of the language of health and mental health. The interest of cybernetics impacted how machines were considered to increase understanding of human functioning in education, in measurement, and in health (McReynolds, 1950; Wenger, 1950). The application of cybernetics to psychiatry was examined on several fronts, including linguistic analysis, schizophrenia, communication, and neural networks (Ashby, 1954; Berne, 1953; Dal Bianco, 1957; MacCarthy, 1955; Hirschfeld, 1957; George, 1958; Gurevich, 1959). From an information searching and resource discovery perspective, researchers added *cybernetics*, *automatic data processing*, and *bionics* to their vocabulary.

The developing importance of high-speed computers was viewed as a critical issue in research design. Problem-solving theory, for example, was examined in terms of information processes. One set of postulates addressed "[a] control system consisting of a number of memories, which contain symbolized information and are interconnected by various ordering relations; a number of primitive information processes, which operate on the information in the memories; a perfectly definite set of rules for combining these processes into whole programs of processing" (Newell, Shaw, & Simon, 1958, p. 151).

The proliferation of types of computers was discussed thoroughly in the literature. It was no longer an issue of *a* computer, but rather of determining *which* computer was the best for one's research—the Psycheac, the UNIVAC, the "701," the ENIAC, or the University of Illinois electronic computer (Iliac)—and determining the computer's effectiveness and cost efficacy of operation (Leavitt, Stone, & Wrigley, 1954; North, 1955; Wrigley & Neuhaus, 1955).

Commonly used in nursing and medical education, as well as in K–12 education, the use of "telecasts" in mental health started in the mid-1950s. Cecil Wittson and staff at the Nebraska Psychiatric Institute first demonstrated the use of this technology in mental health training (Wittson, Affleck, & Johnson, 1961). A small closed-circuit interactive television system (IATV), originally established for lectures and instructional purposes at the Institute, was expanded in 1956 with interactive audio links to hospitals in Nebraska, Iowa, North Dakota, and South Dakota. Therapists led two televised and two non-televised small groups of patients (Wittson et al., 1961). Radio conferences, using two-way radio, were also emerging as educational and diagnostic tools (Meneely & Sands, 1958). With the increased penetration of plain old telephone service (POTS), telephone consultation was considered standard practice (Barr, 1958).

Television, seen as having possible therapeutic value in residential settings, was publicized as a possible mass teaching medium (Babcock, 1951; Warner, 1954; Warner & Bowers, 1954). There were mixed reviews of the media and its effect on pedagogy. On one hand, " … the quality of this TV instruction is such that students taught by this means seem to get at least as much factual information as do those who sit in on conventional lectures" (Aronov, 1955, p. 88). On the other hand, there were concerns about the dehumanizing effect of a non-interactive class: "The technique described recalls to mind the image of the children in Aldous Huxley's *Brave New World* receiving their sterile education via standardized recorded lectures" (Aronov, 1955, p. 88).

Public awareness for mental health issues continued to use television and radio media (Television and Education, 1953; Gordon, 1953; Thompson, 1954). Psychologists had broadcast educational shows that offered a "less dramatized, less spectacular version of the work done by psychologists [than] that presented by newspapers and other popular publications" (Aronov, 1955, p. 88). Psychologists were reporting their own efforts, such as "Child Behavior," a half-hour program sponsored as a public service by the *Boston Globe* and the local television station WBZ-TV (Ames, 1954). City-focused series, such as "Health of Our City" in Grand Rapids, Michigan (Barrett, 1954), or Washington, D.C. (Keesey, 1954), or Denver, Colorado (Pinckney, 1954), became more commonplace. There was continued emphasis on health education using television as a media to reach a broader audience in a more relaxed setting. Studies of the time included assessment efforts to determine the impact of television programs across diverse audiences and content areas, such as child psychology on audiences comprising parents and teachers (Terrell, 1958) and other health education programs in public health and nursing (Knutson & Shimberg, 1955; Spangler, 1955).

THE 1960S

The growing interest in digital computing in the 1950s bore fruit in the next decade (Meehl, 1956; Meehl, 1962). During the 1960s, the use of computers in mental health research was a recurring theme in the literature. *Computers in Behavioral Science*, a Dutch journal, started publication in the late 1950s, providing "provocative summaries of work on learning, perception, information retrieval, and language translation" (Ackoff, 1960). The Mental Health Research Institute at the University of Michigan, Ann Arbor, in concert with the Institute of Management Sciences, published *Behavioral Science,* which examined the uses of computing in the behavioral sciences.

It was no longer necessary to argue the worth of computers and the use of computing. After all, "[c]omputer programs now play chess and checkers, find proofs for theorems in geometry and logic, compose music, balance assembly lines, design electric motors and generators, memorize nonsense syllables, form concepts, and learn to read" (Simon & Newell, 1962, p. 137).

An early adapter predicted that the computer's excellence in binary logic would someday automate the task of data analysis and interpretation (Ax, 1967). Articles on factor analysis using the computer emphasized the possibility of having dozens of variables that could not have been previously handled prior to the advent of the computer (Ivey, 1971). In 1966, a state-of-the-art review of computer use in psychophysiological research recommended an "Ideal-1966" system that would be based on "real-time on-line computer capabilities" (Ax, 1967). When this statement was made, computing instruments were analog (not digital), not programmable, and the IBM 7094 was the state of the art (Kahn, Bowne, & Swint, 1972).

The 1960s also saw the evolution of tape records with batch mode updates and record modification capabilities to newer forms of disk storage with online access for file maintenance (Graham, 1977). Examples of this included *Chemical Abstracts*, a database that linked substance names with their appropriate Chemical Abstracts Service (CAS) chemical compound Registry Numbers.

With the emergence of automated information retrieval systems, research concerns focused on the definition of subject and psychological taxonomies, the issues involved in encoding the information into the database, and query and retrieval issues in selecting relevant files (Fliege, 1966). Developments in abstracting and indexing in computer science and library/information science helped to create workable solutions that evolved as technology evolved (DuBois, 1965; Edmundson & Wyllys, 1961).

Although data analysis was the most popular use of computers, discussions emerged on the use of computers in medical diagnosis (Borke, 1969; Graetz, 1965; Ledley, 1959; Vandenberg et al., 1960), the use of automated information retrieval for literature reviews (DuBois, 1965; Edmundson & Wyllys, 1961), systems analysis and research to assist in decision-making systems (Fliege, 1966; Green, 1963a), and complex problem-solving tasks (Gyr, Thatcher, & Allen, 1962; Newell et al., 1958; Simon & Newell, 1962). The literature reflected an optimistic perspective that a national health computer network would be feasible with then-current computing technology (Ledley & Lusted, 1960).

The early 1960s also saw studies in artificial intelligence begin to improve the ability of computers in specific activities and to better understand the simulation of behaviors (Green, 1963a; Minsky, 1961; Pfeffer, 1962). Work done on medical diagnosis evolved into work on mental measurements and psychological diagnostic tests (Borke, 1969; Graetz, 1965; Ledley & Lusted, 1960). In 1966, ELIZA was created, one of the first computer-assisted interviewing attempts that simulated the behavior of a psychotherapist (Weizenbaum, 1976). Users believed that they were interacting with a human rather than a machine—one of the criteria to pass the "Turing Test," a measure of artificial intelligence (Turing, 1950). It led the way for subsequent computer models that could mimic dysfunctional personalities (Colby, 1975).

Computer-aided learning, also known as computer-based teaching, became an important area of study (Baber, 1965; Cooley & Glaser, 1969; Green, 1963b; Stillerman, 1963). Fliege (1966) suggested that the value of a computer-based teaching machine was its capacity to dynamically vary the presentation of materials to students based upon their performances through "branching." Real-time process control examined performance on single questions, cumulative performance scores, student response, response latencies, and sequencing of presentation (Judd & Glaser, 1969; O'Neil, Spielberger, & Hansen, 1969; Rapoport, 1969; Slack & Van Cura, 1968; Spolsky, 1966). Other issues examined were creativity and the role of personality in learner behaviors (Ripple, O'Reilly, Wightman, & Dacey, 1965; Tobias, 1969). Also during the 1960s, early mental health information systems were developed at Camarillo State Hospital (Graetz, Agan, Arnsfield, Jacobus, & Wells, 1965) and at Fort Logan Mental Health Center (Truitt & Binner, 1969).

In addition, television and microwave technology were initially used in academic settings, with the KUMC television link to the University of Kansas (Geertsma, 1967). Microwave technology was used as a method of consultation between Dartmouth-Hitchcock Mental Health Center and Claremont General Hospital (Solow, 1971). By 1968, Massachusetts General Hospital was providing emergency mental health consults at Logan Airport Medical Station using IATV (Dwyer, 1973). The use of television and videotape for group and individualized instruction became more prevalent (Benschoter, Eaton, & Smith, 1965; Kagan, Krathwohl, & Miller, 1963; Moore, Chernell, & West, 1965). These "audio-visual biopsies" (Wilmer, 1968) were seen as a way for mental health professionals to "see" themselves during the interview so that there would be opportunities to improve their clinical skills and methodologies (Goldman, 1969; Hill & Stoller, 1967; Wilmer, 1967).

New modalities emerged, such as micro-counseling, a video method of training counselors in the basic skills of counseling within a short period of time (Ivey, 1971; Ivey & et al., 1968). Patients were able to see the effects of interactions with counselors and family members and to provide more realistic self-assessments (Beakel & Mehrabian, 1969; Borke, 1969; Dinoff, Clark, Reitman, & Smith, 1969; Geertsma & Reivich, 1965).

The consensus in the field held that video was valuable for both patients and therapists; the literature reflected articles stressing confidentiality, equipment evaluations, and how best to use videotaping with patients (Berger, 1969; Ekman & Friesen, 1969; Poling, 1968). There were predictions that within five years, 25% of practitioners in the United States would be using videotapes in their practices (Berger, 1969) and that new information storage and retrieval systems would help videotapes supplant the current lecture system (Romano, 1967).

THE 1970S

By the 1970s, computer applications fully emerged in the field of mental health. Not only could computers expedite the handling of routine, repetitive tasks, but the speed and flexibility of these new computer information systems could provide reports on patients, patient-doctor interactions, and hospital admissions and discharges. Other administrative data, including length of stay, re-admission statistics, and drug inventory reports were also available using computers.

With the advent of computers in mental health facilities, large clinical databases were waiting to be mined for administrative uses (Chapman, 1976; Cooper, 1973; Halpert, Horvath, & Young, 1970). New applications and programs were built to handle issues in using coded data, such as coding errors. Programs, such as ClinQuery, facilitated exploration and analysis (Berry & Reichelt, 1977) using alternative clinical data, such as discharge diagnoses.

Also during the 1970s, discussion of the use of computer retrieval services was growing in the professional literature (Markley & Adams, 1973; Peper & Toth, 1971). For example, a 1973 examination of 15 mental health journals published between 1960 and 1969 showed approximately 2,500 reports of new measures, with 70% of these measures never cited again after publication (Chun, Cobb, French, & Seashore, 1973). A new computerized information retrieval system, the National Repository of Social Science Measures, was a primary resource in locating psychological measures (Chun, Cobb, & French, 1975). Other literature addressed the use and limitations of online bibliographic resources, as well as the difficulties encountered in staying up to date (Beck, 1977; Knapp, 1979).

The increase in online bibliographic searching, as opposed to manual (or hand) searches, assisted in the development of new areas of research, including range of data coverage, searcher skill levels, and information seeking and gathering tasks, such as question analysis, searching, photocopying, shelving, and output distribution (Elchesen, 1978). The literature also addressed increasing search efficiency in online databases. In a retrospective (3-year) search on drug safety in Excerpta Medica, the researchers discovered that 50% of the references appeared in only 148 journals, or 6% of all journals surveyed (Kitaguchi, Nojiri,

Suzuki, Fukita, & Kawana, 1983). Research continued to address how best to search and how best to strategize.

Although, in most cases, studies showed that online searching was faster than manual searching, for certain types of query/information source combinations, manual searching still offered some advantages in precision and turn-around time (Lorent, 1979; Schneiweiss, 1979). Optimally, manual and online searching would complement each other as far as serendipity, relevance, and uniqueness, all qualities that can be attributed to a "good search." Weekly newsletters from indexing and abstracting resources, such as *Chemical Abstracts*, provided guidelines and tips for users regarding the use of controlled vocabulary or new interface options (Moody & Zahm, 1980).

Abstracts used in medical records abstracting systems also came under examination. The utility of medical records abstracts, used in clinical research, utilization review, and health statistics, is determined primarily by the accuracy of the stored abstracts. For these systems to have face validity, quality control procedures and error identification systems are essential to assure content validity (Gardiner, 1978).

The transmission of vast amounts of data had improved the clinician's ability to make decisions regarding patient care. One such application was biofeedback, based on the premise that individuals could learn to control physiological activity if they could see a recognizable representation of the activity. Since the computer could change analog signals from the body into digital representations, users could be connected to sensing devices and review simple displays (Kantor & Brown, 1970). The widespread use of biofeedback brought about iteration after iteration of computerized equipment and clearly demonstrated that the real-time processing of human physiological signals was feasible (McArthur, Schandler, & Cohen, 1988).

THE 1980S

By the 1980s, use of computing in mental health was entering its fourth generation. This was " ... because the Japanese are already at work on the fifth generation" (Blum, 1983, p. 47). Emphasis was placed upon the information needs of private practitioners, current and future trends in micro-technology for clinical applications, organizational issues in implementing computer systems, automated psychological testing, patient assessment and diagnosis, computer-aided education and treatment, accounting systems, and administrative and clinical information management.

The increased reliance on mental health information databases became critical in the planning, provision, and evaluation of mental health services delivery. The National Institute of Mental Health (NIMH) was busy designing a prototype management information system (MIS) for community mental health centers (National Institute of Mental Health, 1983; Wurster & Goodman, 1981). By the end of the 1970s, more than three-fourths of all community mental health centers were using some form of a computerized management information system (Gorodezky & Hedlund, 1982). Although most of these systems offered "traditional" services (staff activity reporting, patient register, financial and billing systems, and program evaluation) run through a batch process, newer systems included online interactive data entry and retrieval. MIS was viewed as an evolving technology for improving emergency mental health services and decision making, for planning alcohol abuse services, for supporting consultation and liaison mental health services, and for behavioral assessment and diagnosis of children with mental disorders. The potential of using personal and mainframe computer systems in various types of psychiatric care was the focus of many academic and professional texts (Lieff, 1987). However, the question "Should there be a national quality monitoring system for mental health?" was a constant refrain (Iezzoni & Greenberg, 1994).

Computer assisted instruction (CAI) for mental health professionals and for mental health consumers was on the rise. Programs were developed to teach clinicians and nurses basic mental health information. Techniques and methodologies varied. Short simulated patient interviews were created to develop specialized interviewing techniques, such as suicide assessment, based upon diagnosis or discipline, or on the side effects of antipsychotic medications (Santo & Finkel, 1982; Smith, Parmar, & Paget, 1980; Van Donegan, 1984; Wolfman, 1980). Continuing professional education was a growing area (Lynett, 1985). Community mental health public information CAI programs were expanding. For example, CAI allowed the development of an interactive system that asked for basic individual demographics, gave a short quiz on general mental health knowledge, and gave feedback that corrected misconceptions about mental illness and treatment (Abernathy, 1979).

THE 1990S

In 1991, the Institute of Medicine issued a report calling for the development of a computerized patient record system (Dick & Steen, 1991). Much of what the Institute advocated included incorporation of "best practice" guidelines for clinical and pharmaceutical care, patient monitoring data, and medical records. Those same clinical workstations became part of administrative and quality assurance systems targeted to improving patient outcomes and services delivery.

The 1990s also saw the continued evolution of research databases as opposed to record systems designed to support clinical practice (Agency for Health Care Policy and Research, 1991; Ashton, Menke, Deykin, Camberg, & Charns, 1996; Biczyk do Amaral,1993; Buican et al., 1999; Mohan, Muse, & McInerney, 1998; Safran, 1991; Tierney & McDonald, 1991). In geriatric psychiatry, for example, GPSYCH was a supplemental electronic medical record system that provided organization of clinical information with powerful search capabilities. Its primary goal was to support clinical decision making and to facilitate clinical research (Aisen, 1996). Using an SPSS/PC statistical program, clinicians could answer a question such as whether behavioral disturbances in Alzheimer's patients worsen as cognitive function declines, or the number of patients with severe extrapyramidal reactions to neuroleptics (Aisen, 1996).

During the 1990s, computing took a quantum leap forward with the development of the world wide web (WWW). Computing was no longer limited to local area networks (LANs); it now had wide area networks (WANs). Although computer-mediated communication, in various forms, was commonly used in disaster management, this decade saw the emergence of wide area computer networks (i.e., the Internet) in disaster management and prevention (Butler & Anderson, 1992). The first directory file structure, Gopher, was ubiquitous and provided easy access to mental health resources set up by professional associations, colleges, and universities. The types of resources found at these sites included links to job listings, electronic journals, and university psychology departments with Internet directories of information. The first Internet-based journal, initially circulated by electronic mail, was *Psycoloquy*, which was also the first electronic journal indexed in PsycINFO.

The Computers in Teaching Initiative Center for Psychology saw the WWW as a support to mental health education by disseminating information, generating and accessing resource materials, and enhancing knowledge exchange (Trapp, Hammond, & Bray, 1996). The Web also provided a useful forum for dialogue and feedback. For example, Hanover College and the American Psychological Society (APS) developed web-based tutorials in sensation and perception (Krantz, 1995). Other research involved the development and use of a multimedia primer in auditory perception that included instructional material and acoustical experiments conducted over the WWW (Welch & Krantz, 1996).

"Patient informatics" also emerged as an evolution of the patient-centered/consumer-centered focus of health care providers and managed care companies in response to provider "report cards" and the growing availability of health information on the Internet (Bader & Braude, 1998; Burk et al., 2003; Cline & Haynes, 2001; Ellis, Jankowski, Jasper, & Abdul, 1996; Lopez & Prosser, 1999; White, 1998). The shift toward a "person-centered" focus in mental health (recovery paradigm) became an important consideration in the development of satisfaction and quality measures (Buckley, 1993; Dumont et al., 2006).

THE 2000S

With the advent of graphically based browsers, the use of Internet technology accelerated at a dramatic pace. The Internet created opportunities for the use of updated full-text resource literature (Felkey & Buring, 2000). Since the main disadvantage of print resource literature was its lag time, the Internet all but eliminated this disadvantage. Publishers of electronically formatted fee-based literature, previously only available on CDs or network servers, rapidly moved their products into Internet formats, resulting in increased accessibility to updated information from anywhere in the world. Journals, textbooks, medical databases, and media productions, such as video- and audio-casts, became available directly online to researchers, mental health care professionals, and consumers of mental health care services.

The changes in transmission network switching, and information processions through improvements in fiber optic technology, integrated circuits, faster computer hardware, and emergent freeware did not go unnoticed by the U.S. government. The National Science Foundation made available to universities a number of meritorious applications via its Internet2 grants to develop high bandwidth projects. Researchers eagerly developed a number of web-based video projects. One such project was the University of South Florida, Louis de la Parte Florida Mental Health Institute's "Streaming Video Database in Support of Mental Health Education and Training" (http://web.archive.org/web/20060905034937/http://lib.fmhi.usf.edu/projects/internet2-blueline2.pdf). The Institute developed a searchable database of online video archives, viewable across a number of network bandwidths ranging from 56 kb/sec up to 1Mbit/sec (Kearns, 2003). The streaming video database embedded the media viewer within the record, allowing the user to read about the video and then choose to play it. Since part of the Institute's mission is to disseminate knowledge about mental illnesses and to reduce the stigma associated with them, the streaming video format was seen as a way to bring people together by using high-speed Internet technology (Kearns, 2003). This product has been in use continuously since 1999, and was demonstrated nationally at the March 2000 Annual Member Meeting of Internet2 in Washington, D.C. (see Figure 3.1).

Webcasts are "pushed" to users via online mail and distribution lists, RSS feeds, and other online delivery methods. Online symposia, such as the "Mental Health & Rehabilitation eCast," a monthly production of the Center for Psychiatric Rehabilitation at Boston University, and the "Symposia Series on Systems Science and Health," sponsored by the NIH Office of Behavioral and Social Sciences Research and CDC's Syndemics Prevention Network, are freely available online. New technologies address the continued convergence of services and resources, platform/network development, data management trends, and applications designed for "real world" solutions. Computational, spatial, social, and environmental data and resources converge in health services research, especially in the integration of research into practice, the development of "best practices," fidelity in implementation, and the issues surrounding transformational research (Drake, Teague, & Gersing, 2005; Dumont et al., 2006; Medow et al., 2001; Staff, 2002). Data mining large

author : Burr, Diane W.// Mullins, Larry C.//Rich, Thomas, A.//Roorda, James A.//Boucher, Louisette A.//Zuk, Irene M.//Oliver, Kimberly R. Sullivan-Mintz, Judith.
title : Older Homeless Adults in America. Part 9. Law enforcement.
collection : Webcast (1000kb)
date : 1992
location : System requirements: Internet connectivity (1000kb). Web browser software, Microsoft Media Player. If you do not see a viewer in the field below this message, you will need to download Media Player from this site.
extent : 15:34 minutes

pages :
abstract : This nine-part video series was produced by the Institute's Department of Aging and Mental Health in 1992. Funded by the Retirement Research Foundation, the series was developed as a training program to support education efforts in the state of Florida. Part 9 (original title: "A Social Problem, Not a Crime: a video guide for law enforcement") reviews the demographics of the older homeless adults, the effects of deinstitutionlization and economic conditions, medications, physical health problems, and the older homeless adult as a victim of other crime on the streets.
callnumber : In process (In-house collection)
descriptors : webcast 1000/ internet2/ elderly/ staff training/ Roorda, James R. (scriptwriter)/Roorda, James R. (narrator)/streaming video webcast -- educational, training narrative/ homelessness/ mentally ill/ grant/ Retirement Research Foundation/ Aging and Mental Health/ AMH/ Aged/ older homeless adults/ social policy/ vignette/ community mental health services/ homeless persons -- mental health services -- United States/ homeless persons -- services for -- Florida/ housing -- United States/ deinstitutionalization/ law enforcement/ crisis intervention/ stereotypes/ stigma/ labeling

FIGURE 3.1 Screen Shot of Record in Streaming Video Database in Support of Mental Health Education and Training. Permission granted by the Louis de la Parte Florida Mental Health Institute.

quantitative datasets, modeling real-life phenomena, prediction or forecasting of long-term behaviors and activity—all of these activities, and more, comprise what we read and do every day in mental health informatics.

Studies on the clinical efficacy and cost effectiveness of telemental health services abound. Some studies are affirmative in the use of telecommunications technologies, while other studies have given mixed reviews and somewhat less than glowing reports (Hailey, Roine, & Ohinimaa, 2008; Eisen et al., 2002). Costs of such programs and the problems of dealing with an increasing technological practice environment continue to be prevalent in the literature (Barthell et al., 2003; Barrett et al., 2002; Kennedy & Yellowlees, 2000; Kennedy, 2005; Lehoux & Blume, 2000; Lehoux, Denis, Tailliez, & Hivon, 2005; Monnier, Knapp, & Frueh, 2003; Pesamaa et al., 2004).

Obviously, significant progress has been made over the past half century regarding the growth of information technology and its applications for health and mental health services delivery. In addition, the growth of managed care has changed the way in which mental health providers, organizations, and government agencies have used and shared statistical information.

Legislation

Congress was also active in enacting legislation to improve access to the internet. Rapid technological change drives regulatory change. One of the early federal Acts, the Communications Act of 1934 (47 U.S.C. § 151 et seq.), regulated interstate and foreign commerce in communication by wire and radio, replaced the Federal Radio Commission with the Federal Communications Commission (FCC), and transferred regulation of interstate telephone services from the Interstate Commerce Commission to the FCC. However, with the growth of the information economy, changes in market conditions spurred a number of regulatory changes in the telecommunications industry.

The Telecommunications Act of 1996 dramatically altered the communication rates and services potentially available to telehealth and telemental health providers. This federal legislation was the first major overhaul of American telecommunications policy in nearly 62 years. The Act was electronically signed by President Clinton in the Library of Congress Reading Room, making it the first bill signed into law in cyberspace. The signing was also viewable in real-time over the Internet, delivered over a "high speed, fiber-optic synchronous optical network link" (Lamolinara, 1996, pp. 2–3).

Noting the historic nature of the bill, President Clinton suggested that the legislation would "stimulate investment, promote competition, provide open access for all citizens to the Information Superhighway" (Clinton, 1996, February 8). He also drew parallels with the signing of the Interstate Highway Act of 1957, "which met the challenge of change ... and literally brought Americans closer together...." "That same spirit of connection and communication is the driving force behind the Telecommunications Act of 1996." Vice President Albert Gore, an advocate for the Information Highway, said "This legislation will expand and strengthen universal service.... It allows open access to the pipelines of knowledge" (Lamolinara, 1996, p. 3). Approximately $500 million was allocated to health care providers, libraries, and schools in rural areas to offset telephone line charges incurred in connecting to the Internet via the Universal Service Fund (United States General Accounting Office, 2002).

In the Act, the internet is defined as

- "the international computer network of both Federal and non-Federal interoperable packet switched data networks" (47 U.S.C. § 230(f)(1)) and as
- "the combination of computer facilities and electromagnetic transmission media, and related equipment and software, comprising the interconnected worldwide network of computer networks that employ the Transmission Control Protocol/Internet Protocol or any successor protocol to transmit information" (47 U.S.C. § 231(e)(3)).

The Act further states that the policy of the United States is "to promote the continued development of the Internet," "to preserve the vibrant and competitive free market that presently exists for it," and "to encourage the development of technologies" (47 U.S.C.§230).

As technology advances, so do issues of access to technology. The Twenty-First Century Communications and Video Accessibility Act of 2010 was introduced during the 111th Congress and signed into law by President Obama. S. 3304, the Equal Access to 21st Century Communications Act, increased the access of persons with disabilities to modern communications. Also, in 2010, Senators John D. Rockefeller IV, John F. Kerry, and Representatives Henry A. Waxman and Rick Boucher announced their intent to update the 1996 Telecommunications Act. However, since the 1996 Act took several years of hearings and reviews before legislation reached consensus, it was expected that the process of amending the Act would take at least that long.

In 2011, the Senate and the House introduced versions of the proposed Public Safety Broadband and Wireless Innovation Act (S. 28, H.R.2482, and H.R.3509). The Act essentially would ensure the reallocation and deployment of a nationwide public safety interoperable broadband network in the 700 MHz and 700 MHz D block spectrum band for deployment in both rural and urban areas. In addition to the establishment of a public safety advisory board, the act would also establish a network construction fund, a network maintenance/operation fund, and a federal grant program to assist public safety entities in the establishment of the network. It would also amend the National Telecommunications and Information Administration (NTIA) Act and assign additional responsibilities to the FCC in regard to the allocation of broadcast spectrums and licenses.

From a mental health perspective, several important initiatives emerged in 1996. Perhaps the most pertinent legislation, from an informatics perspective, was the signing of the Health Insurance Portability and Accountability Act (HIPAA) by President Clinton. Addressing the security and privacy of health data, Title II of HIPAA requires the establishment of national standards for electronic health care transactions and national identifiers for providers, health insurance plans, and employers.

Legislation created during the Clinton Administration set the foundation for many of the initiatives for subsequent administrations, including the President's New Freedom Commission, signed into existence by a Presidential Executive Order on June 18, 2001

(Bush, 2002, May 3). The first comprehensive study of the U.S. mental health service delivery systems in nearly 25 years, the Commission's purpose was to:

> help Americans with disabilities increase access to innovative new technologies that help them participate fully in society, expand their educational opportunities, better integrate them into the workforce, and promote their full access to community life. (A Blueprint for New Beginnings: A Responsible Budget for America's Priorities, 2001, p. 61)

The President directed the 22 commission members to "study the problems and gaps in the mental health system and make concrete recommendations for immediate improvements that the Federal government, State governments, local agencies, as well as public and private health care providers, can implement" (The President's New Freedom Commission on Mental Health, 2003, p. 3). The Commission stated six goals for America to meet its mandate:

1. Americans understand that mental health is essential to overall health.
2. Mental health care is consumer and family driven.
3. Disparities in mental health services are eliminated.
4. Early mental health screening, assessment, and referral to services are common practice.
5. Excellent mental health care is delivered and research is accelerated.
6. Technology is used to access mental health care and information (The President's New Freedom Commission on Mental Health, 2003, p. 5).

We will learn more about the legislation and its impacts in subsequent chapters.

Implications for Mental Health Informatics

We started this chapter recalling events from the 1950s, with technology gaining world prominence, with Sputnik, cybernetics, and Vannevar Bush's Memex machine (Bush, 1945), a futuristic device that foreshadowed the modern computer, global networks, and "grokking" (to completely understand) the net.

Telecommunication and information technology, including the Internet, holds enormous potential for transforming mental health service delivery systems in America. Central to the application of information science and technology to promote mental health and prevent mental disorders in at-risk populations is the establishment of an infrastructure to develop comprehensive integrated health surveillance and information systems that bridge programmatic boundaries within communities. It would also provide informatics training for both new and existing health and mental health professionals, provide safeguards for confidentiality and privacy for these information systems, and foster improved exchange of information between health and mental health professionals and their patients.

Historically, federal and state budgets appropriated funding for health and mental health programs. However difficult it may have been to administer health programs in rural areas prior to online communications networks, provision of services to rural and frontier areas has become more difficult (Ferguson, 1998; Levin & Hanson, 2001; Smith & Allison, 19998). Criteria for funds often have been based upon criteria relevant to urban areas. Allocation of these funds to rural areas may not cover the administrative requirements of the grant.

From an organizational perspective, a continuing issue in the use of telecommunications technology is the ongoing expense of time and money for staff training. This issue has become more complicated with HIPAA regulations for compliance and training of all staff regarding what their knowledge of HIPAA regulations must be. Training should not be viewed as a "one-time" expense, since infrastructure changes over time to keep pace with new regulations and network updates.

Finally, if the use of technology is to become a tool to improve delivery of and access to services for mental health, then five areas need to be resolved: (1) reimbursement; (2) licensure; (3) expanded coverage area by Medicare and private health plans; (4) adequate infrastructure in rural and frontier areas; and (5) the costs of technology. Reimbursement practices need to be standardized to expedite payment for services and expanded to provide increased access to essential mental health diagnostic, consultative, and clinical services. In addition, federal agencies, such as Medicare, need to move forward to ensure adequate reimbursement for "tele-consultations."

Adequate infrastructure in rural and frontier areas is still a significant problem. Although telecommunications networks are ubiquitous in metropolitan and suburban areas, the efforts and cost of "telefying" rural and frontiers areas mirror those of the rural electrification program in the early twentieth century. Costs of technology must be added to infrastructure development costs. For example, teleconferencing units that cost $300,000 in the early 1990s now cost $10,000. However, for rural and frontier area facilities, single practitioner settings, or practitioners in less-affluent areas, this equipment is still not affordable without subsidies from the federal government. Even with subsidies, the costs of maintenance, training, and upgrades still place tele-technologies beyond the reach of most facilities and providers.

References

Abernathy, W. B. (1979). The microcomputer as a community mental health public information tool. *Community Mental Health Journal, 15*(3), 192–202.

Ackoff, R. L. (1960). Periodicals. *Operations Research, 8*(1), 152–154.

Agency for Health Care Policy and Research. (1991). *The feasibility of linking research-related data bases to federal and non-federal medical administrative data bases: Report to Congress* (AHCPR pub. No. 91–0003). Rockville, MD: The Agency.

Aisen, P. S. (1996). Informatics and geriatric psychiatry. *American Journal of Geriatric Psychiatry, 4*(2), 140–151.

Ames, L. B. (1954). A child behavior program on television. *American Psychologist, 9*(9), 588.

Aronov, B. M. (1955). Aren't we forgetting something? A note on psychology via TV. *American Psychologist, 10*(2), 88.

Ashby, W. R. (1954). The application of cybernetics to psychiatry. *The Journal of Mental Science, 100*(418), 114–124.

Ashton, C. M., Menke, T. J., Deykin, D., Camberg, L. C., & Charns, M. P. (1996). A state-of-the-art conference on databases pertaining to veterans' health: a resource for research and decision making. *Medical Care, 34*(3, Suppl.), 1–8.

Ax, A. F. (1967). Electronic storage and computer analysis. In P. Venables (Ed.), *Manual of psychophysiological methods* (pp. 481–520). Amsterdam: North Holland Publishing Company.

Babbage, H. P. (1899). *Babbage's calculating engines: Being a collection of papers relating to them, their history and construction.* London: E. and F.N. Spon.

Babcock, K. B. (1951). Telecasts offer hospitals a mass teaching medium. *Hospitals, 25*(2), 55–56.

Baber, E. R. (1965). Improving health education through modern technics. *American Journal of Public Health and the Nation's Health, 55,* 404–408.

Bader, S. A., & Braude, R. M. (1998). "Patient informatics": Creating new partnerships in medical decision making. *Academic Medicine, 73*(4), 408–411.

Ball, W. W. R. ([1908] 1960). *A short account of the history of mathematics.* New York: Dover Publications.

Barr, N. L. (1958). Long-distance telephone technic is latest aid to diagnosis. *Modern Hospital, 91*(6), 64–65.

Barrett, J., Goh, S., Todd, C., Barclay, S., Daza-Ramirez, P., & Vardulaki, K. (2002). A description of an intermediate care service using routinely collected data. *Journal of Nursing Management, 10*(4), 221–227.

Barrett, M. (1954). "Health of Our City" in Grand Rapids. *Public Health Reports, 69*(6), 608–610.

Barthell, E. N., Foldy, S. L., Pemble, K. R., Felton, C. W., Greischar, P. J., Pirrallo, R. G. et al. (2003). Assuring community emergency care capacity with collaborative Internet tools: The Milwaukee experience. *Journal of Public Health Management & Practice, 9*(1), 35–42.

Beakel, N. G., & Mehrabian, A. (1969). Inconsistent communications and psychopathology. *Journal of Abnormal Psychology, 74*(1), 126–130.

Beck, C. (1977). Information systems and social sciences. *American Behavioral Scientist, 20*(3), 427–448.

Benschoter, R. A., Eaton, M. T., & Smith, P. (1965). Use of videotape to provide individual instruction in techniques of psychotherapy. *Journal of Medical Education, 40*(12), 1159–1161.

Berger, M. M. (1969). Integrating video into private psychiatric practice. *Voices: The Art & Science of Psychotherapy, 5*(4), 78–85.

Berne, E. (1953). Concerning the nature of communication. *The Psychiatric Quarterly, 27*(2), 185–198.

Berry, V. I., & Reichelt, P. A. (1977). Using routinely collected data for staffing decisions. *Hospitals, 51*(22), 89–90, 92.

Biczyk do Amaral, M., Satomura, Y., Honda, M., & Sato, T. (1993). A design for decision making: Construction and connection of knowledge bases for a diagnostic system in medicine. *Medical Informatics/Medecine et Informatique, 18*(4), 307–320.

A blueprint for new beginnings: A responsible budget for America's priorities. (2001). Washington, DC: U.S. Government Printing Office. Retrieved from http://www.whitehouse.gov/news/usbudget/blueprint/blueprint.pdf.

Blum, B. I. (1983). Mainframes, minis, and micros: Past, present, and future. *Medcomp, 48,* 40–48.

Boole, G. (1854/1951). *An investigation of the laws of thought: On which are founded the mathematical theories of logic and probabilities.* New York: Dover Publications.

Borke, H. (1969). The communication of intent: A revised procedure for analyzing family interaction from video tapes. *Journal of Marriage & the Family, 31*(3), 541–544.

Buckley, S. M. (1993). *Moving MHSIP toward a person-centered paradigm: A concept paper submitted to CMHS and the MHSIP Ad Hoc Advisory Group.* [New York]: New York State Research Foundation for Mental Hygiene under subcontract to the Cosmos Corporation. Retrieved March 2006 from http://www.mhsip.org/library/pdfFiles/movingMHSIP-toapersoncenteredparadigm.pdf.

Buican, B., Spaulding, W. D., Gordon, B., & Hindman, T. (1999). Clinical decision support systems in state hospitals. *New Directions for Mental Health Services, 84,* 99–112.

Burk, K. E., Martin, M. T., Reilly, C. A., & Kuperman, G. J. (2003). An online consumer health information resource: 3-year usage summary. *AMIA Annual Symposium Proceedings/ AMIA Symposium,* (p. 800). Bethesda, MD: American Medical Informatics Association.

Bush, G. W. (2002, May 3). Presidential documents: Title 3—Executive Order 13263 of April 29, 2002: The President President's New Freedom Commission on Mental Health. *Federal Register, 67*(86), 22337–22339.

Bush, V. (1945). As we may think. *Atlantic Monthly, 176*(1), 101–108.

Butler, D. L., & Anderson, P. S. (1992). The use of wide area computer networks in disaster management and the implications for hospital/medical networks. In D. F. Parsons, C. M. Fleischer, & R. A. Greenes (Eds.), *Extended clinical consulting by hospital computer networks* (pp. 202–210). New York: New York Academy of Sciences.

Chamberlain, J. (1954). Machines that think: Electronic computers are becoming big business. *Barron's National Business and Financial Weekly, Dec 27,* 34, 52.

Chapman, R. L. (1976). *The design of management information systems for mental health organizations: A primer.* Rockville, MD: U.S. Department of Health, Education, and Welfare, Public Health Service, Alcohol, Drug Abuse, and Mental Health Administration, National Institute of Mental Health, Division of Biometry and Epidemiology.

Chun, K.-T., Cobb, S., & French, J. R. (1975). *Measures for psychological assessment: A guide to 3,000 original sources and their applications.* Ann Arbor: University of Michigan, Institute for Social Research.

Chun, K.-T., Cobb, S., French, J. R., & Seashore, S. (1973). Storage and retrieval of information on psychological measures. *American Psychologist, 28*(7), 592–599.

Cline, R. J., & Haynes, K. M. (2001). Consumer health information seeking on the Internet: The state of the art. *Health Education Research, 16*(6), 671–692.

Clinton, W. (1996, February 8). *Remarks by the President in signing ceremony for the Telecommunications Act Conference Report.* Washington, DC: Library of Congress.

Colby, K. M. (1975). *Artificial paranoia: A computer simulation of paranoid processes* (Pergamon general psychology series No. 49). New York: Pergamon Press.

Cooley, W. W., & Glaser, R. (1969). The computer and individualized instruction. *Science, 166*(905), 574–582.

Cooper, E. M. (1973). *Guidelines for a minimum statistical and accounting system for community mental health centers: A working handbook with illustrative end-product tables, document forms, and procedures.* Rockville, MD: U.S. Dept. of Health, Education, and

Welfare, Alcohol, Drug Abuse, and Mental Health Administration, National Institute of Mental Health.

Dal Bianco, P. (1957). Schizophasie et cybernetique; etude de statistique linquistique [Schizophasia & cybernetics; a study in linguistic statistics]. *Acta Neurologica et Psychiatrica Belgica, 57*(12), 937–949.

Dick, R. S., & Steen, E. B. (1991). *The computer-based patient record: An essential technology for health care.* Washington, DC: National Academy Press.

Dinoff, M., Clark, C. G., Reitman, L. M., & Smith, R. E. (1969). The feasibility of video-tape interviewing. *Psychological Reports, 25*(1), 239–242.

Drake, R. E., Teague, G. B., & Gersing, K. (2005). State mental health authorities and informatics. *Community Mental Health Journal, 41*(3), 365–370.

DuBois, N. S. (1965). Documents from two sources are reconciled with a digital computer. *Behavioral Science, 10*, 312–319.

Dumont, J. M., Ridgway, P. A., Onken, S. J., Dornan, D. H., & Ralph, R. O. (2006). *Mental health recovery: What helps and what hinders? A national research project development of recovery system performance indicators phase II technical report: Development of the recovery oriented indicators (ROSI) measures to advance health system transformation.* Alexandria, VA: National Technical Assistance Center for State Mental Health Planning; National Association of State Mental Health Program Directors. Retrieved from http://www.nasmhpd.org/general_files/publications/ntac_pubs/Phase%20II%20Mental%20Health%20Recovery.pdf.

Dunlap, K. (1913). Obtaining the mean variation with the aid of a calculating machine. *Psychological Review, 20*(2), 154–157.

Dwyer, T. F. (1973). Telepsychiatry: Psychiatric consultation by interactive television. *American Journal of Psychiatry, 130*(8), 865–869.

Edmundson, H. P., & Wyllys, R. E. (1961). Automatic abstracting and indexing-survey and recommendations. *Commission of the ACM, 4*(5), 226–234.

Eisen, S. V., Wilcox, M., Idiculla, T., Speredelozzi, A., & Dickey, B. (2002). Assessing consumer perceptions of inpatient psychiatric treatment: the perceptions of care survey. *The Joint Commission Journal on Quality Improvement, 28*(9), 510–526.

Ekman, P., & Friesen, W. V. (1969). A tool for the analysis of motion picture film or video tape. *American Psychologist, 24*(3), 240–243.

Elchesen, D. R. (1978). Cost-effectiveness comparison of manual and on-line retrospective bibliographic searching. *Journal of the American Society for Information Science. American Society for Information Science, 29*(2), 56–66.

Ellis, R. D., Jankowski, T. B., Jasper, J. E., & Abdul, A. (1996). Gero-informatics and the Internet: Locating gerontology information on the world wide web (WWW). *Gerontologist, 36*(1), 100–105.

Felkey, B. G., & Buring, S. M. (2000). Using the Internet for research. *Journal of the American Pharmaceutical Association, 40*(4), 546–553.

Ferguson, T. (1998). Digital doctoring-opportunities and challenges in electronic patient-physician communication. *Journal of the American Medical Association, 280*, 1361–1362.

Fliege, S. (1966). Digital computers. In J. B. Sidowski (Ed.), *Experimental methods and instrumentation in psychology* (pp. 699–734). New York: McGraw-Hill.

Gardiner, R. C. (1978). Quality considerations in medical records abstracting systems. *Journal of Medical Systems, 2*(1), 31–43.

Geertsma, R. H., & Reivich, R. S. (1965). Repetitive self-observation by videotape playback. *Journal of Nervous and Mental Disease, 1141*(1), 29–41.

Geertsma, R. H. (1967). TV microwave system: The KUMC television link to the University of Kansas. *Journal of the Kansas Medical Society, 68*(3), 90–95.

George, F. H. (1958). Machines and the brain: Mathematical logic helps design complex nets whose arrangements resemble the structure of the brain. *Science, 127*(3309), 1269–1274.

Goldman, B. A. (1969). Effect of classroom experience and video tape self-observation upon undergraduate attitudes toward self and toward teaching. *Proceedings of the Annual Convention of the American Psychological Association, 4*(Pt. 2), 647–648.

Goode, J., & Greatbatch, D. (2005). Boundary work: The production and consumption of health information and advice within service interactions between staff and callers to NHS Direct. *Journal of Consumer Culture, 5*(3), 315–337.

Gordon, J. (1953). Health education via television. *Public Health Reports, 68*(8), 816–821.

Gorodezky, M. J., & Hedlund, J. L. (1982). The developing role of computers in community mental health centers: Past experience and future trends. *Journal of Operational Psychology, 13* (2), 94–99.

Graetz, R. E., Agan, M. L., Arnsfield, P. J., Jacobus, H. J., & Wells, W. S. (1965). *Psychiatric data automation project: Final progress report.* Camarillo, CA.

Graetz, R. E. (1965). Research utilization of patient data files in clinical drug studies. *Behavioral Science, 10*, 320–323.

Graham, W. (1977). CHEMFILE: An in-house information system for the chemical indexing of Abstracts on Health Effects of Environmental Pollutants (HEEP). *Journal of Chemical Information and Computer Sciences, 17*(4), 200–202.

Greenberg, L., D'Andrea, G., & Lorence, D. (2004). Setting the public agenda for online health search: A white paper and action agenda. *Journal of Medical Internet Research, 6*(2), e18. doi:10.2196/jmir.6.2.e18.

Green, B. F. Jr. (1963a). *Digital computers in research: An introduction to behavioral and social scientists.* New York: McGraw-Hill.

Green, E. J. (1963b). The concept of programmed instruction: An overview. *Transactions of the New York Academy of Sciences, 25*, 919–931.

Gurevich, B. Kh. (1959). Cybernetics and certain modern problems of physiology of the nervous system. *The Journal of Nervous and Mental Disease, 128*(2), 169–178.

Gyr, J., Thatcher, J., & Allen, G. (1962). Computer simulation of a model of cognitive organization. *Behavioral Science, 7* (111–116).

Hailey, D., Roine, R., & Ohinmaa, A. (2008). The effectiveness of telemental health applications: A review. *Canadian Journal of Psychiatry, 53*(11), 769–778.

Halpert, H. P., Horvath, W. J., & Young, J. P. (1970). *An administrator's handbook on the application of operations research to the management of mental health systems.* Chevy Chase, MD: National Clearinghouse for Mental Health Information.

Hartree, D. R. (1946). The ENVIAV, an electronic computing machine. *Nature, 158*(4015), 500–506.

Hill, W. F., & Stoller, F. (1967). Summation: Toward the "ideal" course. *American Behavioral Scientist, 11*(1), 38–43.

Hirschfeld, H. (1957). Schizophrenia and cybernetics. *Folia Psychiatrica, Neurologica et Neurochirurgica Neerlandica, 60*(5), 388–401.

Iezzoni, L. I., & Greenberg, L. G. (1994). Widespread assessment of risk-adjusted outcomes: Lessons from local initiatives. *Joint Commission Journal on Quality Improvement, 20*(6), 305–316.

Ivey, A. E., et al. (1968). Microcounseling and attending behavior: an approach to prepracticum counselor training. *Journal of Counseling Psychology, 15*(5 Pt. 2), 1–12.

Ivey, A. E. (1971). *Microcounseling: Innovations in interviewing training*, 2nd ed. Springfield, IL: C C. Thomas.

Judd, W. A., & Glaser, R. (1969). Response latency as a function of training method, information level, acquisition, and overlearning. *Journal of Educational Psychology, 60*(4), 1–30.

Kagan, N., Krathwohl, D. R., & Miller, R. (1963). Stimulated recall in therapy using video tape: A case study. *Journal of Counseling Psychology, 10*(3), 237–243.

Kahn, S. D., Bowne, G. W., & Swint, E. B., Jr. (1972). A survey of the sources and availability of computer software applicable to psychophysiological research in the periodical literature. *Psychophysiology, 9*(5), 527–532.

Kantor, R. E., & Brown, D. (1970). On-line computer augmentation of biofeedback processes. *Bio-Medical Computing, 1,* 265–275.

Katz, L. (1950). Punched card technique for the analysis of multiple level sociometric data. *Sociometry, 13*(2), 108–122.

Kearns, W. D. (2003). Libraries as publishers of digital video. In A. Hanson, & B. L. Levin (Eds.), *The building of a virtual library* (pp. 37–51). Hershey, PA: IDEA Group Publishing.

Keesey, T. J. (1954). Health education via television: Three TV series in Washington, D.C. *Public Health Reports, 69*(6), 599–605.

Kennedy, C. A. (2005). The challenges of economic evaluations of remote technical health interventions. *Clinical and Investigative Medicine. Medecine Clinique et Experimentale., 28*(2), 71–74.

Kennedy, C., & Yellowlees, P. (2000). A community-based approach to evaluation of health outcomes and costs for telepsychiatry in a rural population: Preliminary results. *Journal of Telemedicine and Telecare, 6* (Suppl 1), S155–S157.

Kitaguchi, T., Nojiri, T., Suzuki, S., Fukita, T., & Kawana, T. (1983). Selection of scientific periodicals to monitor drug safety information using Excerpta Medica and Japicdoc in the post marketing surveillance of drugs. *Drug Information Journal, 17*(3), 177–193.

Knapp, S. D. (1979). Online searching in the behavioral and social sciences. *Behavioral & Social Sciences Librarian, 1*(1), 23–36.

Knutson, A. L., & Shimberg, B. (1955). Evaluation of a health education program. *American Journal of Public Health, 45*(1), 21–27.

Krantz, J. H. (1995). Linked gopher and world-wide web services for the American Psychological Society and Hanover College Psychology Department. *Behavior Research Methods, Instruments & Computers, 27*(2), 193–197.

Lamolinara, G. (1996). President Clinton signs Telecommunications Act of 1996 in Library's Main Reading Room—and in cyberspace. *A periodic report from the National Digital Library Program, March*(6), 1–3, 8. Retrieved June 2007 from http://www.loc.gov/ndl/march-96.pdf.

Leavitt, G. S., Stone, G., & Wrigley, C. (1954). Let's reduce statistical drudgery. *American Psychologist, 9*(10), 645–646.

Ledley, R. S. (1959). Digital electronic computers in biomedical science. *Science, 130,* 1225–1234.

Ledley, R. S., & Lusted, L. B. (1960). Computers in medical data processing. *Operations Research, 8,* 299–310.

Lehoux, P., & Blume, S. (2000). Technology assessment and the sociopolitics of health technologies. *Journal of Health Politics, Policy & Law, 25*(6), 1083–1120.

Lehoux, P., Denis, J. L., Tailliez, S., & Hivon, M. (2005). Dissemination of health technology assessments: Identifying the visions guiding an evolving policy innovation in Canada. *Journal of Health Politics, Policy & Law, 30*(4), 603–641.

Levin, B. L., & Hanson, A. (2001). Rural mental health services. In S. Loue, & B. E. Quill (Eds.), *Handbook of rural health.* (pp. 241–256). New York: Plenum.

Licklider, J. C. R. (1960). Man-computer symbiosis. *Institute of Radio Engineers: Transactions, HFE-9,* 4–11.

Lieff, J. D. (1987). *Computer applications in psychiatry.* Washington, DC: American Psychiatric Press.

Lopez, S. J., & Prosser, E. (1999). Preparing psychologists: More focus on training psychologists for a future in evolving health-care delivery systems. *Journal of Clinical Psychology in Medical Settings, 6*(3), 295–301.

Lorent, J. P. (1979). Outline literature retrieval in poison control. *Veterinary and Human Toxicology, 21 Suppl,* 89–90.

Lynett, P. A. (1985). The current and potential uses of computer assisted interactive videodisc in the education of social workers. *Computers in Human Services, 1*(4), 75–85.

MacCarthy, R. A. (1955). Electronic principles in brain design. *Journal of the Irish Medical Association, 37*(221), 325–329.

Markley, R. P., & Adams, R. M. (1973). The Science Citation Index. *American Psychologist, 28*(6), 534.

McArthur, D. L., Schandler, S. L., & Cohen, M. J. (1988). Computers and human psychophysiological research. *Computers in Human Behavior, 4*(2), 111–124.

McReynolds, P. (1950). Logical relationships between memorial and transient functions. *Psychological Review, 57*(3), 140–144.

Medow, M. A., Wilt, T. J., Dysken, S., Hillson, S. D., Woods, S., & Borowsky, S. J. (2001). Effect of written and computerized decision support aids for the U.S. Agency for Health Care Policy and Research depression guidelines on the evaluation of hypothetical clinical scenarios. *Medical Decision Making: An International Journal of the Society for Medical Decision Making, 21*(5), 344–356.

Meehl, P. E. (1962). *Clinical versus statistical prediction.* Minneapolis: University of Minnesota.

Meehl, P. E. (1956). Symposium on clinical and statistical prediction: The tie that binds. *Journal of Counseling Psychology, 3*(3), 163–164.

Meneely, J. K. Jr., & Sands, W. L. (1958). Two-way radio conference on psychotherapy. *New York State Journal of Medicine, 58*(23), 3831–3838.

Minsky, M. (1961). A selected descriptor-indexed bibliography to the literature on artificial intelligence. *IRE Transactions on Human Factors in Electronics, HFE-2,* 39–55.

Mohan, L., Muse, L., & McInerney, C. (1998). Managing smarter: A decision support system for mental health providers. *The Journal of Behavioral Health Services & Research, 25*(4), 446–455.

Monnier, J., Knapp, R. G., & Frueh, B. C. (2003). Recent advances in telepsychiatry: An updated review. *Psychiatric Services, 54*(12), 1604–1609.

Moody, R. L., & Zahm, B. C. (1980). Chemical Abstracts as a resource for health and safety-related chemical information. *Journal of Chemical Information and Computer Sciences, 20*(1), 12–14.

Moore, F. J., Chernell, E., & West, M. J. (1965). Television as a therapeutic tool. *Archives of General Psychiatry, 12*(2), 117–120.

Moore School of Electrical Engineering. (1944). *The ENIAC (Electronic Numerical Integrator and Computer)*. Philadelphia: University of Pennsylvania, Moore School of Electrical Engineering.

National Institute of Mental Health. (1983). *Implementing the NIMH prototype in a mental health agency* (The NIMH/PROTOTYPE management information system series; DHHS Publication No. (ADM) 83–1299). Rockville, MD: U.S. Department of Health and Human Services, Public Health Service, Alcohol, Drug Abuse, and Mental Health Administration, National Institute of Mental Health.

Newell, A., Shaw, J. C., & Simon, H. A. (1958). Elements of a theory of human problem solving. *Psychological Review, 65*(3), 151–166.

Newland, T. E. (1948). Psychological library of broadcast transcriptions. *American Psychologist, 3*(6), 207.

North, R. D. (1955). Psycheac, Univac, or 701? *American Psychologist, 10*(6), 249–250.

O'Neil, H. F. Jr, Spielberger, C. D., & Hansen, D. N. (1969). Effects of state anxiety and task difficulty on computer-assisted learning. *Journal of Educational Psychology, 60*(5), 343–350.

Owens, L. (1986). Vannevar Bush and the differential analyzer: The text and context of an early computer. *Technology and Culture, 27*(1), 63–95.

Paul, C. (2003). *Digital art*. London: Thames and Hudson.

Peper, E., & Toth, M. (1971). How do you get those references for that review paper? *American Psychologist, 26*(8), 740.

Pesamaa, L., Ebeling, H., Kuusimaki, M. L., Winblad, I., Isohanni, M., & Moilanen, I. (2004). Videoconferencing in child and adolescent telepsychiatry: a systematic review of the literature. *Journal of Telemedicine and Telecare., 10*(4), 187–192.

Pfeffer, J. (1962). *The thinking machine*. Philadelphia, PA: Lippincott.

Pinckney, C. E. (1954). "Your Lease on Life" in Denver. *Public Health Reports, 69*(6), 606–608.

Poling, E. G. (1968). Video tape recordings in counseling practicum: II. Critique considerations. *Counselor Education and Supervision, 8*(1), 33–38.

The President's New Freedom Commission on Mental Health. (2003). *Achieving the promise: Transforming mental health care in America: final report* (DHHS publication No. SMA-03-3832). Rockville, MD: President's New Freedom Commission on Mental Health. Available from http://govinfo.library.unt.edu/mentalhealthcommission/reports/reports.htm.

Rapoport, A. (1969). Optimal and suboptimal decisions in perceptual problem-solving tasks. *Behavioral Science, 14*(6), 453–466.

Rentchnick, P. (1950). [Cybernetics or the analogies between man and machine]. *Medecine et Hygiene, 8*(176), 300–301.

Ripple, R. E., O'Reilly, R., Wightman, L., & Dacey, J. (1965). Programmed instruction and learner characteristics: Preliminary data. *Psychological Reports, 17*(2), 633–634.

Romano, M. T. (1967). Health science education in the space age. *Annals of the New York Academy of Sciences, 142*(2), 348–356.

Safran, C. (1991). Using routinely collected data for clinical research. *Statistics in Medicine, 10*(4), 559–564.

Santo, Y., & Finkel, A. (1982). A computer simulation of schizophrenia. In B. I. Blum (Ed.), *Proceedings of the sixth annual symposium on computer applications in health care* (pp. 737–741). New York: Institute of Electrical Engineers.

Schneiweiss, F. (1979). Alternative sources of drug information: indexing and abstracting systems. *Drug Intelligence & Clinical Pharmacy, 13*(9), 512–517.

Scripture, E. W. (1891). Arithmetical prodigies. *The American Journal of Psychology, 4*(1), 1–59.

Simon, H. A., & Newell, A. (1962). Computer simulation of human thinking and problem solving. *Monographs of the Society for Research in Child Development, 27*(2), 137–150. [Special issue: Thought in the Young Child: Report of a Conference on Intellective Development with Particular Attention to the Work of Jean Piaget].

Slack, W. V., & Van Cura, L. J. (1968). Computer-based patient interviewing: 1. *Postgraduate Medicine, 43*(3), 68–74.

Smith, H. A., & Allison, R. A. (1998). *Telemental health: Delivering mental health care at a distance.* Rockville, MD: Substance Abuse and Mental Health Services Administration and the Health Resources and Services Administration.

Smith, N. J., Parmar, G., & Paget, N. (1980). Computer simulation and social work education: A suitable case. *British Journal of Social Work, 10*(4), 491–499.

Snyder, W. U. (1949). Personal advice over the radio. *American Psychologist, 4*(5), 153–153.

Solow, C. (1971). 24-hour psychiatric consultation via TV. *American Journal of Psychiatry, 127*(12), 1684–1687.

Spangler, R. W. (1955). We're on TV every week. *The American Journal of Nursing, 55*(5), 592–593.

Spolsky, B. (1966). Some problems of computer-based instruction. *Behavioral Science, 11*(6), 487–496.

Staff. (2002). New tools help behavioral health providers boost quality while documenting value. *Disease Management Advisor, 8*(1), 5–8.

Stillerman, M. (1963). A demonstration project in programmed instruction. *Transactions of the New York Academy of Sciences, 25,* 932–937.

Taylor, F. V. (1949). Review of Cybernetics (or control and communication in the animal and the machine). *Psychological Bulletin, 46*(3), 236–237.

(1953). Television and education. *BMQ: The Boston Medical Quarterly, 4*(2), 52–53.

Terrell, G. (1958). Television instruction in child psychology. *American Psychologist, 79*(8), 484.

Thompson, R. C. (1954). Be wise-televise. *Journal of Rehabilitation, 20*(2), 7–9.

Tierney, W. M., & McDonald, C. J. (1991). Practice databases and their uses in clinical research. *Statistics in Medicine, 10*(4), 541–547.

Tippett, L. H. C. (1927). *Random sampling numbers (Tracts for computers, No. XV).* London: Cambridge University Press.

Tobias, S. (1969). Effect of creativity, response mode, and subject matter familiarity on achievement from programmed instruction. *Journal of Educational Psychology, 60*(6), 453–640.

Trapp, A., Hammond, N., & Bray, D. (1996). Internet and the support of psychology education. *Behavior Research Methods, Instruments & Computers, 28*(2), 174–176.

Truitt, E. I., & Binner, P. R. (1969). The Fort Logan Mental Health Center. In C. A. Taube (Ed.), *Community mental health center data systems: A description of existing programs* (pp. 22–38). Rockville, MD: National Institute of Mental Health.

Turing, A. M. (1950). Computing machinery and intelligence. *Mind, 59*, 433–460.

United States General Accounting Office. (2002). *Telecommunications: Federal and state universal service programs and challenges: Report to the Ranking Minority Member, Subcommittee on Telecommunications and the Internet, Committee on Energy and Commerce, House of Representatives* (GAO No. 02–187). Washington, DC: United States General Accounting Office. Retrieved November 2006 from http://www.gao.gov/new.items/d02187.pdf.

Vandenberg, S. G., Silberman, H. F., Uhr, L., Wrigley, C. F., Holtzman, W. H., & Smith, P. A. (1960). Computers in behavioral science: The impact of computers on psychological research. *Behavioral Science, 5*, 170–187.

Van Donegan, C. J. (1984). CAI applications in mental health nursing. *Computers in Psychiatry/Psychology, 6*(1), 25–26.

von Foerster, H., Mead, M., & Teuber, H. L. (1953). *Cybernetics: Circular causal and feedback mechanisms in biological and social systems: Transactions of the eighth conference.* New York: Josiah Macy, Jr. Foundation.

Warner, R. S., & Bowers, J. Z. (1954). The use of open-channel television in postgraduate medical education. *Journal of Medical Education, 29*(10), 27–33.

Warner, R. S. (1954). New audio-visual methods in postgraduate medical education. *Journal of the Biological Photographic Association, 22*(4), 150–160.

Weiner, N. (1948). *Cybernetics.* New York: John Wiley & Sons.

Weizenbaum, J. (1976). *Computer power and human reason.* San Francisco: Freeman.

Welch, N., & Krantz, J. H. (1996). The world-wide web as a medium for psychoacoustical demonstrations and experiments: Experience and results. *Behavior Research Methods, Instruments & Computers, 28*(2), 192–196.

Wenger, M. A. (1950). Mechanical emotion. *The Journal of Psychology, 29*(1), 101–108.

White, E. B. (1998). Outcomes: essential information for clinical decision support: an interview with Ellen B. White. Interview by Melinda L. Orlando. *Journal of Health Care Finance, 24*(3), 71–81.

Wilmer, H. A. (1968). Television as participant recorder. *American Journal of Psychiatry, 124*(9), 1157–1163.

Wilmer, H. A. (1967). The role of the psychiatrist in consultation and some observations on video tape learning. *Psychosomatics: Journal of Consultation Liaison Psychiatry, 8*(4 Pt. 1), 193–195.

Wittson, C. L., Affleck, D. C., & Johnson, V. (1961). Two-way television in group therapy. *Mental Hospital, 12*(10), 22–23.

Wolfman, C. (1980). Microcomputer simulated psychiatric interviews used as a teaching aid. *Journal of Psychiatric Education, 4*(3), 190–201.

Wrigley, C., & Neuhaus, J. O. (1955). The use of an electronic computer in principal axes factor analysis. *Journal of Educational Psychology, 46*(4), 31–41.

Wurster, C. R., & Goodman, J. D. (1981). NIMH prototype management information system for community mental health centers. In J. T. O'Neill (Ed.), *Proceedings, the Fourth Annual Symposium on Computer Applications in Medical Care: November 2–5, 1980, Washington, D.C.* (pp. 907–912). New York: Institute of Electrical and Electronics Engineers: Long Beach, CA.

Part 2 Standards and Implementation

Do not forget that an electronic health record (EHR) represents a unique and valuable human being: it is not just a collection of data that you are guarding. It is a life....

OFFICE OF THE NATIONAL COORDINATOR FOR HEALTH INFORMATION TECHNOLOGY, 2011, p.1

4   Data and Standards

Hogan and Essock (1991) suggest that the integration of patient care, human resources, financial services (a.k.a. event), and organizational databases will create a foundation for both clinical and administrative data-based decision support, as well as for evaluation, program planning, and research. However, to accomplish this, we need to understand the importance of standards and the data elements necessary to create such a system.

This chapter provides an overview of the development of a national electronic health record, the issues involved in developing data sets for a variety of uses within mental health organizations, current standards development, and the implications and future of the electronic health record in mental health.

Evolution of the Electronic Health Record

The Institute of Medicine (Committee on Data Standards for Patient Safety, 2003) defines an electronic health record (EHR) as having four components. The first component is "the longitudinal collection" of patient information. The second component is immediate and 24/7 electronic access to that information by all *authorized* parties. The third component is the use of that information to improve clinical decision making and quality of care. The last component is to improve health care efficiency.

New data standards, which have emerged from the increased (Aspden, 2004) for services and the inclusion of consumers (Office of the National Coordinator for Health Information Technology, 2007) in outcomes discussions for mental health services, also have changed in terms of what is measured, what is counted, what is assessed, and what the outcomes are to establish quality and effectiveness of services and care (Committee on Quality of Health Care in America, 2001). To further complicate information management, the federal Health Insurance Portability and Accountability Act (HIPAA, 1996) requires administrative simplification of health information data for all print or online administrative transactions (including forms) and standardization of the health record, also in print and online formats.

A health record holds many types of information. Some of this information may be coded to specific diagnostic or billing schedules, some of it may be in a narrative format, and some of it may be notations by health care professionals. At a minimum, a health record contains data that is organized by dates, times, and a patient identification number. Data that may be found in a patient record includes the following:

- Patient registration data;
- List of diagnoses and problems that tracks these events over time (patient history);
- Medications that a patient may have received over time;
- Allergies to specific medications;
- Test results (laboratory, radiology, psychiatric tests, etc.);
- Appointment-related data;
- Clinical notes; and
- Billing information.

The notion of an electronic health record is not new. Moor (1946) discussed the evolution of the medical record and urged standardization to increase the use of the record in decision making. In the 1960s, with the emergence of computers, there was renewed interest in creating electronic health records to help with treatment decisions and to streamline administrative functions, such as appointment making, billing, payroll, and human resources. With the convergence of networking standards in health care, Harrington (1990) suggested that a significant goal was the "life-long, longitudinal electronic medical record." Such a record would include data in all formats, including text, voice, images, and numeric data. In 2004, the Office of the National Coordinator for Health Information Technology (ONC) was established by Executive Order No 13335 to coordinate the development of a national health network for the electronic exchange of health information (also see National Coordinator for Health and Information Technology, 2009, 2010).

Why do we need an electronic health record? First, clinical practice is a data intensive process, and poor or inconsistent data communication causes errors that may adversely affect a client's quality of life, treatment, and care. Second, although humans are good at recognizing patterns, they are not as adept at remembering lists or quickly evaluating complex decision-making pathways. Further, in theory, an EHR is available 24/7, can be viewed by multiple users, is legible, and is available from any location. Finally, an EHR helps to organize data among providers and clinicians, as well as other members of a health care team. It also enhances decision making and patient outcomes. Thompson and Brailer (2004) offer additional reasons for the creation of a national EHR: "readiness for change in health care, avoid medical errors, improve use of resources, accelerate diffusion of knowledge, reduce variability of care, advance consumer role, strengthen privacy and data protection, and promote public health and preparedness" (p. 2).

In addition to the basic information on the traditional medical record, an EHR has a number of value-added features, such as a clinical knowledge hierarchy (term dictionary). The term "dictionary" ties clinical concepts together, such as confounding effects of preexisting conditions, lists of current clinical recommendations (medication indications, doses, adverse effects and interactions, test utility, and cost of procedure). An EHR may link data from other reporting and diagnostic systems, such as a laboratory database, which uses specialized laboratory coding; a radiology system, which stores test reports and images; a pharmacy system; a billing system, which uses specialized diagnostic codes (e.g., ICD, International Classification of Diseases; and CPT, Current Procedural Terminology), and patient registration systems. In addition, an EHR may also link to an order entry system (where health care professionals enter orders, prescriptions, and notes online) and a decision support system, which the health care professional may access at point of care for information regarding clinical knowledge, guidelines, list of medication indications, and doses. Current EHR models include all of the above types of data, as well as additional features that allow synchronization of master files between systems and medical records document management.

The Mental Health Record Then and Now

A mental health record is part of a medical record. Just as the medical record has been redefined over time, so has the mental health record. There is extensive literature on the definitions and manners of recording psychiatric histories, the importance of complete and scientific patient records to improve patient care, and suggested simplification of patient clinical records.

The mental health record serves a number of purposes. It documents the evaluation and treatment course of a patient's illness during each episode and serves as a historical basis for planning patient care and recovery. It also serves as a vehicle for documenting communication between all staff assigned to provide care to a specific patient. The record also serves as a basis for review and evaluation of the care/services rendered to the patient for fiscal and research purposes. In addition, the record coordinates activities and events at various locations and times, linking the activities of staff without the need for real-time, face-to-face interaction. Finally, the record meets the legal and confidentiality requirements of the facility and/or provider.

Another way to look at the patient record is to see the record as part of a data accumulation system that results in a powerful "external memory" (Nygren & Henriksson, 1992). However, this "external memory" is not passive. Since the record provides a specific structure and context for the data, the format of the record can be said to enhance the information content of these data. Berg and Toussaint (2003) suggest that the information system (whether paper or electronic) is only one active element in the accumulation and coordination of patient information. Since the individuals inputting the data also play their part in constituting memory and coordinating the work, the record reflects only a part of the work process. So, the record is more than just the sum of its parts.

One of the earliest examples of computerizing the medical record in mental health was the program developed at the Institute of Living in Hartford in 1964 (Glueck, 1965). Not only did the medical record contain the medical evaluation and the behavior analysis of the patient, it also included admission data, demographic information, nursing and administrative data, and costing procedures. A standard personality survey was also developed to provide a behavioral profile of the patient.

Unlike most medical organizations, it was not uncommon for each type of mental health program to create its own content for clinical records and its own information system, which may be based on standards required by its funding agency or accreditation authority (Zinober & Leginski, 1984). In addition, mental health data collection emphasized measurement of disease prevalence and health utilization for use in comparison with other state mental health organizations and agencies.

From the 1960s to the 1980s, with deinstitutionalization and the implementation of the Community Health Centers Act, mental health service systems grew in their complexity and diversity of services and available programs. However, there appeared to be a lack of standards for data content, terminology, and definitions to keep up with the changes in statistical reporting from the standards developed in the 1950s.

In 1976, the Mental Health Statistics Improvement Program (MHSIP) was created to develop guidelines, definitions, and standards for mental health records for a national mental health reporting system, with a focus on its use in decision support systems (which will be covered more in depth in Chapter 5 of this volume). This was a complex task, considering the many programs or service pathways that a person in a single mental health system may take. Consider that in a typical organization chart, programs within a single mental health organization may look like the array depicted in Table 4.1.

If an individual was receiving substance abuse services, there would be an additional organizational chart linked to the mental health organizational chart, indicating entry into those specialized treatment/case management programs. In addition, a client in a mental health care organization may fail to provide identifying information due to confidentiality concerns, the emergency nature of the intervention, or the manifestation of a psychotic or delusional episode.

Another problem area for the mental health record is the inclusion of interviews with relatives or friends of the patient, or the inclusion of family members or friends as part of a patient/client's treatment plan, which may be counted as individual, group, or family sessions. Finally, continuity of care documentation may be problematic as patients/clients move through a multiservice organization, across multiple service sectors (e.g., health, criminal justice, and mental health), or re-enter into a service organization in the future. Hence, a minimum mental health patient data set would have included 29 items (see Table 4.2).

This patient data would have been in addition to minimum data sets established for event data, human resources data, financial data, and assessment data, in addition to any additional reporting data for a funding organization or state agency. This creates many levels of complexity when we view a patient's history from longitudinal, temporal, and spatial perspectives, especially as we count what activities are performed in mental health services delivery, such as event and service data.

TABLE 4.1

Typical Mental Health Program Organizational Chart

Inpatient		Community Support Programs		Ambulatory Care			Remote Sites
Admissions	Treatment Units →	Transitional Living Program	Supervised Apartments →	Program A →	Program B →	Program C →	Inpatient →
	Emergency/Crisis Unit		Rehabilitation Workshops →	Testing →	Treatment & Rehabilitation →	Treatment Research →	Ambulatory Care →
			Mobile Teams →	Consultation →	Emergency Services and Crisis Teams →	Day Activities Program →	Case Management
			Case Management →	Client Liaison		Peer-Run Programs →	Rehabilitation Workshops →
			Peer-Run Programs →				Mobile Teams →
			Hotline/Crisis Services				Peer-Run Programs

TABLE 4.2

Minimum Mental Health Patient/Client Data Set

1. Organization identifier
2. Client status
3. Unique patient/client identifier
4. Date of most recent admission
5. Date of discontinuation/discharge/death
6. Program element activity
7. Gender
8. Date of birth
9. Race
10. Hispanic origin
11. Current marital status
12. Veteran status
13. Legal status
14. Coded area of residence prior to admission to organization
15. Current coded area of residence
16. Presenting problems at time(s) of admission
17. Diagnosis
18. Severity of condition or level of functioning at admission
19. Chronicity of mental illness
20. Eligibility determination
21. Source of referral
22. History of use of mental health services prior to most recent admission to this organization
23. Residential arrangement
24. Living arrangement
25. Expected payment source
26. Discontinuation status
27. Referral upon discontinuation
28. Current primary therapist of case manager
29. Date of report

Reprinted from: Leginski, W. A. et al. (1989). *Data standards for mental health decision support systems* (Mental health service system reports Series FN: Information systems, no.10). Rockville, MD: National Institute of Mental Health, p. 49. This report is in the public domain.

Event data comprises three types of actions:

- A transaction between a staff member of a mental health organization and a client in which a significant activity occurs;
- A significant action between a staff member on behalf of a client, interviewing a collateral, providing various kinds of adjunctive services, and many case management activities; or
- Other actions by staff that facilitate the provision of services to or on behalf of patients, i.e., activities that support the continued operation of the organization (Leginski et al., 1989, p. 50).

Consider, too, that providers document every event to leave behind an audit trail, which can track the provision of services, may be subject to a treatment review, or may used in a variety of other ways.

Event data differs from unit of service data. A unit of service categorizes and/or measures production outputs and/or capacities that are associated with the financing and economics of care. Hence, a billed unit of service includes both clinical costs and overhead costs. For example, a unit of service may bill for a two-hour group therapy session with 20 clients and a single therapist. However, the event data is then collected and documented for each individual in the group by the professional. Both are different ways of looking at the activities conducted by professionals and staff at mental health settings. A minimum data set for event data reporting would comprise ten data elements: (1) organizational identifier; (2) date of event; (3) staff member reporting; (4) program element identifier and attendance logs; (5) patient(s) involved in the event; (6) type of event; (7) scheduled event; (8) event duration; (9) presence of other staff members; and (10) location of event.

Human resources data covers all individuals who work for an organization, contractually provide a service to an organization's patients, provide administrative services, or provide other support services on a full-time, part-time, or volunteer basis. Human resources data would include information on the education, training, licensing, and credentialing of staff, which would then inform administration and oversight agencies regarding the composition of staff to provide X services to Y number of clients, professional development needs, personnel assessment, retention and recruitment of staff, managing staff burnout, provision of in-service training, opportunities for case consultations, fostering the growth or development of new programs, or retooling existing programs to better meet patient needs. A minimum human resources data set would comprise 23 items (Leginski et al., 1989, p. 76).

Financial data addresses an organization's assets, liabilities, revenue and support, and expenses. Financial data is used to assess (1) the financial solvency and security of an organization; and (2) how well it manages its programs. Program management is usually assessed using the cost per unit of service in conjunction with patient data and human resources data. There are 15 elements in a minimal financial data set (Leginski et al., 1989).

Assessment data help management and administration assess the impact of their services. Typical questions include the following: Are services adequate? Do we have sufficient resources? Are we spending our resources wisely? Is the distribution of service equitable to our population base and our service centers in comparison to other agency programs? How efficient are we in the provision of services? How effective are our programs? Is one program more effective in terms of clinical outcomes? Assessment data consists of patient data, event data, human resources data, financial data, as well as other qualitative and quantitative measures, including surveys, interviews, external reviewers, and accreditation and credentialing reports.

All of this data is the result of a single patient interaction. It is crucial to understand the effectiveness of mental health services and program utilization both from the individual perspective and from a national perspective (see Figure 4.1).

From a micro-level (individual) perspective, the mental health record is linked to a patient's physical health record, which is part of the larger local health delivery system. From a meso-level perspective, this information is part of the networked delivery of services at a state and national level, which leads us to a macro-level perspective: the U.S. public health system, which is responsible for the well-being of the nation. Further, certain of these data elements may be coded to multiple specific coding schema and specialized clinical or administrative vocabularies.

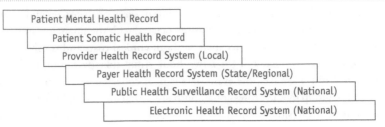

FIGURE 4.1 Types of Patient Records: Local to National.

In 2003, the President's New Freedom Commission on Mental Health (2003) stated six critical goals to transform mental health care in America. Goal 6 emphasized the use of technology to access mental health care and information:

6.1 Use health technology and telehealth to improve access and coordination of mental health care, especially for Americans in remote areas or in underserved populations. 6.2 Develop and implement integrated electronic health record and personal health information systems. (p. 15)

The Commission recognized that integrated electronic health record and personal health information systems can promote quality, coordinated services across numerous service delivery areas and among providers, including psychiatrists, physicians, psychologists, social workers, nurses, and other health and human service providers.

The Veterans Health Information Systems and Technology Architecture (VistA) Electronic Health Record (EHR) is used throughout the U.S. Department of Veterans Affairs Veterans Health Administration (VHA). The VHA EHR, which supports both ambulatory and inpatient care, is a collection of approximately 100 integrated software modules (U.S. Department of Veterans Affairs, 2011), much more complex than the discrete 29 data elements from the earlier patient health records mentioned above. However, those same data elements are still part of its EHR.

In 2004, the Institute of Medicine (IOM) described the components of a national health information infrastructure (NHII) as "(1) electronic health record (EHR) systems with decision support for clinicians, (2) a secure platform for the exchange of patient information across health care settings, and 3) data standards that will make shared information understandable to all users" (IOM, 2004, p. 259).

In 2006, the IOM completed a study on the quality of care and problems in mental health and substance abuse treatment systems. The IOM (2006) pointed out that the NHII was not addressing the needs of behavioral health clients as well as it did for those patients with general health care needs. It urged the development of specialized information systems for behavioral health service users, practitioners, and providers to meet their needs and to integrate the HIT across behavioral and somatic health. The IOM emphasized the importance of information technology in coordinating care and improving the quality of care across mental health and substance abuse service delivery systems.

In 2004, the IOM specifically addressed the need for standards in the collection, coding, classification, and exchange of clinical and administrative data for behavioral health in the areas of terminology, data interchange, and knowledge representation. A terminology is like a controlled vocabulary, in that specific terms and concepts are used to describe, classify, and code health care data. In addition, terminology also defines the processes that describe the relationships among the terms and concepts. A data interchange is a standard format for electronically encoding and structuring health care data elements as they are exchanged. Data interchange also creates the information models that define the relationships among data elements. Knowledge representation codifies the methods for electronically representing health care literature, clinical guidelines, and other information for decision support within the EHR or linked to other electronic clinical or administrative documents also from the EHR. These guidelines and reports can be called upon by the clinician or health care professional as necessary (IOM, 2004).

Standards

The success of a national health record depends on the development of a series of standards for a national health infrastructure. A health record is more than just client data, which represents just one small element of an EHR. An EHR is just one component of a national health infrastructure, which includes hardware and physical facilities to store, process, and transmit information; software applications and software allow access, structure, and manipulation of information; and network standards and transmission codes facilitate inter-organizational and cross-system communication. Each of these components must meet a number of standards in order to function effectively.

Why are there standards? Standards and interoperability are integral factors in the implementation of any electronic health record in a national health infrastructure. Standards are widely used throughout the government, public, and private sectors in the United States. Standards exist for numerous actions and products, including programming languages, operating systems, data formats, communications protocols, applications interfaces, services delivery, record formats, and so on. The purpose of standards is to ensure compatibility and interoperability between independent (discrete) systems and compatibility of data for comparative statistical or analytical purposes, to reduce duplication of effort and redundancies, and to create taxonomies, ontologies, and classifications to aid in analysis and review. Standards establish a common ontology, in which the "world of knowledge on X" is conceptualized.

Standards also ensure conformity assessment and usability. Standards for conformity assessment represent an international consensus on best practices and provide a reference framework, or a common technological language, between suppliers and their customers. This ensures that a product, material, service, system, or process measures up to the specifications of a relevant standard or specification. Standards on usability address "the extent to which a product can be used by specified users to achieve specified goals with effectiveness, efficiency, and satisfaction in a specified context of use" (ISO, 1998). Standards on accessibility ensure that any IT system works for all of the people who must use it. In short, standards must be *"relevant,* meeting agreed criteria and satisfying real needs by providing added value ... *responsive* to the real world; they use available, current technology and do not unnecessarily invalidate existing products or processes ... [and] *performance-based,* specifying essential characteristics rather than detailed designs" (American National Standards Institute, 2000, p. 4, italics in original).

Numerous governmental and nongovernmental organizations are involved in the development of the national health infrastructure within the United States. Some of the technical standards in use for the electronic health record include the Health Care Standards Landscape (HCLS), the Health Care Information Technology Standards Panel, the ASTM (American Society for Testing and Materials) Committee E31 on Health Care Informatics, Health Level 7 (HL7), and the ISO (International Organization for Standardization) Technical Committee on Health Informatics.

Developers

The National Institute of Standards and Technology (NIST) is an agency of the U.S. Department of Commerce. Founded in 1901, NIST conducts research to advance our national health technology infrastructure, with a focus on measurement science and standards development. NIST plays a major role in the 2008–2012 Federal Health Information Technology (IT) strategic plan and partners with the Office of the National Coordinator for Health Information Technology (Office of the National Coordinator for Health Information Technology, 2009, 2010). In the Health Information Technology for Economic and Clinical Health Act (HITECH Act), NIST was charged with advancing information enterprise integration, issues in HIT adoption and implementation, voluntary certification programs, and pilot testing of HIT systems. Health Care Standards Landscape (HCLS) is the repository of information on HIT standards and organizational development, promotion, and use, as maintained by NIST.

Founded in 1918, the American National Standards Institute (ANSI) is a private sector voluntary standards organization composed of government agencies, organizations, corporations, academic and international bodies, and individuals. Although ANSI does not create American National Standards (ANS), it oversees the creation, promulgation, and use of voluntary consensus standards for personnel, processes, products, and services systems in the United States (ANSI, 2010, 2012). It sponsors the Health Care Information Technology Standards Panel, a cooperative partnership between U.S. public and private sectors to achieve standards—specifically, to enable and support widespread interoperability among health care software applications. DICOM (Digital Imaging and Communications in Medicine), for example, is a subsidiary of the Association of Electrical and Medical Imaging Equipment Manufacturers (NEMA), which develops HIT standards for digital imaging and communication and partners with ANSI.

In addition, ANSI accredits organizations that carry out product or personnel certification in accordance with requirements defined in international standards. ANSI is a member of the ISO and the International Electrotechnical Commission (IEC), both of which are involved in the creation and adoption of international standards. ANSI has representatives on a number of ISO technical advisory groups (ANSI, 2011).

Formerly known as the Hospital Management Systems Society, Health Care Information and Management Systems (HIMSS) was founded over 50 years ago to improve the use of health information technology and management systems. HIMSS has over 540 corporate members, 120 not-for-profit organizations, and 38,000 individual members. Over two-thirds of its members work in health care provider, governmental, and not-for-profit organizations (HIMSS, 2011). In addition, HIMSS is working with ANSI and two other corporate partners on the Health care Information Technology Standards Panel (HITSP). The priorities for the panel are provided by the American Health Information Community (AHIC), a federally chartered advisory committee to the Department of Health and Human Services (HHS), concerning how to make health records digital and interoperable while assuring the privacy and security of those records. From 2006 to 2009, HITSP created 27 use cases, such as Consumer Access to Clinical Information and Public Health Case Reporting, and 18 interoperability specifications, such as Consumer Empowerment (IS03), Consumer Empowerment and Access to Clinical Information via Media (IS05), Quality (IS06), and Medication Management (IS07), to name just a few.

Founded in 1898, the American Society for Testing and Materials (ASTM), now known as ASTM International, is a globally recognized leader in the development and delivery of over 12,000 international voluntary consensus standards. ASTM has over 141 technical standards writing committees. Of most interest is the ASTM Committee E31 on Health Care Informatics. E31 develops HIT standards used within health care and health care decision making. These communication-based standards are related to the architecture, content, storage, security, confidentiality, functionality, and communication of information, including the Continuity of Care Record (CCR) standard.

Founded in 1987, HL7 (Health Level 7), is a nonprofit ANSI-accredited standards developing international organization, which produces health care information technology (HIT) standards in the domain of clinical and administrative data, with a focus on record and systems interoperability. "Level Seven" refers to the seventh level of the ISO seven-layer communications model for Open Systems Interconnection (OSI) at the application level (see Table 4.3).

Each of these layers addresses a different need in the transmission and receipt of electronic data (to be discussed more completely in Chapter 5). The HL & EHR Committee is one of 60 standards groups, and it works closely with related groups, such as Clinical Decision Making, Architecture Review, Implementable Technology Specifications, and Infrastructure and Messaging. Its goals are to create and promote standards that include the functional requirements for both electronic health records (EHR) and systems (EHRS) and personal health records (PHR) and systems (PHRS), to define the framework to support the interoperability requirements and life cycles, and to identify existing and emerging information requirements (HL7, 2010). HL7 is closely linked to a technical committee within the ISO TC 215, which specifies communication contents and exchange formats.

ISO is the world's largest developer and publisher of international standards. Headquartered in Geneva, Switzerland, it coordinates the network of the national standards institutes of 163 countries and has a portfolio of over 18,000 standards (ISO, 2010). An ISO International Standard represents "a global consensus on the state of the art in the subject of that standard" (ISO, 2010, p. 2). The ISO Technical Committee on Health Informatics (ISO TC215) is a nongovernmental, international organization that generates standards in the field of health information to achieve compatibility and interoperability (see Table 4.4).

TABLE 4.3

OSI Model Data Unit Layer Function

	Data unit	Layer	Function
Host Layers	Data	Application	Network process to application
		Presentation	Data representation, encryption and decryption, convert machine dependent data to machine independent data
		Session	Interhost communication
	Segment	Transport	End-to-end connections, reliability and flow control
Media Layers	Packet	Network	Path determination and logical addressing
	Frame	Data Link	Physical addressing
	Bit	Physical	Media, signal and binary transmission

TABLE 4.4

Selected Health Information Standard Development Organizations

1. American National Standards Institute; http://www.ansi.org/
2. Health Information Technology Standards Panel (HITSP); http://hitsp.org
3. International Organization for Standardization Technical Committee 215: Health Informatics (ISO/TC215) http://www.iso.org/iso/standards_development/ technical_committees/list_of_iso_technical_committees/iso_technical_committee. htm?commid=54960
4. Health Care Standards Landscape; http://www.itl.nist.gov/div897/docs/hc_roadmap.html
5. Standard Setting Organization and Standards List; http://www.consortiuminfo.org/ links/health
6. Military Health System Technology Management Integration & Standards (TMIS); http://www.tricare.osd.mil/tmis_new/IA.htm
7. Consolidated Health Informatics Initiative (CHI); http://www.hhs.gov/healthit/chi.html

(*continued*)

TABLE 4.4

Selected Health Information Standard Development Organizations (*continued*)

8. ANSI Health Level Seven (HL7): http://www.hl7.org/
9. ANSI Data Interchange Standards Association; http://www.disa.org/
10. ANSI The Accredited Standards Committee X12; http://www.x12.org/
11. ANSI National Council for Prescription Drug Programs (NCPDP); http://www.ncpdp.org/
12. ANSI American Society of Testing and Materials (ASTM); http://www.astm.org/
13. ANSI Institute of Electrical and Electronic Engineers (IEEE); http://standards.ieee.org/
14. Integrating the Health Care Enterprise (IHE); http://www.ihe.net/
15. Workgroup for Electronic Data Interchange; http://www.wedi.org/
16. Digital Imaging and Communications in Medicine (DICOM); http://medical.nema.org/
17. Clinical Data Interchange Standards Consortium (CDISC); http://www.cdisc.org/
18. Logical Observation Identifiers Names and Codes (LOINC); http://loinc.org/
19. International Health Terminology Standards Development Organization (IHTSDO); http://www.ihtsdo.org/(Systemized Nomenclature of Medicine: SNOMED)
20. World Health Organization (WHO) International Classification of Disease (ICD); http://www.who.int/classifications/icd/en/
21. United States Health Information Knowledgebase; http://www.ushik.org

Office of the National Coordinator for Health Information Technology

In 2004, the Office of the National Coordinator for Health Information Technology (ONCHIT) was established by Executive Order No. 13335 within the Office of the Secretary of the Department of Health and Human Services (DHHS) to coordinate nationwide efforts to implement the most advanced health information technology and the electronic exchange of health information. In 2009, the office was legislatively mandated in the Health Information Technology for Economic and Clinical Health Act (HITECH Act) of 2009. One of its most important projects is the Consolidated Health Informatics (CHI) Initiative, a collaborative effort to adopt health information interoperability standards for implementation in over 20 federal departments and agencies, including the Department of Health and Human Services, the Department of Defense, and the Department of Veterans Affairs (see Table 4.5). The CHI Initiative also coordinates a number of related initiatives and projects (see Table 4.6).

However, one of the most important roles that the ONCHIT CHI Initiative plays in the Federal Health Architecture (FHA) Program is the standardization of existing clinical vocabularies and messaging standards into an interoperable federal health data system; all are essential to the design and utilization of an electronic health record.

TABLE 4.5

Consolidated Health Informatics Federal Partner Departments and Agencies

Department-Level	Agency-Level
Veterans Affairs	Veterans Health Administration
Defense	
Health & Human Services	Office of the Secretary
Health & Human Services	Centers for Medicare & Medicaid Services
Health & Human Services	Centers for Disease Control & Prevention
Health & Human Services	Indian Health Service
Health & Human Services	National Institutes of Health
Health & Human Services	National Library of Medicine; National Cancer Institute
Health & Human Services	Agency for Health Research & Quality
Social Security Administration	
General Services Administration	
Office of Management & Budget	
Environmental Protection Agency	
Department of Energy	Los Alamos National Laboratories
	National Institute of Standards & Technology
	US Agency for International Development

Reprinted and adapted from http://www.hhs.gov/healthit/chiinitiative.html.

TABLE 4.6

CHI Initiative: Related Initiatives and Projects

Related Initiatives	Project/Product
Cybersecurity	Meaningful Use Criteria
Innovations	Investing in Innovations (i2)
	Startup America
	Health Data Initiative
	AHRQ Innovations Exchange
	popHealth
	MedlinePlus Connect
Nationwide Health Information Network	The Direct Project
	CONNECT Open Source Software
	Medicare & Medicaid Electronic Health Records Incentive Programs
Federal Health Architecture	E-Government Line of Business initiative

(continued)

TABLE 4.6

CHI Initiative: Related Initiatives and Projects (*continued*)

Related Initiatives	Project/Product
Rural Health IT: DHHS, U.S. Department of Agriculture	Community Facilities Program
	Distance Learning and Telemedicine Grant Program
State-Level Health Initiatives	State Health Policy Consortium
	State Alliance for eHealth
	Health Information Security and Privacy Collaboration (HISPC)
	State-level Health Information Exchange Consensus Project
Health IT Adoption	CDC National Ambulatory Medical Survey (NAMC) [The survey can be used to define two levels of electronic health record: basic and full]
	American Hospital Association (AHA) annual survey
	[The survey can be used to define two levels of electronic health record: basic and full]
Clinical Decision Support	Inventory of Federal Clinical Decision Support Activities
	CDS Government Collaboratory
	Roadmap for National Action on Clinical Decision Support
	American Health Information Community (AHIC) workgroups

Standardizing Vocabularies

Standard or controlled vocabularies are used to create subject headings, index terms, and thesauri. Standard vocabularies are composed of words and phrases that are defined with a structured description to indicate that X = X. These vocabularies also group synonymous terms so that X_1, X_2, and X_3 also mean X. The purpose of such vocabularies is to provide conceptual access to terms and phrases that are the same definitionally and conceptually but may be named differently based upon nomenclature used by different disciplines. These terms may be "pre-coordinated" (i.e., established before the vocabulary is published) or "post-coordinated" (i.e., established after the vocabulary is published). Each term is assigned a unique code or number. Two concepts can be added together, such as the use of the adjective *severe* and the noun *affective disorder* to qualify a disorder by severity. Three terms combined together, such as *elderly* with *alcohol abuse* with *epidemiology,* may qualify the extent of a disorder in a population.

In mental health, two common standard vocabularies are found in the *Diagnostic and Statistical Manual* (DSM) and the *International Classification of Disorders* (ICD). The DSM is the standard for psychiatric diagnosis in the United States and the ICD is the international standard diagnostic classification for epidemiological coding, health management procedures, and clinical use for mental health. Consider for a moment that the ICD classification for mental disorders consists of 10 main groups, and the DSM consists of five axes of disorders. In the creation of a national EHR, there must be a map or crosswalk between the two standard vocabularies to simplify the clinical or administrative decision-making process. Magnify this across the many specialized vocabularies in medicine and mental health, and there is a clear need for standards to fill the gaps in coverage, definition, and implementation of content and vocabulary standards.

As the central coordinating body for clinical terminology standards for the Department of Health and Human Services, the National Library of Medicine (NLM) works closely with the Office of the National Coordinator for Health Information Technology (ONC) to ensure the nationwide implementation of an interoperable health information technology infrastructure. It is also the U.S. representative to a number of national and international organizations, such as the International Health Terminology Standards Development Organisation (IHTSDO).

One might wonder why the NLM would be a member of teams working in health information technology infrastructure. The answer is simple. Clinically specific vocabularies facilitate the exchange of clinical data and improve the retrieval of health information. Health care providers must produce billing and statistical data using the HIPAA code sets. However, coding records is time- and labor-intensive. The use of standard clinical vocabularies will help to improve the clinical workflow and decision-making processes if required HIPAA code set data can be generated from health care information recorded using standard clinical vocabularies.

The National Committee on Vital and Health Statistics (NCVHS) sees the mapping from standard clinical terminologies, regulatory terminologies, and interface terminologies to the HIPAA code sets as a critical component to the success of the electronic health record. NLM has been recommended as the appropriate body to coordinate and/or develop and disseminate the mappings within the Unified Medical Language System (UMLS) Metathesaurus. The UMLS Metathesaurus is a set of files and software that brings together many health and biomedical vocabularies and standards to enable interoperability between computer systems (NLM, 2009). The UMLS is used to enhance or develop applications, such as electronic health records, classification tools, dictionaries, and language translators. It is used to link terms and codes between doctors, pharmacies, and insurance companies and to strengthen patient care coordination among several departments within a hospital. The UMLS is also utilized in search engine retrieval, data mining, public health statistics reporting, and terminology research (NLM, 2009).

In addition to developing mappings between HIPAA code sets and standard clinical, regulatory, and interface vocabularies, the NLM also contracts with Health Level 7 (HL7), the global authority on standards for interoperability of health information technology mentioned above, to align HL7 message standards with CHI standard vocabularies and to create implementation guides for exchange of entire EHRs.

The NLM has developed or supports the Systematized Nomenclature of Medicine-Clinical Terms (SNOMED CT), Logical Observation Identifiers Names and Codes (LOINC), and RxNorm. The SNOMED CT is maintained by the International Health Terminology Standards Development Organization (IHTSDO). Mapping the SMOMED CT to the ICD is a priority for the IHTSDO and the World Health Organization (WHO) (Berg & Campbell, 2008), and it was released for review in 2011 (WHO, 2011).

Produced by the Regenstrief Institute, the Logical Observations Identifiers, Names, Codes (LOINC®) is a clinical terminology important for laboratory test orders and results. One of the designated standards for use in U.S. federal government systems for the electronic exchange of clinical health information, LOINC was identified by the HL7 Standards Development Organization as a preferred code set for laboratory test names in electronic transactions between health care facilities, laboratories, laboratory testing devices, and public health authorities (Clement et al., 2003). The Clinical Data Interchange Standards Consortium (CDISC), which includes all of the major pharmaceutical manufacturers and the Food and Drug Administration, uses LOINC codes for identifying laboratory tests and EKG results in new drug submissions (CDISC, 2011).

RxNorm is the NLM's standardized nomenclature for clinical drugs and drug delivery devices derived from the Unified Medical Language System (UMLS) Metathesaurus. RxNorm also includes the Veterans Health Administration National Drug File—Reference Terminology (NDF-RT) used to code clinical drug properties, including mechanism of action, physiologic effect, and therapeutic category.

RxNorm maps and normalizes names for clinical drugs across the National Drug Codes (NDCs) and standard nonproprietary names of medications used in pharmacy management and drug interaction software. NDCs are product identifiers assigned by manufacturers and packagers of drugs in the United States. Each time a manufacturer produces the same medication in packages of different sizes, each package size of medication receives a unique NDC. RxNorm creates standard names and identifiers for the combinations of ingredients, strengths, and dose forms that doctors include on the prescriptions they write. Since doctors do not know the specific product that will be used to fill the prescription, RxNorm provides the connection between the medication/strength/dose in an electronic health record (see Table 4.7).

Creating defined relationships among the generic and branded normalized forms and the names of their individual components allows precision and consistency in the electronic prescribing by health care professionals without undue complication or burden on their normal workflow process.

The work by NLM is used by the HIMSS Standards Task Force (2008) Taxonomy of Standards, part of the work program of the ISO/TC215. Its Workgroup on Semantic Content focuses on terminology and knowledge representation, and uses the SNOMED-CT,

TABLE 4.7

Standardizing Clinical Drugs	
Generic	Individualized Components
For generic drug name	Acetaminophen 500 MG Oral Tablet
For a branded drug name	Acetaminophen 500 MG Oral Tablet [Tylenol]
For a generic drug pack	{5 (Aspirin 325 MG Oral Tablet)/5 (Pravastatin 20 MG Oral Tablet)} Pack
For a branded drug pack	{30 (Aspirin 325 MG Oral Tablet)/30 (Pravastatin 20 MG Oral Tablet [Pravachol])} Pack [Pravigard 325/20]

Adapted from http://www.nlm.nih.gov/research/umls/rxnorm/overview.html.

LOINC, and the ICD as part of their standards toolbox. Let's take a look at a practical example of how these standards are used by the Centers for Medicare and Medicaid.

EXAMPLE: NURSING HOME MINIMUM DATA STANDARDS

The nursing home Minimum Data Set (MDS) data is used by the federal government to establish payment rates for Medicare skilled nursing facilities and quality measures and quality indicators for Medicare and Medicaid nursing facilities and in-patient rehabilitation facilities. To integrate the nursing home MDS with the HIT and to modernize the Medicare and Medicaid programs, the Centers for Medicare and Medicaid Services (CMS) sponsored a study to standardize the nursing home Minimum Data Set (MDS). The nursing home MDS consists of questions and answers that are in natural (human) language. The responses to the questions, however, were to be created in computer language for use by regulatory and reimbursement agencies. To facilitate the transition, the Consolidated Health Informatics (CHI) Initiative endorsed the Health Level Seven Version 2 (HL7v2+) as the standard to send coded clinical information electronically, using the SNOMED-CT for nursing content, the HL7 vocabulary for demographics, and RxNorm as one of the standards for medications.

Extending the Use of the Electronic Health Record

When one discusses data and standards for an electronic health record, it is not enough to only consider clinical use. It is important to see how this data may be able to work in counting and assessing real-world situations, especially for those involved in public mental health services delivery. The national *Healthy People 2020* initiative, which focuses on improving the overall health of persons living in the United States, relies upon data from a number of external sources, such as surveillance data, national censuses, and nationally representative sample surveys, such as the Health Information National Trends Survey, the Collaborative Psychiatric Epidemiology Surveys, and the Behavioral Risk Factor Surveillance System. Used to plan health programs addressing health behaviors and chronic disease, these data are national baseline data for measurable objectives in *Healthy People*.

In *Healthy People*, there are 13 objectives specifically designated under health communication and health information technology (HC/HIT). Two objectives specifically address electronic health records: HC/HIT-5 Electronic personal health management tools, and HC/HIT-10 Electronic health records in medical practices. Both objectives require the development of standards for data interchange, standard vocabularies, and security protocols currently under development in the national health information infrastructure. It is possible that data from the personal health record and the EHR will become national baseline data for *Healthy People*.

Another extension of the EHR may be to track the impact of violence from a public health perspective. The Violence Against Women Health Initiative Act of 2011 explicitly added the use of health information technology to improve documentation, identification, assessment, treatment, and follow-up care to strengthen the response of health care systems to victims of domestic violence, dating violence, sexual assault, and stalking.

Linking surveillance methods to EHRs first requires the standardizing of interview protocols, instruments, and measures of behavior and disease. This would make comparing community- and state-level initiatives easier. The next step is to significantly widen data collection within the national health information infrastructure. Colpe et al. (2010) suggest that a national health information infrastructure should include substance use disorders; should use different interval reference periods, such as the appropriateness of dichotomous versus continuous variables; and should rethink current approaches to data collection. Surveillance efforts also should be more relevant to the needs of state mental health and substance abuse programs and initiatives. Child health measurement, for example, could benefit greatly from more considered and integrated data collection and analyses. A significant opportunity exists in innovative and translational use of survey data to improve knowledge dissemination of best practice and evidence-based practices.

The National Institute for Occupational Safety and Health (NIOSH) also is interested in incorporating work history information into patient electronic health records by 2015. Working with the IOM, NIOSH plans a series of public meetings to examine the potential benefits from a public and individual health perspective; to determine which, if any systems, currently incorporate work history into the EHR, with application to clinical decision making and public health reporting activities; and to address the technical issues, barriers, and alternatives involved in the creation of a work history module in the EHR (IOM, 2011). Two significant issues have emerged from these discussions. First, coding and standard vocabulary also come into play in this initiative, since NIOSH uses its own coding system for industry, product, and occupation data. This may require normalization of data as well as crosswalks between the many different taxonomies currently in use across the diverse disciplines involved in the EHR. Second, NIOSH, working with its governmental and nongovernmental partners, will need to construct protocols and procedures that will make such an effort successful.

Implications for Mental Health Informatics

Ackoff (1989) suggested that data are just symbols. Information is data that are processed to answer "who, what, when, where" questions. Knowledge of the application of data and information is needed to answer the "how" question. Understanding is synthesizing data, information, and knowledge to appreciate the "why" question. Finally, he suggested that wisdom is evaluating what it is one understands (Ackoff, 1989).

From a mental health informatics perspective, the first four categories document events that have occurred, such as visits for care, services delivered, staff involvement, time spent, and outcomes achieved. Data does not have meaning outside a strictly defined context. A represents A; if it also represents D, the next question is to make sense of that relationship. Information creates that relation. However, the information may not yet make sense. Knowledge is cognitive and analytic activity in which information and data are determined to be useful and to be contextually situated. Understanding takes situational knowledge and views it within interpolative and probabilistic frameworks. As one continues on to wisdom, discernment occurs, decisions are made, judgments are passed, principles are known, and new questions are generated that require data. And so the processes continue, as one understands relations, patterns, and principles that build from data to wisdom.

Now consider these activities not just by ones or twos, but by thousands and tens of thousands of actions performed daily by tens of thousands or hundreds of thousands of providers. Now the importance of common data elements, crosswalks, definitions, portability, interoperability, and taxonomy becomes clear. This chapter has provided a small slice of what it means to collect and share mental health data, which in itself encompasses health data, which then generates public health/mental health data across the individual, the workplace, community, and nation.

References

Ackoff, R. L. (1989). From data to wisdom. *Journal of Applies Systems Analysis, 16,* 3–9.

American National Standards Institute (2011). *ANSI Accredited US TAGs to ISO.* Retrieved from http://www.ansi.org/standards_activities/iso_programs/tag_iso.aspx American National Standards Institute (2012). *ANSI essential requirements: due process requirements for American National Standards.* Retrieved from http://publicaa. ansi.org/sites/apdl/Documents/Standards%20Activities/American%20National%20Standards/Procedures,%20Guides,%20and%20Forms/2010%20ANSI%20Essential%20Requirements%20and%20Related/2010%20ANSI%20Essential%20Requirements.pdf.

American National Standards Institute. (2000). *National standards strategy for the United States.* New York: ANSI. Retrieved from http:// http://web.archive.org/web/20071017214205/http://publicaa.ansi.org/sites/apdl/Documents/News%20and%20Publications/Brochures/national_strategy.pdf.

Aspden, P., Corrigan, J. M., Wolcott, J., Erickson S. M. (2004). *Patient safety: Achieving a new standard for care.* Washington, DC: The National Academies Press. Retrieved from http://www.nap.edu/catalog.php?record_id=10863.

Berg, L., & Campbell, J. R. (2008). *Mapping SNOMED CT to ICD-10: A joint task of IHTSDO and WHO-FIC (WHO-FIC 2008/00-3).* Retrieved from http://www.tc215wg3.nhs.uk/docs/isotc215wg3_n362.pdf.

Berg, M., &Toussaint, P. (2003). The mantra of modeling and the forgotten powers of paper: a sociotechnical view on the development of process-oriented ICT in health care. *International Journal of Medical Informatics, 69*(2–3), 223–234.

Clement. C. J., Huff, S. M., Suico, J. G., Hill, G., Leavelle, D., Aller, R.... & Maloney, P. (2003). LOINC, a universal standard for identifying laboratory observations: A 5-year update. *Clinical Chemistry, 49*(4), 624–633. doi: 10.1373/49.4.624.

Clinical Data Interchange Standards Consortium. (2011). *Submissions data domain models v3.1.* Round Rock, TX: The Consortium. Retrieved from http://bbs.cdisc.org/bbs/forums/forum-view.asp?fid=106&bookmark= 21&displaytype=flat.

Colpe, L. J., Freeman, E. J., Strine, T.W., Dhingra, S., Mcguire, L. C., Elam-Evans, L. D., & Perry, G. S. (2010). Public health surveillance for mental health. *Prevention & Chronic Disease, 7*(1), A17. Retrieved from http://www.ncbi.nlm.nih.gov/pmc/articles/PMC2811512/.

Committee on Data Standards for Patient Safety. (2003). *Key capabilities of an electronic health record system.* Washington, DC: The National Academies Press. http://www.nap.edu/catalog.php?record_id=10781.

Committee on Quality of Health Care in America (2001). *Crossing the quality chasm: A new health system for the 21st century*. Washington, DC: National Academy Press. Retrieved from http://www.nap.edu/catalog.php?record_id=10027.

Glueck, B. S. (1965). The use of computers in patient care. *Mental Hospitals, 16*, 117–120.

Harrington, J. (1990). The networking standards evolution: toward a real electronic medical record. *Computers in Health care, 11*(2), 18–21.

Health Level Seven International. (2010). Electronic health records. Retrieved from http://www.hl7.org/Special/committees/ehr/overview.cfm.

HIMSS Standards Task Force. (2008). *Taxonomy of standards*. Retrieved from http://www.himss.org/content/files/2008_Taxonomy_of_Standards_STF_law.pdf.

HIMSS. (2012), About HIMSS. Retrieved from http://www.himss.org/ASP/aboutHimssHome.asp

Hogan, M. F., & Essock, S. M. (1991). Data and decisions: Can mental health management be knowledge-based? *Journal of Mental Health Administration, 18*(1), 12–20. doi: 10.1007/BF02521129.

Institute of Medicine. (2006). *Improving the quality of health care for mental and substance-use conditions: Quality Chasm Series*. Washington, DC: The National Academies Press. Retrieved from http://www.nap.edu/catalog.php?record_id=11470.

Institute of Medicine. (2011). *Occupational information and electronic health records*. Washington, DC: IOM. Retrieved from http://www.iom.edu/Activities/Environment/OccupationalHealthRecords.aspx.

International Organization for Standardization. (1998). *ISO 9241-11:1998: Ergonomic requirements for office work with visual display terminals (VDTs): Part 11: Guidance on usability*. Geneva: IOS.

International Organization for Standardization (2010). *ISO strategic plan: 2011–2015*. Geneva. Retrieved from http://www.iso.org/iso/iso_strategic_plan_2011-2015.pdf.Leginski, W. A., Croze, C., Driggers, J., Dumpman, S., Geertsen, D, Kamis-Gould, E., … Wurster, C. R. (1989). *Data standards for mental health decision support systems* (DHHS: Pub. No. (ADM) 89-1589. Washington, DC: Supt. of DOCs., U.S. Govt. Print. Office.

Moor, H. B. (1946). The evolution of the medical record. *Rhode Island Medical Journal 29*, 523.

National Library of Medicine. (2009). *UMLS® reference manual*. Bethesda, MD: National Library of Medicine. Retrieved from http://www.ncbi.nlm.nih.gov/books/NBK9676/.

Nygren, E., & Henriksson, P. (1992). Reading the medical record. I. Analysis of physicians' ways of reading the medical record. *Computer Methods and Programs in Biomedicine 39*(1–2), 1–12.

Office of the National Coordinator for Health Information Technology. (2007). *Consumer empowerment: Consumer access to clinical information detailed use case*. Washington, DC: U.S. Department of Health and Human Services. Retrieved from http://healthit.hhs.gov/portal/server.pt/gateway/PTARGS_0_10731_848105_0_0_18/UseCaseCACI.pdf.

Office of the National Coordinator for Health Information Technology. (2009). *Office of the National Coordinator for Health Information Technology: Health Information Technology*. Retrieved from http://www.hhs.gov/recovery/reports/plans/onc_hit.pdf.

Office of the National Coordinator for Health Information Technology. (2011). *Why should health care practices worry about security?* Retrieved from http://healthit.hhs.gov/portal/server.pt/community/healthit_hhs_gov__cybersecurity/3696.

President's New Freedom Commission on Mental Health. (2003). *Achieving the promise: Transforming mental health care in America*. Rockville, MD: The Commission. Retrieved from http://govinfo.library.unt.edu/mentalhealthcommission/reports/FinalReport/downloads/FinalReport.pdf.

Thompson, T., & Brailer, D. M. (2004). *The decade of health information technology: Delivering consumer-centric and information-rich health care: Framework for strategic action.* Retrieved from http://www.providersedge.com/ehdocs/ehr_articles/The_Decade_of_HIT-Delivering_Customer-centric_and_Info-rich_HC.pdf.

U.S. Department of Health and Human Services, Office of the Secretary (2009, December 1). Statement of organization, functions, and delegations of authority; Office of the National Coordinator for Health and Information Technology. *Federal Register, 229*(74), 62785–62786. Retrieved from http://edocket.access.gpo.gov/2009/pdf/E9-28755.pdf.

U.S. Department of Health and Human Services, Office of the Secretary (2010, August 13). Statement of organization, functions, and delegations of authority; Office of the National Coordinator for Health and Information Technology; Correction, *Federal Register, 75*(156), 49494. Retrieved from http://edocket.access.gpo.gov/2010/pdf/2010-19999.pdf.

U.S. Department of Veterans Affairs. (2011). *VistA: Description.* Retrieved from http://www.virec.research.va.gov/DataSourcesName/VISTA/VISTA.htm.

World Health Organization. (2011). SNOMED CT to ICD-10 Cross Map Preview Release. Retrieved from http://www.who.int/classifications/icd/snomedCTToICD10Maps/en/index.html.

Zinober, J. W., & Leginski, W. A. (1984). Availability of comparable data in state mental health programs, *Community Mental Health Journal, 20*(1), 14–26.

5   Management Information Systems

The delivery of mental health services is information-based as well as knowledge-based. Mental health providers have relied on information technology to acquire, manage, analyze, and disseminate information on treatment, research, and practice. The Committee on Engaging the Computer Science Research Community in Health Care Informatics (Computer Science and Telecommunications Board, 2009) emphasized the need for cognitive support for health care providers in the development, adoption, implementation, and utilization of computer-based tools and systems. This is particularly critical in the development of a national health information infrastructure (NHII) and the implementation of a national electronic health record (EHR).

The EHR is an important element in clinical decision making, outcomes assessment, and quality management. It should also increase the patient's participation in his or her individual health care. Just as the paper health record is one important component of providing guidelines and knowledge in the treatment of mental and substance use disorders, the electronic health record is also one component in the use of the management information system (MIS) and the clinical decision support system (CDSS) in mental health. In the literature, the term EHR is now used in place of MIS and CDSS. In this chapter, the term MIS refers to the system and the EHR refers to the individual patient record (unless EHR is used in quoted text from another source). It is equally important to note that there are thousands of MISs and CDSSs that will be integrated into the national health information infrastructure, and each will have to incorporate an EHR, national standards, and protocols into the workplace.

This chapter will examine the emergence of management information systems in mental health, with a focus on decision making, operations management, cognitive support, and usability. It will also review comparative effectiveness research, patient portals, and report cards as key components and products in mental health management information systems.

Emergence of Management Information Systems

A management information system (MIS) is a commercially available integrated software application to support health and mental health organizations, whether it is as a provider of mental health services or as an administrator for a network of contracted mental health service providers. It commonly handles client data, scheduling, authorization tracking, billing, accounts receivable management, the client medical record, reporting, compliance, and financial data. Each of these elements also plays a crucial role in the treatment, outcomes assessment, and program evaluation of a mental health organization.

There are many advantages to an MIS. From a clinical perspective, it provides improved access to clinical information for service providers from any location on a 24/7 basis. It increases the availability of clinicians to patients, since it reduces provider paperwork and improves workflow processes. It also provides improved clinical outcomes, since client history, treatment protocols, and reference information are available to support clinical treatment decisions. Client information can be viewed from a larger system of care perspective, enhancing program evaluation and developing long- and short-term goals to improve the quality of patient care.

From an efficiency perspective, an MIS significantly reduces the amount of time spent on handling, storing, and retrieving paper records and reduces the amount of physical space necessary to store medical records. It improves a clinician's ability to schedule, plan, and document the delivery of services and creates a longitudinal view of services for staff or external agencies. An MIS also improves regulatory and board reporting to its many credentialing, licensing, and funding agencies. Finally, it enhances an organization's ability to strategically plan and implement management decisions which impact quality of care, services delivery, and staff development partnerships (Cesare-Murphy, McMahill, & Schyve, 1997; Persell et al., 2011).

MISs are not new. The history of mental health information systems actually begins with the first recording of the admission and discharge registers and annual statistical summaries of state mental health programs and admission characteristics in the early 1800s. These records evolved over time and often noted the following data: (1) patient name; (2) gender; (3) age; (4) marital status; (5) date of admission or discharge; and (6) county of residence. Additional information included to whom the patient was discharged, remarks, type of commitment or discharge order(s), and general mental and physical condition when discharged. Information given may also include the total number of admissions per year, ward number, first admission/readmission, financial arrangement, patient case book volume and page number, period of treatment, duration of symptoms previous to admission, form of "insanity," and the cause of death if the patient died in the asylum.

In 1840, the U.S. Census Bureau began a national reporting program for mental health statistics. Forty years later, a diagnostic classification system was created that described and coded seven distinct forms of insanity. In 1946, the National Institute of Mental Health

(NIMH) began collecting and preparing consolidated (aggregated) reports on mental health information. In 1951, NIMH established a Model Reporting Area for Mental Health Statistics Program (MRAP), which established and standardized definitions for the states and "set up a mechanism for the exchange of information" (National Institute of Mental Health, 1962, p 3). The 1956 MRAP Conference recommended several changes in the collection of mental health statistics, including the need to justify current expenditures, to show the need for additional funds in view of the large national mental hospital population, to document the increase in usage of medications in U.S. mental hospitals, and to develop scales for quantifying the degree of mental illness (Current Reports Section, 1956).

By 1960, the introduction of computing in data processing, clinical studies, and hospital diagnoses was initiated (Ledley & Lusted, 1960). Automated systems and the use of those systems to improve mental health care delivery were underway. By the early 1970s, NIMH had published several guidelines on the design of management information systems (Cooper, 1973; Chapman, 1976). Nevertheless, today, many information system concerns remain for mental health providers, including quality improvement; program evaluation; outcomes assessment; patient-centered recovery planning; and financial and budgetary issues. Therefore, the question remains, how are decisions best made in mental health service settings?

Decision Making in Mental Health

Within health and mental health care environments, many activities need to be managed and many decisions need to be made. When important decisions must be made frequently, information systems can help to manage this process. Coiera (2003) has suggested a five-step process for activity management:

1. Defining a set of management goals;
2. Establishing a model of the system;
3. Collecting measurement data;
4. Evaluating the measurements taken in relation to the model of the system; and
5. Taking action(s) based upon the original management goals.

Once the action has been taken (e.g., administering treatment to an individual), one must assess the outcome of that decision (Has the patient improved as a result of the treatment?). This cycle of establishing a model of a system, measuring data, and taking action to improve the management of the system forms an integral part of information systems.

However, decision making in clinical care is compounded by its complexity and lack of system transparency; constant interruptions; lack of documentation of protocols, procedures, and processes; and poorly defined expectations and outcomes at both the patient and the provider organizational levels. Further, many health information technology (HIT) applications simply automate tasks and/or organizational processes, providing little cognitive support for the knowledge-based tasks that clinicians perform. In the following sections, we will examine both the management and knowledge processes involved in the creation of an MIS.

Linking Data in Mental Health: Operations Management

Mental health and substance abuse organizations have numerous internal and external requests for information. As the scale and complexity of such delivery systems have increased, the use of computer-based information systems has become a necessity. However, the migration from legacy systems to second-generation systems has also become more complicated. The development of second-generation information systems to meet current reporting and information needs illustrates the unique data structure and analysis problems of mental health delivery systems. These problems are further complicated by federal and state regulatory agencies' external reporting requirements.

Squire et al. (2002) maintain that linking client data from different health and behavioral health care sectors and agencies is necessary to assure the continuity of care, evaluation, and planning of mental health services. Hogan and Essock (1991) suggest that integration of client, human resources, finance, services, and organizational databases will create a foundation for both clinical and administrative data-based decision support and for evaluation, program planning, and research.

Overall, there are several reasons to implement an MIS, including improving the quality and consistency of client care and documenting the outcomes of services provided. An MIS may also serve to aggregate data at the state and local levels for accountability, external and internal reporting, reports to funding sources and state legislatures, policy and program planning, and for quality improvement systems. Finally, an MIS will help to identify and document gaps in access to critical health services, using tracking data (as required by public health standards and surveillance), and will improve program efficiency.

Therefore, what kind of information is needed? Let's start with a snapshot of a client data module. In a client data module, there are data (demographic) on the client, the client address, phone number, and registration information. There are also four additional sub-modules that address (1) screenings, (2) visits, (3) plans for care, and (4) outcomes (Table 5.1a). If we examine the four data elements more closely, each has a "collection" of data attached to that module. Further, several of these "collections" are "instrument collections" mirrored across three of the sub-modules.

If we examine the "instrument data" (Table 5.1b), we can see how each data element is named and how it is linked to a sub-module. Further, instruments are a key diagnostic tool in mental health services and can help assess outcomes overall at both a client and system level of care. The information from this client data module links to other modules within the MIS that deals with patient care, outcomes assessment, and recovery planning. This information is required for each client in a mental health services agency, organization, or facility.

When looking at how services are delivered in mental health (e.g., regardless of private or public sector care), an MIS has to deal with multi-facility designs and multiple patient numbers as patients move across facilities and systems of care. Persons receiving care in the mental health system are not like most individuals receiving general medical care. Persons receiving mental health services may be enrolled simultaneously in inpatient and outpatient hospital-based or community-based mental health programs, supported services programming (e.g., employment, housing, or education), assistance programs (e.g., Medicaid, SSDI, food stamps), and may be receiving medical care for a physical illness.

TABLE 5.1A

Sample Client Data Module in an EHR

Client	
Client Address	
Client Phone	
Client Registration	
Client Screenings	Instrument Answer Collection
	Instrument Intervention Collection
Client Visits	Instrument General Collection
	Instrument Follow-Up Collection
	Instrument Intervention Collection
	Instrument Notes Collection
Client Plan for Care	Plan Data
	Risk Factor Collection
Client Outcomes	Instrument General Collection
	Instrument Intervention Collection
	Instrument Notes Collection

TABLE 5.1B

Instrument Data in Sample Client Data Module in an EHR

Instrument General	Instrument Intervention	Instrument Outcome
Instrument Id	Intervention Id	Outcome Id
Visit Type Id	Intervention Answer Text	Intervention_Answer_Text
Others Present Text	Intervention_Other_	Intervention_Other_
Instrument Taken Date	Description	Description
Instrument Start Time	Screen Answer_Date	Screen Answer Date
Instrument End Time	Screen Clinician	Screen Clinician
Client Birth Date		
Doctor_ Name		
Client_ Care_Start_Date		
Care_Plan_Flag		
Care_Plan__Name		
Other_Services_Flag		
Other_Services_Name		
Instrument_Notes		
Staff_Names		

Tracking an individual's use of services across systems of care can be a nightmare. Take, for example, Figure 5.1. It documents "an emotional chain of custody" through the many service delivery systems where children who have suffered a traumatic event may end up for a significant length of time. Note that the chart does not subdivide all of the various

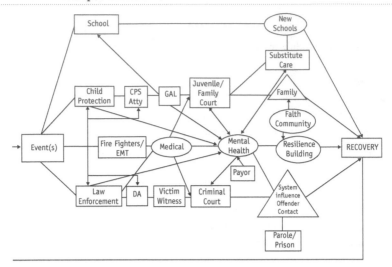

FIGURE 5.1 Emotional Chain of Custody.

The National Child Traumatic Stress Network. Emotional chain of custody. Child Welfare Trauma Training Toolkit (p. 83), March, 2008. Retrieved from http://www.nctsnet.org/nctsn_assets/pdfs/CWT3_ Supplementals.pdf.

sub-units within the larger agencies/settings. Further, each area (e.g., Child Protection, Juvenile/Family Court) has its own data collection and its own MIS that collects data from each of its sub-units.

To be most useful, an information system should link data from each of these sources to allow for an individual's history of care (from all health and mental health providers) to be available in one place. One of the challenges is that various programs do not "speak the same language" in terms of treatments, outcomes, and client characteristics (Manos, 2009). This suggests the need for integrated systems that require a standard data collection system and shared definitions across all sources/organizations.

Meanwhile, coding and classification occurs in each system of care. Consider that, *at a minimum*, there may be four coding systems (again federally approved) used within one system of state providers (health): (1) *International Classification of Diseases*, 10th edition, Clinical Modification (ICD-CM10); (2) *Common Procedural Terminology*, 4th edition (CPT-4); (3) Health Care Finance Administration Common Procedural Coding System (HCPCS); and (4) National Drug Codes (NDC). In addition, there may be a "crosswalk" that matches local (state) codes to federal codes for purposes of comparative data across states and within the nation (Table 5.2).

In addition to the clinical data stored within an MIS, financial data is stored in the general ledger. However, the general ledger, in some MIS programs, may be modified to allow users to input data on anything that users can count (e.g., number of patients served by program X) or scale (e.g., ratings 1 to 5 for service satisfaction). This might include the amount of floor space devoted to specific programs, staffing, or the level of functioning of a patient.

TABLE 5.2

Local to Federal Codes Crosswalk

Current Code	National Code	Modifier	Notes
Z9986	Z99861		Crisis Stabilization
Y0300	90804	HF	Refer to CPT manual for national code description. This substance abuse service is covered for FAMIS recipient's only. Focus must be on substance abuse.

From the Virginia Local Codes Crosswalk, Report run on: May 19, 2004 2:55 pm. Available online at http://www.dmas.virginia.gov/downloads/pdfs/hpa-local_codes_crosswalk.pdf.

Linking Data in Mental Health: Cognitive Support

It has been projected that over the next 15 years, incorporating the EHR into existing or new MIS may result in a net savings of $371 billion for hospitals and $142 billion for physician practices (Venkatraman et al., 2008). These savings are expected from increased safety and efficiencies in health care. In addition, it has been suggested that the EHR may double these savings due to more effective management of chronic diseases and increased opportunities for prevention. However, from a provider perspective, " ... very little systematic evidence has been gathered on the usability of EHRs in practice and the implications of their design on cognitive task flow, continuity of care, and efficiency of workflows" (Armijo, McDonnell, & Werner, 2009).

A number of federal agencies, including the Agency for Healthcare Research and Quality (AHRQ) and the Institute of Medicine (IOM), have made cognitive support a key factor in the design of the systems using the EHR in the NHII. In addition to the need for "comprehensive data on patients' conditions, treatments, and outcomes," cognitive support would assist health care professionals to "integrate patient-specific data where possible and account for any uncertainties that remain" and "to integrate evidence-based practice guidelines and research results into daily practice" (IOM, 2009, pp. 21–22). The Committee on Engaging the Computer Science Research Community in Health Care Informatics (Computer Science and Telecommunications Board, 2009) emphasized the need for cognitive support for health care providers in the development, adoption, implementation, and utilization of computer-based tools and systems.

Why is cognitive support such an issue? After all, the EHR (a.k.a. MIS) promises efficiencies in work, cost savings, and strategic planning. The question of how we integrate health transaction data and related raw data to create a conceptual model of the patient and his or her care, without losing the patient among all the data, is not an easy question to answer (Computer Science and Telecommunications Board, 2009).

Hence, a human-centered approach to design is critical. Cognitive support refers to the assistance that tools provide to humans in their decision-making processes and problem solving. The goal of cognitive support within an MIS application/system is to transfer to software some of the user's cognitive processes involved in performing a task.

Since this reduces the number of items that a user must internally track and process, the user is able to concentrate his or her expertise on other parts of the task. By understanding the decision-making processes used in the mapping of tasks, cognitive support can be introduced to reduce the cognitive load experienced by users. However, "[t]o develop a human-centered product for a work domain, we first need to understand the nature of the work" (Zhang, 2005). Understanding both the human and systems side of work process and decision making requires a new way of conceptualizing the ways of working, from the perspectives of all those who may use the MIS.

Let's first look at a very simple mapping of the patient-provider interaction (Figure 5.2). Something happens that disturbs the well-being of the patient. This disturbance is recorded as an "event" in an MIS. This "event" changes the previous understanding of the health of the patient. To understand the current state of health, consultations and tests are performed. The provider(s) (together) construct a new definition of the health of the patient through the results of the tests, consultations, or with additional research. They each provide input based upon their level of involvement. After consolidating this information, the clinician determines what needs to be done to return the patient to his or her previous state of health. This leads to a plan of care (intervention), which produces a change in the status of the patient's health. This change provides feedback as to whether the plan of care was successful. In an MIS, all of those steps to the success (or not) of treatment then signify a change in the understanding of that specific event. The work processes and information to understand that event are now linked in the MIS. Over time, that one event may be linked to other patients' care, used as part of a larger surveillance of disease, or even as an example to support a new protocol for treatment.

Within each of these actions (e.g., event, change in patient status), there are numerous decisions and activities for each specific action. The change in the patient's health status results in a phone call to the clinician's office to schedule an appointment. His or her patient record is updated to reflect an incidence of illness. The patient comes in for the appointment. He or she is checked in. Health insurance information is updated and scanned or photocopied for the records. The nurse takes his or her vitals (blood

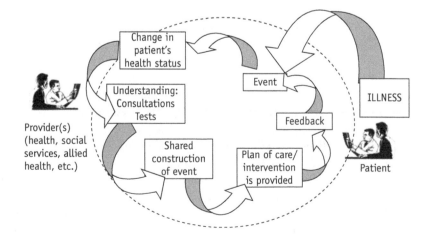

FIGURE 5.2 Simple Event Map for Diagnosing Illness.

pressure, temperature, weight) and updates the paperboard and/or the electronic record as to history of the event that caused the visit (symptoms, duration, patient administered tests, e.g., temperature-taking), existing medication history and additional medication (over-the-counter), or other efforts to feel better. The nurse may briefly update the doctor verbally before he or she enters the room.

The doctor may review the nurse-collected information before having the patient again recite the reasons for the visit. The doctor may then perform some basic physical checks on the patient, noting them in a paper or e-record. Based upon the data the doctor has collected, he or she may decide to write a prescription and ask for a follow-up visit (in so many days) if symptoms do not go away. The doctor may decide to request additional tests, which may require a referral script to another clinician or a prescription for laboratory tests.

All of these decisions are recorded in the EHR and are coded according to type of diagnostic tests performed, treatment decisions made, referrals authorized, tests requested, and need, if any, for follow-up. Each decision as to preliminary diagnosis and treatment is part of a diagnostic algorithm: determining disease/disorder, severity, treatment protocol, and knowledge of the patient as to understanding of the diagnosis and compliance to have the tests completed or to take medication. Some of the EHR transactions are business operations (scheduling and billing). However, the diagnosis and decision on treatment paths are clinical decision making.

Clinical workflows consist of complex clinical processes, which by definition are not linear. Further, these clinical workflows often are performed under time constraints and may require adjustments as conclusions are reached and decisions made. Further, clinicians use information from a variety of sources, from laboratory results to drug interactions, behavioral or physical symptoms, and expected or predicted outcomes. This information may be generated by providers who are in-house or external to the clinician's current workplace. Intuitively based decisions that can be made by humans require complex, relational programming if done by a machine.

One way to counter this is to use expert-oriented cognitive engineering tools to study organizational routines to develop effective interface designs, evaluation, and vendor practices. Bowens et al. (2010), Unertl et al. (2009), and Vishwanath et al. (2010) examine user perspectives and individual, group, and organizational workflow processes to inform and facilitate the development of "context appropriate" clinical informatics tools. These types of studies reduce cognitive load by considering the breadth of data necessary in clinical decision making, the complexity of relationships among people and processes, how to deal with uncertainty in decision making, and how to improve a shared cognition among clinicians, again stressing individual and team levels.

Usability in MIS Systems (People and Processes)

The National Institute of Standards and Technology (NIST, 2007) defines usability as the " … effectiveness, efficiency and satisfaction with which the intended users can achieve their tasks in the intended context of product use." There are numerous examples in the literature which describe negative consequences of MIS that can be attributed directly to usability and design (Ash, Berg, & Coiera, 2005; Crabtree et al., 2005; Tang & Patel, 1994).

To counter negative consequences, MIS design and usability must address both the independent and interdependent nature of professional providers and clinical teams. With the increasing emphasis on client-centered models and medical homes (Amiel & Pincus, 2011), an MIS must support and coordinate care across multiple health professionals, social services professionals, and clients using personal health records integrated with an MIS. Further, usability testing will need to take into consideration typical settings of care, as well as the professionals within those settings, which include acute care, intensive care, emergency rooms, home care, skilled nursing facilities, and long-term care facilities.

One usability challenge concerns the synthesis of information, which occurs in acute and chronic care coordination, such as patient hand-offs (one health care provider takes responsibility for health care from another health care provider), medication administration, and after-discharge care. Clinicians need to understand the whole client, not just his or her specialty "slice." This is particularly critical in mental health and substance abuse treatment. A client may have multiple comorbidities: two or more mental disorders; a mental and substance use disorder; or a mental and/or substance use disorder with a physical disorder. The client may be released from acute care to a community-based care facility with changes in medication and requirements to see a primary care physician for follow-up laboratory work. At each step, the clinician will need different information that will ensure that the client can move to the next level of care.

In the acute care setting, questions revolve around the current medication, treatment, and behaviors, with inquiries regarding what changes have occurred since the last time the clinician was on shift. As a client transitions to less intensive settings, the current clinician needs to be aware of the client's progression. Upon discharge to aftercare, again the referring clinician needs to ensure that the referral clinician has the same information (medication, treatment, and behavioral) to ensure continuity of care. These kinds of data can be difficult to locate in a client EHR, much less to have a user-friendly, "at a glance" type of display, with easily understood icons, support for tasks, such as creating a missed medications list, or rationale for changes in medication.

For an MIS to function effectively from a usability standpoint, it must serve four functions: (1) memory aid; (2) computational aid; (3) decision support aid; and (4) a collaboration aid (Armijo, McDonnell, & Werner, 2009). As a memory aid, it reduces the cognitive need for the clinician to rely upon his or her memory of how to complete a task. As a computational aid, it reduces the need to cognitively group, compare, and analyze information. As a decision support aid, it enhances the clinician's ability to integrate information to make evidence-based decisions. Finally, as a collaboration aid, it assists clinicians in the effective communication of information and decisions among and between providers and patients (Armijo, McDonnell, & Werner, 2009).

So, how does one design a system to reflect real-world needs and expectations? Software application developers create use cases to categorize and organize user interface and related functional requirements. A use case is a description of a system's behavior and appearance as it responds to a stimulus. The system responses are then used to conceptually define the requirements to achieve the specified task, whether it is an administrative function or to provide a cognitive support function (see Figure 5.3). A use case also evaluates compliance with user requirements during testing and evaluation activities. For example, a client signs into a clinic for HIV testing. Rather than ask the client if he or she has consented to the test, the MIS should display a consent form on record. If there is no form, then the consent form is automatically generated for the client to fill out and is stored in the MIS.

Armijo and colleagues (2009) recommended the establishment of certification requirements for EHRs. These requirements include the specifications of usability and/or information design as an essential part of the certification process, address EHR design and functionality in standards and guidelines, and provide documentation that these programs have been tested at both individual and process levels. These steps should enhance the integration of cognitive support into the development of EHRs.

Key Tasks	EHR Role			
	Memory	Computation	Decision Support	Collaboration
Review patient history	Displays available history and demographics	Provides contextual view of overall patient health	Recommends care based on patient characteristics	Incorporate information from outside sources
Conduct patient assessment	Prompt for required information	Compute statistics (BMI, etc.)	Action oriented clinical reminders	Coordinate care across multiple providers
Determine clinical decision	Relate assessment to patient history	Display trends, reference ranges	Support based on outside research or recommendations	Staff view and/or instructions
Develop treatment plan	Standards of care, care plans, evidence-based guidelines	Apply standards of care based on patient characteristics	Evidence-based care adjusted by patient characteristics	Patient summary, educational tools
Order additional services	Review previous services and/or results	Determine appropriate provider and/or location	Alignment with insurance requirements	Create referrals. Facilitate provider communication
Prescribe medications	Medication, dose, history, allergies, formulary	Dose calculation	Interactions, contraindications, effectiveness	Patient instructions, side effects, and warnings
Document visit	Diagnosis and treatment codes	Prompts and/or automatic population	Insurance guidelines	Patient education, coordination with multiple providers

FIGURE 5.3 Expected EHR Tasks.

Adapted from Armijo, D., McDonnell, C., & Werner, K. (2009). *Electronic health record usability: Interface design considerations* (AHRQ Publication No. 09(10)-0091-2-EF; page 3). Rockville, MD: Agency for Healthcare Research and Quality. Document in the public domain.

Principles and Goals ↓	Goals and objectives	Conceptual:
Framework ↓	Reporting requirements	WHAT WHOM
Domains ↓	Service/Support criteria	WHERE WHENE
Indicators ↓	(What is measured, counted, assessed)	
Measures ↓	(How is it measured)	Technical: HOW
Product ↓	Analysis and Report	Program/Outcomes Evaluation

FIGURE 5.4 Mental Health Accountability.

Implementing Evidence-Based Practice in Mental Health MIS

With the continued emphasis on evidence-based practice in mental health, Sim, Sanders, and McDonald (2002) suggest that there are four major difficulties in taking research to practice:

1. Obtaining evidence that is relevant to the clinical activity;
2. Having a systematic review of the evidence;
3. Applying this evidence to a decision-based context; and
4. Supporting and measuring how effective the change has been in practice.

This has important implications for the skills that one has in using computerized databases for clinical decision making.

New data standards, which have emerged from the increased accountability for services and the inclusion of consumers in outcomes discussions for mental health services, have also changed what is being measured, what is counted, what is assessed, and what the outcomes are to establish quality and effectiveness of services. In order to ensure accountability, consistent service/support criteria, performance indicators and measures, and reporting requirements for those measures are needed. Performance measures for each indicator will be used to measure progress toward the goals and objectives (see Figure 5.4). To further complicate information systems management, the Federal Health Insurance Portability and Accountability Act (HIPAA) requires administrative simplification of health information data for all print or online administrative transactions (including forms) and standardization of health records (in print and online formats).

Outcomes Data

Historically, research and evaluation occurred at the conclusion of program planning and implementation. However, in today's managed care environment, evaluation is now discussed during initial planning stages of new programs. Evaluation is no longer just "counting" things; evaluation has moved to outcomes assessment with continuous quality improvement. This requires an integrated or holistic look at not just services provided or the number of the clients treated but the quality of the programming and the quality of life enhancement for the recipients of these services. From a patient perspective, any information that is collected should lead to improved quality of care and services delivery, regardless of whether the information is about patient-based clinical reports or system-wide report cards. From a staff perspective, information should also lead to a better quality of care for patients, a better workplace environment for staff (and patients), and better staff productivity.

There has been an increasing demand for outcomes data from both purchasers of health care as well as providers. This is especially true within the managed behavioral health care industry. As consumers become more educated about health care and participate more actively in treatment decisions, providers will need to provide "report cards" so that consumers may assess the quality of health and mental health care and make informed decisions on which treatment provider to use. Therefore, when creating outcomes components in mental health information systems, system designers need to build in patient-reported outcomes data, clinical information, and functional status as components of the system. Many existing report cards measure organizational arrangements and/or provider activities, that is, the structure and process of care, respectively. Outcomes data in mental health services can be difficult to define and, since they are subject to the interpretation of the user, can vary widely in interpretation.

One of the advantages of an MIS is the ability to generate comparative data on services delivery, outcomes, and programs. Originally for use by administrators and oversight agencies, comparative data, known as report cards, are used to create information for consumers and providers to compare services options and interventions across and within provider settings and networks. Report cards track performance over time, identify areas for improvement, improve allocation of resources and staff, facilitate operational and clinical decision making, and determine priorities for new health initiatives. Further, it is important for performance measures to be administratively feasible, that is, data collection and management costs should be offset by the value of the information obtained. These report cards are not new; however, the development of standards is an important component when examining provider performance data.

MENTAL HEALTH STATISTICS IMPROVEMENT PROGRAM

Located within the Center for Mental Health Services (CMHS), a federal agency in the U.S. Substance Abuse and Mental Health Services Administration (SAMHSA), the Mental Health Statistics Improvement Program (MHSIP) develops and improves the reporting of mental health statistics and the use of information systems. Since 1976, MHSIP has supported the use of statistical information in the management and study of mental health programs. An MHSIP advisory group report emphasized the person-centered paradigm (MHSIP Ad Hoc Advisory Group, 1992) and suggested that MHSIP "systematically expand the scope and coverage of mental health organizations that are involved"; "reinforce decision support especially at the system or auxiliary level"; and "highlight the person as the crucial level for data integration, and the managed system as the crucial level for data analysis" (pp. 22–24). A second report (Buckley, 1993) noted that "quality-through-participation techniques that rely heavily on data to promote informed participation in decision making" suggest that MHSIP's natural evolutionary step is to develop a person-centered orientation, with "accountability to a broader range of stakeholders' decision support needs; adding a focus on consumer preferences and satisfaction; emphasizing consumer outcomes over time" (pp. 10–11).

The Mental Health Statistics Improvement Program (MHSIP) developed a "report card" in 1996 that was consumer-based. MHSIP's working group decided that an effective and quality mental health system should reduce symptom distress, help an individual increase independent functioning, improve performance and productivity at work or school, develop a system of natural supports, and gain access to physical health services. Outcomes assessment requires providers and practitioners to understand exactly who the patients are, what their lives are like, and how their lives may be improved by a specific facility or agency.

JCAHO AND ORYX

The Joint Commission on Accreditation of Healthcare Organizations (JCAHO) is a national leader in the accreditation and credentialing of health care organizations. Its standards focus on important patient and organizational functions that are essential to providing safe, high-quality care. Like MHSIP, it prepares draft standards using input from external stakeholder groups (task forces, focus groups, and experts) and solicits reviews and comments nationally. ORYX® was created to assist hospitals, home- and long-term care organizations/networks, and behavioral health organizations to integrate outcomes and performance data into the accreditation process. Many of JCAHO's core performance measures mirror the measures required by the Centers for Medicare and Medicaid Services (CMS).

JCAHO also published the National Library of Healthcare Indicators (NLHI; JCAHO, 1997), containing individual profiles for over 200 performance measures used to assess the performance of health plans, integrated delivery networks, and provider-sponsored organizations. The NLHI contained the Health Employer Data Information Set (HEDIS), developed by the National Committee for Quality Assurance (NCQA).

NCQA AND HEDIS

Like JCAHO, the National Committee for Quality Assurance (NCQA) reviews and accredits all types of managed care organizations, as well as point-of-service health plans and certain physician-hospital organizations. Its Health Plan Data and Employer Set (HEDIS) is essentially a report card for managed health care plans, with standardized performance measures designed to ensure that purchasers and consumers may compare the performance of managed health care plans. It has over 70 measures evaluating eight domains of care: (1) effectiveness; (2) access/availability; (3) satisfaction with experience of care; (4) service utilization; (5) cost of care; (6) description of health plan; (7) stability of health plan; and (8) informed health care choices (NCQA, 2011). Measures are reviewed annually to keep current with best practices and new assessment protocols.

Healthcare Effectiveness Data and Information Set (HEDIS) date are collected through administrative data, including surveys, medical charts, and insurance claims for hospitalizations, medical office visits and procedures. Quality Compass is NCQA's interactive, web-based comparison tool that allows users to view plan results and benchmark information using a four-star rating system. It is grouped by the domains of Access and Service, Qualified Providers, Staying Healthy, Getting Better, and Living with Illness. Included in HEDIS is the Consumer Assessment of Healthcare Providers and Systems (CAHPS®) 4.0 survey, which measures members' satisfaction with their care.

AHRQ AND CAHPS

The Agency for Healthcare Research and Quality (AHRQ), a division within the U.S. Department of Health and Human Services, began a multi-year initiative known as the CAHPS program in 1995. CAHPS surveys ask users to report on their experiences with health care services. As with JCAHO's ORYX® and HEDIS, CAHPS surveys are also standardized as to the contents and format of the instrument, field protocols for administering the survey and collecting data, conducting the data analysis, and presentation of the final reports. The CAHPS Health Plan Survey addresses many types of coverage (Medicaid, Medicare, commercial insurance) across a variety of managed care systems, and captures information on the experiences of special populations (e.g., children and adults with chronic conditions and disabilities).

Of special interest is the CAHPS health information technology set, which assesses the patient-centeredness of physician practices and groups that have adopted different kinds of health information technologies, such as secure electronic messaging, electronic medical records, medication lists, personal health records, and appointment scheduling. The CAHPS HIT set produces four patient experience measures (three composite measures plus one single item about access to appointments) (1) helpfulness of provider's use of computers during a visit; (2) getting timely answers to medical questions by e-mail; (3) helpfulness of provider's website in giving you information about your care and tests; and (4) getting timely appointments through e-mail or a website (AHRQ, 2011).

These four organizations are known for being early adopters of technology in the development and deployment of assessment measures. As shown, their MIS not only collect a wide variety of data but also have developed crosswalks across oversight agencies, such as the Centers for Medicaid and Medicare Services, and standards, such as the ICD-10. The performance data collected by agencies and organizations are used in additional comparative research on effectiveness and quality reporting and to meet meaningful use criteria for federal monies to update provider HIT infrastructure.

COMPARATIVE EFFECTIVENESS RESEARCH

Comparative effectiveness research (CER) examines treatments and interventions to determine which evidence-based treatments are effective and beneficial and which ones are not. Comparative effectiveness research is conducted generally through systematic reviews of existing clinical trials, studies, and completed research or by conducting new studies to prove the effectiveness or comparative effectiveness of a test, treatment, procedure, or health care service. By 2005, interest in CER as a standard review practice to establish best practices was growing, and the Agency for Healthcare Research and Quality (AHRQ) was charged with developing CER information. With the passage of the American Recovery and Reinvestment Act of 2009 and the establishment of the Federal

Coordinating Council for CER, comparative effectiveness research became a core evaluation protocol and practice (Roundtable on Value & Science Driven Care, 2011). Since data collected in registries, databases, data networks, EHRs, and provider MIS are critical to CER reviews to substantiate cost, efficacy, and outcomes claims, developing infrastructure, workforce, and new methodologies are key to improving national health care.

MEANINGFUL USE

The 2011 implementation of "meaningful use" legislation for certified electronic health records (EHRs) may overcome data capture issues affecting quality measurement. The Health Information Technology for Economic and Clinical Health Act of 2009 (HITECH) legislation provided financial incentives for Medicare and Medicaid providers (organization and individual) to implement electronic health records systems in their work environments. However, it is not enough to install an EHR. Providers must also use it for daily operations, such as e-prescribing; must demonstrate that electronic exchanges of health information improves the quality of care that they provide to their patients; and must submit information on clinical quality measures to required reporting entities.

Meaningful use includes both a core set and a menu set of objectives that are specific to eligible professionals or eligible hospitals and care facilities. Professionals have 25 meaningful objectives, of which 15 are core objectives and 10 are menu objectives. Professionals must meet 20 of the 25 meaningful objectives. Hospitals and other care facilities have a total of 24 meaningful objectives (15 core objectives and 9 menu objectives), of which 19 of the 24 must be met (see Table 5.3). In addition, professionals must report on

TABLE 5.3

Comparison of the Eligible Professional and Hospital/CAH Core Objectives

Eligible Professional Core Objectives	Eligible Hospital and CAH Core Objectives
(1) Use CPOE for medication orders directly entered by any licensed health care professional who can enter orders into the medical record per state, local and professional guidelines.	(1) Use CPOE for medication orders directly entered by any licensed health care professional who can enter orders into the medical record per state, local and professional guidelines.
(2) Implement drug-drug and drug-allergy interaction checks	(2) Implement drug-drug and drug-allergy interaction checks
(3) Maintain an up-to-date problem list of current and active diagnoses.	(3) Maintain an up-to-date problem list of current and active diagnoses.
(4) Generate and transmit permissible prescriptions electronically (eRx).	
(5) Maintain active medication list.	(4) Maintain active medication list
(6) Maintain active medication allergy list.	(5) Maintain active medication allergy list.
(7) Record all of the following demographics: Preferred language, Gender, Race, Ethnicity, and Date of birth	(6) Record all of the following demographics: Preferred language, Gender, Race, Ethnicity, and Date of birth

(continued)

TABLE 5.3

Comparison of the Eligible Professional and Hospital/CAH Core Objectives (*continued*)

Eligible Professional Core Objectives	Eligible Hospital and CAH Core Objectives
(8) Record and chart changes in the following vital signs: Height, Weight, Blood pressure Calculate and display body mass index (BMI), Plot and display growth charts for children 2–20 years, including BMI.	(7) Record and chart changes in the following vital signs: Height, Weight, Blood pressure Calculate and display body mass index (BMI), Plot and display growth charts for children 2–20 years, including BMI.
(9) Record smoking status for patients 13 years old or older.	(8) Record smoking status for patients 13 years old or older.
(10) Report ambulatory clinical quality measures to CMS or, in the case of Medicaid EPs, the States.	(9) Report hospital clinical quality measures to CMS or, in the case of Medicaid eligible hospitals, the States.
(11) Implement one clinical decision support rule relevant to specialty or high clinical priority along with the ability to track compliance with that rule.	(10) Implement one clinical decision support rule related to a high priority hospital condition along with the ability to track compliance with that rule.
(12) Provide patients with an electronic copy of their health information (including diagnostics test results, problem list, medication lists, medication allergies) upon request.	(11) Provide patients with an electronic copy of their health information (including diagnostics test results, problem list, medication lists, medication allergies) upon request.
(13) Provide clinical summaries for patients for each office visit.	(12) Provide patients with an electronic copy of their discharge instruction at time of discharge, upon request.
(14) Capability to exchange key clinical information (for example, problem list, medication list, allergies, and diagnostic test results), among providers of care and patient authorized entities electronically.	(13) Capability to exchange key clinical information (for example, problem list, medication list, medication allergies, and diagnostic test results), among providers of care and patient authorized entities electronically
(15) Protect electronic health information created or maintained by the certified EHR technology through the implementation of appropriate technical capabilities.	(14) Protect electronic health information created or maintained by the certified EHR technology through the implementation of appropriate technical capabilities.

Adapted from the Centers for Medicare and Medicaid Services (2011). *Eligible Professional Meaningful Use Table of Contents Core and Menu Set Objectives* (https://www.cms.gov/EHRIncentivePrograms/Downloads/EP-MU-TOC.pdf) and *Eligible Hospital and CAH Meaningful Use Table of Contents Core and Menu Set Objectives* (https://www.cms.gov/EHRIncentivePrograms/Downloads/Hosp_CAH_MU-TOC.pdf). Document in public domain.

6 clinical quality measures, while hospitals (and other care facilities) must report on 15 clinical quality measures (Centers for Medicare and Medicaid Services, 2012). This will allow assessment of the health IT infrastructure regarding data collection, data exchange, and systematic improvements in technology and care provision.

Based upon Table 5.3, the reporting requirements for individual providers and organizations mirror each other in many respects. The major differences deal with point of entry and exit, who receives information, and level of reporting. It is important to note that the requirements share many of the same data elements or build upon the elements of individual providers and patient events. The next section describes how data collected by a local mental health center was used to assess and allocate resources to improve patient outcomes.

Case Illustration: A Community Mental Health Center Project

Chinman et al. (2002) described the "Patient Profile Project" at the Connecticut Mental Health Center (CMHC). The CMHC is a state-funded agency providing comprehensive clinical and rehabilitative services to persons with mental illnesses. To gain a better understanding of their clients and their use of services in the effort to improve services and outcomes, a Patient Task Force was established. The Task Force, comprising multiple stakeholders (administrators, practitioners, and clients), was charged to develop a service needs index as part of a continuous evaluation process the CMHC wanted to implement.

Data came from an acuity scale developed by the CMHC and additional data from the state Department of Mental Health and Addiction Services (DMHAS). The acuity scale measured twelve items: (1) appointment compliance; (2) suicidality; (3) medication compliance; (4) homicidality; (5) substance use; (6) medical needs; (7) legal issues; (8) housing status; (9) entitlement issues; (10) social supports; (11) symptomatology; and (12) adjustment to community living. Additional demographic information (age, gender, race, ethnicity, education level, and marital status) on each of the patients was provided by the common clinical information system from the DMHAS. Clinician rating scales for alcohol and drug use, a multi-axial diagnostic form, and the Global Assessment of Functioning Scale (modified) were included in diagnostic measures. In addition to the demographic and clinical information collected, the Patient Care Committee developed a "service need index," which incorporated the patient's average acuity, the GAF-m score, and his or her drug or alcohol use.

Chinman et al. (2002) found that almost 53% of the clients were women. A quarter of the clients were African American, a quarter were of Hispanic origin, and less than half were Caucasians. Approximately 75% of the clients were not in a relationship. Only half earned a high school education or higher. The most common diagnoses were schizophrenia or related psychoses (36%) and affective disorders (26%). Most of the clients had mild to moderate symptoms. However, almost half of the clients had experienced some form of violence, while 25% had been sexually abused (Chinman et al., 2002).

What did the CMHC do with the information it collected? As the data were interpreted and reported, the CMHC invested a significant amount of effort in disseminating the findings to its staff. A grand rounds presentation was conducted at a system-wide level, covering all five treatment sites. It also summarized the results in an in-house newsletter as well as in meetings of senior management and team directors. Instead of generating a single summary report, numerous reports were generated to all stakeholders to receive feedback and comments. In addition, each program director and the clinical providers within the treatment teams received information targeted to their individual program/treatment areas.

How did the CMHC take the data and apply it to client treatment outcomes? The data indicated a significant number of individuals who lacked significant relationships with other individuals. The CMHC determined that expansion of social rehabilitation services should be a priority, so it expanded its collaboration with the local clubhouse and created several projects to expand community, recreational, and social activities. The data also indicated that monolingual Hispanic clients had low levels of educational achievement. The CMHC developed more programs for these clients to expand high school equivalency opportunities, "English as a second language" classes, and adult education classes at their clinics. The data on the amount of violence to which clients had been exposed or experienced led to incorporation of a "street safe" skills training module and a trauma-sensitive orientation into clinical practice across the CMHC. Program data also indicated that certain programs had caseloads that were not in proportion with their clients' service needs. The evaluative data provided important information to reallocate staff and resources to improve caseload/service mix. The fact that data existed and that this data had been incorporated into an ongoing dissemination effort reduced resistance to allocation. Finally, the data indicated that there was overrepresentation of African Americans in the dual diagnosis, assertive community treatment, and outreach/engagement programs. The CMHC explored the possibility that these patients needed programs that were more responsive to the needs of African American patients.

This project shows the value of linking decisions in clinical administration and program development to improve client outcomes, create an invested evaluation-stakeholder feedback loop, and integrate a continuous quality improvement framework within an organization.

Implications for Mental Health Informatics

With the continued development and implementation of online health information management applications and tools, there are a number of implications for practitioners, researchers, and consumers. With the continued commercialization of e-health, international developers and information providers in the e-health market will increase the number of outsourced and off-shore services. This will require greater scrutiny and oversight regarding privacy, security, and quality assurance for all health and mental health information users.

Peer-to-peer (P2P) services are replacing the traditional client-server model. Unlike the client-server model in which servers send information and clients receive information, P2Ps are simultaneously senders and receivers of resources. Since P2Ps are decentralized, the model supports group collaboration, peer governance, and universal access of its information for its users (Taylor & Harrison, 2009). This technology model is mirrored by social P2P processes, which aim to share ownership of information as widely as possible. As P2Ps grow in more sophisticated search protocols and provide more relevance for information seekers, they may supplant the current web portal model (Schnipper et al., 2008).

As broadband applications better address quality of service issues and traffic congestion, clinical services, such as real-time medical consultations, will be in greater demand. In addition, wireless Internet service has revolutionized the use of mobile e-health applications, expanding potential markets for clinical decision-making apps (applications) for handheld devices and formats. Health and mental health professionals can download mobile apps for a number of the National Library of Medicine databases, including Mobile MedlinePlus (clinical information); PubMed for Handhelds; Reuniting families after a disaster (ReUnite); Wireless System for Emergency Responders (WISER); Radiation Emergency Medical Management (REMM); toxicology, hazardous chemicals, environmental health and toxic releases (TOXNET); and federally approved treatment guidelines for adults, pregnant women, and children with HIV/AIDS (AIDSinfo; Conuel, 2010).

There are application development trends that must be considered when working with MIS. For example, personalization and tailoring dynamically alters content according to the profile, preferences, or usage patterns of the individual user. A common component of e-health sites and tools, the online collection and use of sensitive personal health information increases risk, leading to privacy and data security issues, and the subsequent development of new protocols and applications. Nanotechnologies, such as cellular or sub-cellular sensors or computers, are generating innovative methods and tools for collecting, storing, and analyzing Internet-accessible health and mental health data.

MIS development in mental health is evolving rapidly. Considering the complexity of health information applications and systems, there are some elements that we see as common for most MIS/EHRs. Personalization of health information is progressing to the point where templates in turn-key systems will easily create HIPAA and other reporting-compliant progress notes based upon clinical specialization or setting. Automatic prompts will suggest the proper codes, such as ICD or evaluation and management (E/M) to enter into the patient chart. MISs may even be able to populate charts with trends noted based upon event and diagnostic coding and/or free-text entries. One particularly effective feature would be automated task management to update and complete lab results, authorizations, referral, and health maintenance. One critical component will be an authentication feature, using date/time stamps, to create permanent, non-editable notes for legal documentation of patient care.

Additional features would include drug and coding databases with medical necessity warnings and drug interactions, as well as the ability to electronically scan, store, and index paper-based reports and charts. Secure, real-time wireless access to mobile, tablet, and desktop PCs commonly used by health and mental health practitioners would be compatible with voice recognition software, scanners, and digital cameras. Of course, these systems will integrate seamlessly with industry standard HL7 interface with practice management and laboratory information systems.

References

Agency for Healthcare Quality and Research. (2011). *About the CAHPS® health information technology item set* (Document no. 1313). Rockville, MD: AHRQ. Retrieved from http:// www.cahps.ahrq.gov/Surveys-Guidance/Item-Sets/~/media/Files/SurveyDocuments/ CG/12%20Month/Get_Surveys/1313_about_hit.pdf.

Amiel, J. M., & Pincus, H. A. (2011). The medical home model: New opportunities for psychiatric services in the United States. *Current Opinion in Psychiatry, 24*(6):562–568.

Armijo, D., McDonnell, C., & Werner, K. (2009). *Electronic health record usability: Interface design considerations* (AHRQ Publication No. 09(10)-0091-2-EF). Rockville, MD: Agency for Healthcare Research and Quality.

Ash, J., Berg, M., & Coiera, E. (2005). Some unintended consequences of information technology in health care: The nature of patient care information system- related errors. *JAMA, 11*(2):104–112.

Bowens, F. M., Frye, P. A., & Jones, W. A. (2010). Health information technology: integration of clinical workflow into meaningful use of electronic health records. *Perspectives in Health Information Management, 7*(fall), 1d. Retrieved from http://www.ncbi.nlm.nih.gov/pmc/articles/PMC2966355/?tool=pubmed.

Buckley, S. M. (1993). *Moving MHSIP toward a person-centered paradigm: A concept paper submitted to CMHS and the MHSIP Ad Hoc Advisory Group.* Albany, NY: New York State Research Foundation for Mental Hygiene. Retrieved from http://www.mhsip.org/library/pdfFiles/movingMHSIPtoapersoncenteredparadigm.pdf.

Centers for Medicare and Medicaid Services (2012). *Electronic specifications.* Retrieved from https://www.cms.gov/QualityMeasures/03_ElectronicSpecifications.asp.

Cesare-Murphy, M., McMahill, C., & Schyve, P. (1997). Joint commission evaluation of behavioral health care organizations. *Evaluation Review, 21*(3):322–329.

Chapman, R. L., (1976). *The design of management information systems for mental health organizations: A primer.* Rockville, MD: U. S. Dept. of Health, Education, and Welfare, Public Health Service, Alcohol, Drug Abuse, and Mental Health Administration, National Institute of Mental Health, Division of Biometry and Epidemiology.

Chinman, M. J., Symanski-Tondora, J., Johnson, A., & Davidson, L. (2002). The Connecticut Mental Health Center Patient Profile Project: Application of a service needs index. *International Journal of Health Care Quality Assurance Incorporating Leadership in Health Services, 15*(1):29–39.

Coiera, E. (2003). *Guide to health informatics,* 2nd ed. New York: Oxford University Press, 2003.

Committee on Data Standards for Patient Safety. (2003). *Key capabilities of an electronic health record system: Letter report.* Washington, DC: National Academies Press. Retrieved from http://www.nap.edu/catalog.php?record_id=10781.

Computer Science and Telecommunications Board. (2009). *Computational technology for effective health care: Immediate steps and strategic directions.* Washington, DC: National Academies Press. Retrieved from http://http://www.nap.edu/openbook.php?record_id=12572.

Conuel, T. (2010, May 21). Going mobile: Information when and where you need it. *NLM in Focus.* Retrieved from http://infocus.nlm.nih.gov/2010/05/going-mobile-information-when.html.

Cooper, E. M. (1973). *Guidelines for a minimum statistical and accounting system for community mental health centers: A working handbook with illustrative end-product tables, document forms, and procedures.* Rockville, MD: U. S. Dept. of Health, Education, and Welfare, Public Health Service, Alcohol, Drug Abuse, and Mental Health Administration, National Institute of Mental Health, Division of Biometry and Epidemiology.

Crabtree, B. F., Miller, W. L., Tallia, A. F., et al. (2005). Delivery of clinical preventive services in family medicine offices. *Annals of Family Medicine, 3*(5), 430–435.

Current Reports Section, Biometrics Branch, National Institute of Mental Health. (1956).
Progress in reporting mental hospital statistics. *Public Health Reports, 71*(10), 1033–1036.
Retrieved from http://www.ncbi.nlm.nih.gov/pmc/articles/PMC2031001/pdf/
pubhealthreporig00154-0083.pdf.Hogan, M. E., & Essock, S. M. (1991). Data and
decisions: Can mental health management be knowledge-based? *Journal of Mental
Health Administration, 18*(1), 14–15.

Institute of Medicine (2009). *Computational technology for effective health care: Immediate
steps and strategic directions.* Washington, DC: National Academies Press.Joint Commission
on Accreditation of Healthcare Organizations. (1995). *National Library of Healthcare
Indicators (NLHI): Health plan and network edition.* Oakbrook Terrace, IL: JCAHO.

Ledley, R. S., Lusted, L. B. (1960). The use of electronic computers in medical data
processing: Aids in diagnosis, current information retrieval, and medical record keeping.
IRE Transactions in Medical Electronics, ME-7, 31–47.

Manos D. (2009). Obama launches White House Office of Health Reform. *Healthcare
Finance News,* April 13. Retrieved from http://www.healthcarefinancenews.com/news/oba
ma-launches-white-house-office-health-reform.

MHSIP Ad Hoc Advisory Group. (1992). *Mental Health Statistics Improvement Program:
Current status and directions for the future.* Bethesda, MD: MHSIP.

National Committee for Quality Assurance. (2011). What is HEDIS? Retrieved from http://
www.ncqa.org/tabid/187/Default.aspx

National Institute of Mental Health (1962). *The Model Reporting Area for Mental Hospital
Statistics: Development, purpose and program.* Washington, DC: National Institutes of
Health.

National Institute of Standards and Technology. (2007). Common industry specification
for usability requirements: NISTIR 7432 (Publication number IUSR:CISU-R v0.90).
Gaithersburg, MD: NIST.

Persell, S. D., Kaiser, D., Dolan, N. C., Andrews, B., Levi, S., Khandekar, J., Gavagan, T.,
Thompson, J. A., Friesema, E. M., & Baker, D. W. (2011). Changes in performance after
implementation of a multifaceted electronic-health-record-based quality improvement
system. *Medical Care, 49*(2):117–125.

Roundtable on Value & Science Driven Care. (2011). *Learning what works: Infrastructure
required for comparative effectiveness research: Workshop summary.* Washington,
DC: National Academies Press. Retrieved from http://www.nap.edu/openbook.
php?record_id=12214&page=57.

Schnipper. J. L., Gandhi, T. K., Wald, J. S., Grant, R. W., Poon, E. G., Volk, L. A., Businger, A.,
Siteman, E., Buckel, L., & Middleton, B. (2008). Design and implementation of a
web-based patient portal linked to an electronic health record designed to improve
medication safety: the Patient Gateway medications module. *Informatics in Primary
Care, 16*(2), 147–155.

Sim, I., Sanders, G. D., & McDonald, K. M. Evidence-based practice for mere mortals: The
role of informatics and health services research. *Journal of General Internal Medicine, 17*(4),
302–308. doi: 10.1046/j.1525-1497.2002.10518.x

Squire, L, Bedard, M, Hegge, L., & Polischuk, V. (2002). Current evaluation and future needs
of a mental health data linkage system in a remote region: A Canadian experience. *Journal
of Behavioral Health Services & Research, 29*(4), 476–480.

Tang, P. C., & Patel, V. L. (1994). Major issues in user interface design for health professional workstations: Summary and recommendations. *International Journal of Biomedical Computing, 34*(1–4), 139–148.

Taylor, I. J., & Harrison, A. B. (2009). From P2P and grids to services on the web evolving distributed communities. London: Springer. doi: 10.1007/978-1-84800-123-7

Unertl, K. M., Weinger, M. B., Johnson, K. B., & Lorenzi, N. M. (2009). Describing and modeling workflow and information flow in chronic disease care. *Journal of the American Medical Informatics Association: JAMIA, 16*(6), 826.

Venkatraman, S., Balqa, H., Venkatesh, V., & Bates, J. (2008). Virtual extension: Six strategies for electronic medical records systems. *Communications of the ACM, 51*(11), 140–144.

Vishwanath, A., Singh, S. R., & Winkelstein, P. (2010). The impact of electronic medical record systems on outpatient workflows: A longitudinal evaluation of its workflow effects. *International Journal of Medical Informatics, 79*(11), 778–791.

Zhang, J. (2005). Human-centered computing in health information systems Part 1: Analysis and design. *Journal of Biomedical Informatics, 38*(1), 1–3.

One kind of uncertainty is generated by an **innovation**, defined as an idea, a practice, or object that is perceived new by an individual or another unit of adoption. An innovation presents an individual or an organization with a new alternative or alternatives, as well as new means of solving problems. However, the probability that the new idea is superior to previous practices is not initially known with certainty by individual problem solvers. Thus, individuals are motivated to seek further information about the innovation in order to cope with the uncertainty that it creates.

EVERETT M. ROGERS, 2003

6 Adoption and Implementation of Mental Health Information Technology

There is a real need for improvement in organizational capability for and the delivery of mental health services. The diffusion, adoption, and implementation of health information technologies continues to be an issue today, more than 20 years after the development of the Internet, more than 50 years since the introduction of computers in the workplace, and more than a century since the introduction of telecommunications. In this chapter, we explore a number of issues that affect the adoption and implementation of mental health information technology, including the nature of teamwork in health and mental health and its routinization.

Background

In 2003, the President's New Freedom Commission concluded that the nation's mental health service delivery system is ill equipped to meet the complex needs of persons with serious mental illnesses. One of the major issues affecting service quality is attributed to the lag time from research to practice, which may be as long as 15 to 20 years for actual implementation (President's New Freedom Commission, 2003). A second issue is the rapid change in behavioral health technology, which, over the past decade, has brought even more change to research and practice settings. Behavioral health service technologies, known as "soft" technologies, are particularly vulnerable to problems with fidelity in implementation (Aarons, 2005). Fidelity in implementation is critical to the implementation of evidence-based practices in clinical practice. Theoretically, these problems are preventable with effective communication among the teams or groups working with these technologies. A third issue is the impact of technology on workplace processes and practice, especially with rapid technology changes and national mandates to implement health information technology (HIT).

President Bush set a goal to have electronic health records (EHR) for the majority of Americans by 2014 (Committee on Ways and Means, 2008). This was reiterated by President Obama, who considered large-scale adoption of HIT a priority to meet President Bush's 2014 goal (Jones, 2009). President Obama's economic stimulus plan established the Health Information Technology for Economic and Clinical Health (HITECH) Act, which supported the electronic sharing of clinical data among health and mental health stakeholders. The central feature of this data sharing is the EHR (also known as the EMR, or electronic medical record), "a longitudinal electronic record of patient health information generated by one or more encounters in any care delivery setting" (Healthcare Information and Management Systems Society, HIMSS, 2010, p. 1).

A basic EMR/EHR system contains patient history and demographics, a patient problem list, physician clinical notes, and a comprehensive list of patient's medications and allergies. In addition, physicians may place computerized orders for prescriptions and may view laboratory and imaging results electronically (Hsai et al., 2011). However, preliminary estimates from the Centers for Disease Control and Prevention (Hsai et al., 2011) suggest that the overall number of physicians using a basic EHR was 34%. Further, to increase the adoption and utilization of HIT in the United States, the Centers for Medicare & Medicaid Services (CMS, 2010) instituted e-prescribing and EHR programs. However, many health care and safety net providers feel that there are significant gaps in their understanding of how the implementation of HIT and EHR will improve health and mental health care. This perception of the value of HIT and EHR creates critical challenges for the development of policies aimed at speeding up adoption.

Barriers to Adoption

Unlike physicians, an EHR provides unique challenges for non-physician mental health practitioners. Unlike medical data, which often comprises medical test results, mental health data often consists of handwritten notes by practitioners, taken during a session, which are later transcribed or converted into electronic format (Levin & Hanson, 2011). Further, prior diagnoses, assessment reports, and termination summaries may only appear in handwritten formats, which have been transferred from office to office over a period of time. In addition, if a practitioner is using an automated billing system, the notes may be converted into diagnostic or administrative categories (DSM or ICD codes). Finally, many mental health practitioners (solo practitioners or small group practice) who may utilize a minimum record to track visits still rely primarily on paper-based records. However, the purpose of the EHR is to provide a legible, quickly accessible record, standard assessment and diagnostic criteria, and a common language in mental health in order to make mental health data quantifiable for additional stakeholders (Gask et al., 2008; Greenfield & Wolf-Branigin, 2009; Meredith, 2010).

INTEROPERABILITY AND STANDARDS DEVELOPMENT

Interoperability was cited more often as a barrier than as a facilitator to EHR implementation (McGinn et al., 2011). A major barrier to adoption is the selection of a system that will work with the numerous "flavors" of EHRs, legacy systems, and other HIT applications, as well the numerous data collection and reporting requirements of local, state, regional, and federal health and mental health care organizational settings. Not only are there numerous highly decentralized information management, infrastructure, technology, and operations to meet the needs of state agencies independent of one another, health and mental health data are combinations of numerous agency, regulatory, administrative, oversight, and financial data sets, which are required for Medicaid, Medicare, and other public entitlement programs (Hanson & Levin, 2010). Much of this data comes from the day-to-day work activities and behaviors that occur in daily practice, such as scheduling, billing, diagnosis, treatment, follow-up, assessment, and outcomes. These activities are not only reported into EHR/EMR systems, but how the activities are performed may be changed with the adoption of a new system and attendant technologies. Further, depending on the standards upon which the EMR/EHR system is created, interoperability may be affected, requiring the use of multiple paper- and electronic systems.

Standards development affects address interoperability as well as usability issues. There are thousands of HIT systems, ranging from a basic EMR/EHR to fully functional systems, designed to handle numerous types of care settings, with permutations available for every size (e.g., solo, group, state), type of partnership, clinical decision making, and evidence-based practice. Nevertheless, what works for a large urban, multi-group medical practice may not work as well for the solo mental health practitioner in a rural or frontier setting.

USABILITY

Usability is often cited as a central factor in the adoption and implementation literature (Walker, 2005; Campbell, et al., 2007; Armijo, McDonnell, & Werner, 2009; Coons et al., 2009; Yen & Bakken, 2011). Usability evaluation usually involves not only hardware, but also the information and work processes in a given environment. In addition, usability requires an understanding of the clinical, organizational, sociological, and/or technical points of view of members of an organization. The International Organization for Standardization (ISO) proposes two definitions of usability in their standards ISO 9241–11 and ISO/IEC 9126. ISO 9241–11 defines usability within the context of user performance and satisfaction as "the extent to which a product can be used by specified users to achieve specified goals with effectiveness, efficiency and satisfaction in a specified context of use" (ISO, 1998, p. 6). It is a process-oriented standard.

In ISO/IEC 9126, on the other hand, is a product-oriented standard, where usability, functionality, reliability, efficiency, maintainability and portability are product quality standards (ISO, 2001). ISO/IEC 9126 defined usability in a contextual manner, as "the capability of the software product to be understood, learned, used and attractive to the user, when used under specified conditions" (Bevan, 1999). The phrase "when used under specified conditions" clearly denotes that a product, in itself, has no intrinsic usability, only a capability to be used in a particular context by a user to achieve a specific goal to the satisfaction of the user. Although 9126 is now superseded by ISO/IEC 25010:2011, the key elements of usability remain constant.

Under usability are a number of sub-components: learnability; understandability; operability; attractiveness; and compliance. Learnability, defined as "the capability of the software product to enable the user to learn its application," has three attributes to make a system "learnable": (1) comprehensible input and output; (2) instructional readiness; and (3) messages readiness (Bran et al., 2003, pp. 326–327). Bran et al. (2003) suggest that it is critical to evaluate usability through the interaction of user, system, and task in a specified setting, that is, the technical features of HIT and the social features of the work environment. Hence, any review of the usability of an item should address the user, the tool, the task, and the environment. It is not enough to ask the question "Can the user accomplish his or her goal?" (usability), but to ask it concurrently with the question "How easy is it for a user learn the system?" (learnability).

Systematic reviews on interactive health information systems show mixed methodological results. Yen and Bakken (2011), in their review of over 660 studies on HIT implementation, found ambiguity in the types of HIT identified in the studies. This ambiguity was due often to overlapping and complex functions of the types of HIT mentioned in the studies. The three most common types of studies examined (1) decision support systems or other applications with decision support features; (2) computer-based provider order entry within hospital information systems; and (3) electronic health records. They also found a number of methodological issues in the studies, including lack of a theoretical framework and/or model, lack of details regarding qualitative study approaches, a single evaluation focus, a lack of reporting environmental factors in the early stages of development, and use of guideline adherence as a primary outcome. This last issue, found in studies on clinical support systems, also determined a number of workflow problems (such as the failure to receive reminders when not with a patient), affected implementation of recommendations, and contributed to a lack of interaction with the system interface.

Shekelle, Morton, and Keeler (2006) found few individual studies or collection of studies that allowed readers to generalize a study's reported benefit. Peute et al. (2008) examined applied usability studies of health information systems conducted during 1990 to 2006. They, too, found a number of different evaluation methodologies used, with the majority of the studies being summative (73%) and the remainder formative (27%). While the summative studies addressed barriers to adoption issues, the formative studies failed to address iterative development research. O'Malley and colleagues (2010) were able to identify several issues that affected adoption and implementation. One issue was the inability to support care coordination among other clinicians and settings. This is especially problematic with the number of legacy systems and lack of standardization in design and data elements across systems. A second issue was the lack of effective filters for data to reduce cognitive and information overload. A third issue was primarily a perceptual issue regarding the lack of effectiveness of EMR/EHRs in the medical decision-making process and care coordination (O'Malley et al., 2010).

ECONOMICS AND COST OF IMPLEMENTATION

Clinicians may hesitate to adopt EHRs for a number of financial reasons, including initial start-up costs, developmental funding, and delays in return on investment (ROI) (Balfour et al., 2009). Another major concern is whether EHRs can be implemented and maintained as a sustainable business model. Studies within the literature are mixed; however, there are several areas of agreement. First, improved documentation and methodological designs of HIT studies, which describe in greater depth the intervention, disbursement of funds and projects, and the organizational and economic environment in which HIT is implemented, would be of greater value in determining the scope of an HIT implementation (Shekelle et al., 2006; eHealth Initiative, 2009). This would allow clearer documentation of projects that are generalizable, are replicable across settings, and that result in best practices.

ORGANIZATIONAL AND MANAGEMENT BARRIERS

In her systematic review, Lluch (2011) examined organizational and management barriers to HIT adoption. She was able to categorize the barriers under five major headings: (1) organizational structure; (2) tasks; (3) people policies; (4) incentives; and (5) information and decision processes. Autonomy, accountability, and changing ways of work were found across all five categories. Organizations with strong hierarchies, for example, hospitals or large clinical settings, often create forced work distributions, resulting in loss of clinician autonomy and control. Another consequence was the lack of HIT to effectively link articulation of care in the community with accountability by the discharging organization. Further, given the intra- and inter-organization of health and mental health care, HIT models were perceived *not* to enhance care coordination among primary, secondary, tertiary, and community care providers. Again, new ways of working across organizations, disciplines, and teams within a virtual health system must account for issues surrounding autonomy and accountability. Changes in work processes and routines were seen as inevitable consequences; however, underlying such changes are issues of trust, liability, support, training, career development, and use of incentives and rewards. Lluch (2011) suggests that there is a need for further research providing evidence of HIT cost-effectiveness and the development process for optimal HIT applications.

However, the EMR/EHR is seen as a single point of entry into a longitudinal review of a patient. Success stories on its ability to automate and streamline clinician's workflow continue to be published. In addition, there are numerous reports on EMR/EHRs supporting other care-related activities directly or indirectly, including evidence-based decision support, quality management, risk assessment, and outcomes reporting. Much of the uneasiness with adopting EHRs lies in the uncertainty of such a major change and how new technologies are chosen as best practice.

Uncertainty as Change Mechanism

Diffusion of innovations is a model of how new ideas, opinions, or products spread through an organization or society. Diffusion of innovations is not a new idea (Tarde, 1903). Approximately 5,000 published studies have been conducted on the diffusion of innovations over the past 60 years (Haider & Kreps, 2004). However, unlike other models of change that require persuading individuals to change (Valente, 1995), diffusion of innovations conceptualizes change as an evolution or reinvention of behaviors and products to better fit the needs of individuals or an organization (Rogers, 1995, 2003). When examining the factors involved in diffusion (the innovation, the communication channels, temporality, and the social system (Rogers, 2003)), diffusion of innovation is best viewed as a process rather than a distinct event, with different factors affecting diffusion at different stages (Hornik, 2004). So how does change come about?

There are five factors that determine the success or failure of an innovation. The first factor is relative advantage. Relative advantage is the degree to which an innovation is perceived as better than the current situation or product by the persons involved. Measures may include convenience, improvement in the workflow or workplace, economic and/or cost benefits, and overall satisfaction of the users. The higher the advantage of an innovation is perceived, the quicker its adoption.

A second factor is how compatible the innovation is with existing practices and values. An innovation that requires users to completely discard their ways of working together and start from scratch is less likely to be adopted than an innovation that can be implemented using existing behaviors and routines.

A third factor is the simplicity and ease of use of the innovation. If an innovation is perceived as too complex to understand and too difficult to use, successful adoption will be hampered, if not stymied.

A fourth factor is the ability of an innovation to go through a trial period. The "trialability" of an innovation gives users the opportunity to experiment and to become accustomed to new ways of doing and interacting with the innovation.

The final factor is whether or not the innovation provides observable results. "Seeing" the results of the innovation reduces uncertainty about adoption and allows users to talk about their experiences and questions more openly, freeing the group to actively decide to change workflow or behaviors to incorporate the innovation into everyday practice.

Rogers (2003) also suggests that there are five levels of adopters: (1) innovators; (2) early adopters; (3) early majorities; (4) late majorities; and (5) laggards. Innovators ("venturesome") comprise 2.5% of the population, early adopters ("respectable") comprise 13.5%, early majority ("deliberate") comprise 34%, late majority (skeptical) comprise 34%, and laggards (traditional) comprise 16% of the population (p. 291). Each group plays an important role in the success or failure of a technology in an organization. An important consideration is the process, and at which stage of the process an individual agrees to adopt an innovation. The process starts with knowledge, when an individual knows about an innovation and has some understanding of how it functions. It progresses to persuasion, when an individual decides how he or she feels about the innovation. Depending on whether the impression is favorable or unfavorable affects the third step, which is the decision to adopt or reject the innovation. Once a favorable decision is made, the individual actively uses the innovation. The final step, confirmation, is an evaluative step, in which the individual decides if the decision to adopt the innovation has benefited him or her (Rogers, 2003, p. 162). Adoption typically follows an S-shaped curve. After a relatively small number of persons adopt the innovation, there is a relatively rapid adoption by other members of the group, with the laggards eventually joining.

Again, uncertainty drives the reluctance of many individuals and organizations to adopt new technologies. It boils down to the perceived cost of the proposed change. How can someone know *for certain* that there are benefits? To what degree will the innovation disrupt other aspects of their daily life? Is it compatible with existing routines, habits, and values? Is it hard to use? How much new information does someone need to acquire, and how quickly do they need to acquire it? It's new, it's uncertain, and what happens if users don't understand how to use it or use it incorrectly?

The effect on the user is often seen as the major hurdle. The more learnable a system is, the less time a user takes in order to understand how to do a specific task. The more training and documentation a user needs to understand how to perform a task reduces the sense of accomplishment, effectiveness, and satisfaction with a system. Therefore, the more learnable a system, the more usable the system is. In addition to learnability, systems should be flexible (the many ways one may interact with a system), robust (level of support in the system to handle errors), and efficient (How quickly can users perform tasks after they have learned the system?). In addition to satisfaction, memorability is an often neglected aspect of system design. Memorability addresses how easily users reestablish proficiency after they return to the system after a period of time not using it. Drawing on Nielsen and Schneiderman, Table 6.1 lists the core components of a learnable, efficient, and usable system.

For example, in 1994, Nielsen reported that a 6% budget investment on usability provides returns of 200% to 500%. Those figures still hold true today. Benefits of effective health information systems include enhanced patient and staff safety, productivity and work quality, staff satisfaction and acceptance, and ease of learning and use. Further, consider the impacts of a decrease in the number of adverse events, fewer system problems, and, from a user perspective, even less need for continual modifications and "workarounds."

TABLE 6.1

Rubric for Assessing Technology Displays

1. Consistency: Users should know that similar actions lead to similar results.
2. Visibility: Users should be informed about what is going on in the system.
3. Match: Users should have a mental model that matches the state of the medical technology.
4. Minimalist: Users should not be exposed to unnecessary information.
5. Memory: Users should not be required to memorize a lot of information to use the medical technology.
6. Feedback: Users should be provided prompt and informative feedback.
7. Flexibility: Users should have the ability to customize or create shortcuts.
8. Message: Users should receive an informative error message.
9. Errors: Users should be insulated from error occurrence by the design of the medical technology.
10. Closure: Users should be informed of task completions.
11. Undo: Users should have the ability to recover from errors.
12. Language: Users should be presented information in an understandable form.
13. Control: Users should not have the impression that the medical technology is in control.
14. Document: Users should be provided help by the medical technology when necessary.

Nielsen-Schneiderman Heuristics, page 32 from Shaver, E. F., & Braun, C. C. (2008). Assessing devices from the user's perspectives. *Materials Management in Health Care*, September, 30–34.

Of the many issues to focus on in adoption and implementation of health information technology, the integration of technology into work teams is the most interesting.

Routinization and Teams

There are many reasons that widespread adoption and implementation of EHR have not occurred. These range from related costs, resistance to change, fear or avoidance of technology, and patterns of day-to-day work behaviors. It is critical to remember that most individuals have a number of organizational routines which they follow at a subconscious level. Hence, any new *and* sustainable change may require significant effort on the part of both the individual and the organization (Levin & Hanson, 2011). This is particularly true in the adoption and implementation of new health information technology, which extends the incorporation of evidence-based practices into clinical decision-making tools embedded within these technologies.

Evidence-based practice (EBP) in mental health is grounded in large, well-controlled randomized trials, with research designs that minimize bias and maximize generalizability, and effectiveness studies that emphasize their relevance to routine practice settings. However, it is difficult for routine practice settings to adopt and implement evidenced-based mental health interventions and technologies. The literature suggests that there is a lack of understanding and research related to factors critical for implementation. Lambooij, Engelfriet, and Westert (2010) suggest that the context (societal structures, characteristics, and economics) in which professionals operate affects the problems they face and influences how HIT decisions made. Organizational culture, structure, climate, and work attitudes affect the adoption of both EBPs and technology, as well as adherence to treatment protocols (Glisson, 2002; Ganju, 2003; Brooks, Pilgrim, & Rogers, 2011). An important component of the workplace is the conscious and unconscious routines followed every day by its members. Routinization is the "habitual, taken-for-granted character of the vast bulk of the activities of day-to-day social life; the prevalence of familiar styles and forms of conduct, both supporting and supported by a sense of ontological security" (Giddens, 1984, p. 376).

When organizations adopt new technologies, they must also develop new procedures to incorporate the technology into daily activities, workflow, and process. This requires establishing new task-based frameworks, more formalized identification of task processes, or changes to operational requirements, policy, or *modus operandi* (Rogers, 2003). Fixsen et al. (2005) identified six core components critical to the initiation and sustainability of proven programs in new locations and environments. These include first selecting the staff who can implement the program. The next two components address the effective training of staff and ongoing coaching to decrease uncertainty and anxiety. Supervisors should closely supervise staff and use fidelity assessments to provide performance feedback to staff. Performance feedback provides ongoing quality, behavioral, and technological information to ensure successful adoption and to reduce staff uncertainty. Evaluation of how well the program functions overall is key. This provides staff, administration, and client feedback and helps to fine-tune the intervention to ensure fidelity and operational efficiencies. Finally, administrative supports need to be put into place to facilitate implementation and sustainability of the intervention or technology.

A key concept to remember is that learning and practice are both dependent upon routinization, that is, incorporating new knowledge into existing knowledge to create integrated professional frameworks. Routines are divided into two types: ostentive and performative. An ostentive routine is the ideal routine, which is the level of operational and practical knowledge necessary to optimally use a new technology. Ostentive routines are guided by procedural knowledge, that is, the rules of the system. However, especially with technology adoption, rules created for a system built for a larger audience may not take into account the behaviors and knowledge currently in use within an organization. It is through performance of a rule or routine, with the specific actions by specific people in specific places and times, that ostentive routines become a routine in practice. The transition from ostentive to performative routines is often filled with the tension and uncertainty that comes from change. Hence, the social organization of work has a substantial effect on both "the cognition that is the task and the cognition that governs the coordination of the elements of the task" (Hutchins, 1995, p. 176).

In mental health services, clinical, professional, and allied health teams may also be a part of a team or a larger group of teams across governmental, organizational, agency, community, and home settings. Teams work as inter-, intra, and trans-disciplinary, both in- and out-of-house. As teams are composed of multiple levels of social and organizational structures, team solidarity is a crucial component. The more interdependence a group has (its perception of itself as being a group), the more trust among its members and the degree of motivation to participate in the group in shared knowledges and in daily interaction, the easier it is for the group to build consensus and take risks. Howard-Grenville (2005) suggests that there are three basic questions when examining routines of teams. The first question asks how many structures are involved when a routine is performed. The second question examines the types of structures that are affected. Structure types range from technology, control, and administration, to coordination. These types may shape the performance of a routine. The final question is: how aligned are the products, processes, and expectations of each structure?

In their examination of the national dissemination and replication of Blueprint Model Violence Prevention Programs (42 sites) and Life Skills Training (a drug prevention program; 105 sites), Elliott and Mihalic (2004) determined which factors contributed to the fidelity and sustainability of the programs. They found that organizational-level routinization was an essential component of adoption, fidelity, and successful implementation. Moreover, they suggested that perhaps a better question to ask is how a *local context* may need to change to allow successful implementation of a program (Elliott & Mihalic, 2004, p. 50).

Therefore, implementing innovations in behavioral health services must address the relative novelty of the intervention vis-à-vis the existing attitudes, knowledge, or skills of the service providers. In addition, the organization's relationship with its external environment, including supportive services, integrated care providers, and payers, must be clearly defined and examined. After all, any change in internal routines may require organizational retrofitting to its internal and external structures.

In the following section, we briefly discuss two implementation projects to illustrate the complexity of implementing new technologies in mental health service settings.

Wisdom et al. (2008) described the challenges that substance abuse treatment agencies face in the adoption of health technology. The Oregon Practice Improvement Collaborative

(OPIC) provided technical assistance to five community-based drug treatment agencies as the agencies moved to computerized practices during a four-year period. The five agencies varied widely regarding their size, number of staff, level of technology support, and levels of care provided. Three of the programs (A, B, C) wanted to implement self-administered, computerized measures (one of the three focused on residential youth involved in treatment). The remaining two programs, both large comprehensive treatment agencies, wanted to convert existing systems to electronic systems (D, E). Program D wanted to convert its existing client progress monitoring programs to electronic data collection, analysis, and outcomes assessment for its adolescent residential facilities. Program E wanted to adopt an integrated, electronic medical records system, managing client records and tracking outcomes, to increase communication between multiple clinicians who served the same clients. In addition, three of the agencies (A, B, C) were located in urban settings, one was in a rural setting (D), and the last setting was a suburban area (E). At the end of the project period, three of the implementations were successful (A, B, E), one was partially successful (D), and one was unsuccessful (C).

Facilitators and barriers to adoption were identified at each site. For the successful sites, gaining consensus was essential. Although consensus building may delay a more rapid implementation, it is a key component to having a team function effectively. During its consensus process, Agency A chose to revise the electronic Addiction Severity Index instrument to a multimedia format, to capture more data from clients. In addition, Agency A utilized the OPIC team the most, meeting with the OPIC staff monthly during the first year of the implementation, receiving feedback from the OPIC staff, and attending two training sessions on using the computerized measure. Agency A was a mid-sized urban agency with a small staff, limited treatment services, and strong leadership. Staff buy-in was achieved through the focus on a collaborative decision-making process, as well as strong training and coaching.

Agency D, a rural facility, wanted to create an electronic version of the Teaching Our Youth Social Skills (TOYSS) program. This project is considered partially successful. Although Agency D had strong leadership, which facilitated adoption, there was little staff input during the development process. There was staff support for the conversion, but a major barrier was the lack of internal technical support for the new system during the study period. Additional barriers included the lack of assistance requested from the OPIC staff (15 hours over 2 years) and the lack of technological capacity by staff to conduct advanced analysis of the data. The departure of the director also dampened the sustainability of the project, although some of the technological issues were resolved by the agency after the project period.

The project for Agency C was considered an unsuccessful implementation of the Outcome Rating Scale as a feedback tool for its adolescent clients. A small, residential urban facility, it took little advantage of the OPIC staff's technical support. Agency C conducted its training itself and had limited coaching. One of the greatest barriers to implementation, however, was the departure of the director, which effectively stopped all internal communication, performance feedback, and work on the conversion of the intervention. In addition, there was significant employee turnover during the study period.

Child welfare workers are responsible for referring children and adolescents with mental illnesses, substance use disorders, and other behavioral health issues to a wide array of services. Further, the referral process itself can be fraught with difficulties since child welfare services are provided across numerous settings and with other health providers. Therefore, poor assessment of treatment needs and limited access to behavioral health services are seen as major barriers in the provision of child welfare services (Leslie et al., 2005).

Clinical decision support systems (DSS) are designed to reduce the complexity of clinical decision making, rapidly integrate and analyze the clinical literature, and assist in systematic recall of guidelines and protocols. These systems have been shown to improve practice, reduce errors, and improve adherence to evidence-based guidelines and protocols in practice settings. Since DSS provide relevant clinical information at the point of care, they are currently being adapted to other health care settings.

Foster and Stiffman (2009) examine the adoption of the Intervention for Multisector Provider Enhancement (IMPROVE) system, funded through the National Institute on Mental Health, among a sample of state child welfare workers. A decision support system available on personal computer and handheld formats, IMPROVE contains a database of over 2,000 agencies and programs used by child welfare workers. In addition, IMPROVE contains assessment checklists for depression, conduct disorder, attention deficit hyperactivity disorder, and substance abuse problems. The selection of three or more checklist items in an assessment triggers a referral list directly related to observed behaviors and/or identified problems. Since training and coaching are considered two key facilitators of successful implementation, training sessions and shadowing were used to address in-office and in-the-field situations.

Foster and Stiffman (2009) found high correspondence between worker reports of service receipt (Service Assessment for Children and Adolescents, SACA) and administrative data (billing records) in the provision of services. Workers' assessment of mental health and their connectivity to referred agencies and organizations affect child and adolescent access to services. Since children and adolescents in the child welfare system have multiple behavioral health and environmental problems requiring services from multiple service sectors, the more service sectors involved in their care increases the likelihood that children receive the best care available, which reduces service fragmentation and increases inter-agency coordination. Understanding how child welfare workers become aware of *and* become connected to community resources requires an understanding of worker characteristics, practices, and skills. Implementing a new technology, such as IMPROVE, and new models, such as the Gateway Provider Model, opens the door to further adaptation of decision support systems to enhance decision making for other health and mental health professionals.

Clearly, infrastructure and process challenges affect adoption and implementation. What qualities make an innovation spread successfully throughout an organization? The importance of peer-peer conversations and peer networks cannot be underestimated in the adoption, implementation, and sustainability of technologies. Understanding the needs of different user segments, internal and external to an organization, is also key. Identifying, defining, and mapping routines (i.e., knowledge processes) show which knowledge structures affect the performance of a team's work. Explicit knowledge, such as the procedure necessary to enter a prescription for a patient, can be codified and communicated without much difficulty. However, tacit knowledge, which encompasses decision making, judgment in the absence of data, or interpersonal skills, is not so easily defined (Polyani, 1966).

Leadership is also critical, whether it comes from administrative or peer leaders. At least one member of the team must be able to understand the relevance and key elements of the technology or intervention in order to be a change agent within the team (Anand et al., 2003). Consider that teams may be the most common and efficient way of creating knowledge. Not only do teams contextualize each other's expertise and perspectives, teams interpret and construct a shared understanding of the reasons that change may be necessary in existing processes and protocols, and, most importantly, establish credibility criteria for the routines they adopt, implement, and sustain. Since teams vary in the degree to which their pace and activity cycles are internally coordinated, teams with low levels of internal coordination may have difficulty integrating new knowledge and new ways of doing into current routines. Further, as workplace environments become more differentiated due to new technologies, it is essential that new knowledge is successfully integrated with existing knowledge. Yes, change happens, but effective knowledge alignment to new ways of thinking and functioning helps teams and team members more easily transfer the old routines to the new way routines.

Implications for Mental Health Informatics

Routinization is one of the major barriers to adoption of a new practice. After all, "routines create inertia and resist change as long as possible, until exogenous forces overwhelm the structure and revolutionary change occurs" (Feldman & Pentland, 2003, p. 114). To improve the diffusion, adoption, and implementation of EBP, whether it is an intervention or a health information technology, we recommend several next steps.

First, there needs to be a better understanding of diffusion, adoption, and implementation processes, especially in complex services settings. Clarifying the steps involved in these processes will identify the infrastructure necessary to support change as well as the necessary measures for building the supports to create successful adoption, implementation, and sustainability.

Second, support for technology that makes sense in the specific setting is critical. Employing a graduate student to create a home-grown access database for an organization is a fine idea. However, a database used for outcomes assessment requires more knowledge than how to enter data or run simple pre-defined queries. If a homegrown system is built, then staff should be trained in how to use it as a query and analysis tool. The same holds true for off-the-shelf or turn-key systems. Not only does support also mean additional, ongoing, or refresher training, it also requires staff buy-in and involvement in the process, from initial discussions to feedback on operational and coordination issues to an evaluation and outcomes assessment protocol to ensure that the technology/intervention is effective, efficacious, and fits the work environment.

Finally, it's not just talk. Persuasion is effective if the product or behavior change results in improved workflow, services delivery, team coordination, patient care, productivity, and patient and organizational outcomes. It is useful to remember that one size does not fit all.

References

Anand, V., Clark, M. A., & Zellmer-Bruhn, M. (2003). Team knowledge structures: Matching task to information environment. *Journal of Managerial Issues, 15*(1), 15–31.

Armijo, D., McDonnell, C., & Werner, K. (2009). *Electronic health record usability: Evaluation and use case framework* (AHRQ Publication No. 09(10)-0091-1-EF). Rockville, MD: Agency for Healthcare Research and Quality. Retrieved from http://healthit.ahrq. gov/portal/server.pt/gateway/PTARGS_0_1248_907504_0_0_18/09(10)-0091-1-EF.pdf.

Balfour, D. C. 3rd, Evans, S., Januska, J., Lee, H. Y., Lewis, S. J., Nolan, S. R., et al. (2009). Health information technology: Results from a roundtable discussion. *Journal of Managed Care Pharmacy: JMCP, 15*(1 Suppl A), 10–17. Retrieved from http://www.amcp.org/data/jmcp/Jan09a%20Suppl_S10-S17.pdf.

Bevan, N. (1999). Quality in use: meeting user needs for quality. *Journal of Systems and Software, 49*(1), 89–96.

Bran A, Khelifi A, Suryn W, & Seffah, A. (2003). Usability meanings and interpretations in ISO standards. *Software Quality Journal, 11*(4), 325–338.

Brooks, H., Pilgrim, D., & Rogers, A. (2011). Innovation in mental health services: What are the key components of success? *Implementation Science, 6*, 120. doi:10.1186/1748–5908-6-120.

Campbell, E. M., Sittig, D. F., Guappone, K. P., Dykstra, R. H., & Ash, J. S. (2007). Overdependence on technology: An unintended adverse consequence of computerized provider order entry. *AMIA Annual Symposium Proceedings, 2007,* 94–98).

Centers for Medicare & Medicaid Services. (2010). *Federal Register, 75*(8), 1850–1870. Retrieved from http://edocket.access.gpo.gov/2010/pdf/E9–31217.pdf.

Committee on Ways and Means (2008, July 24). *Hearing on promoting the adoption and use of health information technology* (Serial No. 110–93). Washington, DC: GPO. Retrieved from http://www.gpo.gov/fdsys/pkg/CHRG-110hhrg58278/pdf/CHRG-110hhrg58278.pdf.

Coons, S. J., Gwaltney, C. J., Hays, R. D., Lundy, J. J., Sloan, J. A., Revicki, D. A., et al. (2009). Recommendations on evidence needed to support measurement equivalence between electronic and paper-based patient-reported outcome (PRO) measures: ISPOR ePRO Good Research Practices Task Force report. *Value in Health: the Journal of the International Society for Pharmacoeconomics and Outcomes Research, 12*(4), 419–429.

Dix, A., Finlay, J., Abowd, G., & Beale, R. (2004). *Human-computer interaction*, 3rd ed. Upper Saddle River, NJ: Prentice Hall.

eHealth Initiative. (2009). *Migrating toward meaningful use: The state of health information exchange.* Washington, DC: eHealth Initiative. Retrieved from http://www.ehealthinitiative.org/sites/default/files/file/2009%20Survey%20Report%20FINAL.pdf.

Elliott, D. S., & Mihalic, S. (2004). Issues in disseminating and replicating effective prevention programs. *Prevention Science, 5*(1), 47–53.

Feldman, M. S., & Pentland, B. T. (2003). Reconceptualizing organizational routines as a source of flexibility and change. *Administrative Science Quarterly, 48*(1), 94–118.

Fixsen, D. L., Naoom, S. F., Blase, K. A., Friedman, R. M., & Wallace, F. (2005). *Implementation research: A synthesis of the literature* (FMHI Pub. No. 231). Tampa, FL: University of South Florida, Louis de la Parte Florida Mental Health Institute, The National Implementation Research Network.

Foster, K. A., & Stiffman, A. R. (2009). Child welfare workers' adoption of decision support technology. *Journal of Technology in the Human Services, 27*(2), 106–126.

Ganju, V. (2003). Implementation of evidence-based practices in state mental health systems: Implications for research and effectiveness studies. *Schizophrenia Bulletin, 29*(1), 125–131.

Gask, L., Klinkman, M., Fortes, S., & Dowrick, C. (2008). Capturing complexity: The case for a new classification system for mental disorders in primary care. *European Psychiatry: The Journal of the Association of European Psychiatrists, 23*(7), 469–476.

Giddens, A. (1984). *The constitution of society.* Cambridge: Polity Press.

Glisson, C. (2002). The organizational context of children's mental health services. *Clinical Child and Family Psychology Review, 5*(4), 233–253.

Greenfield, L., & Wolf-Branigin, M. (2009). Mental health indicator interaction in predicting substance abuse treatment outcomes in Nevada. *The American Journal of Drug and Alcohol Abuse, 35*(5), 350–357.

Haider, M., & Kreps G. L. (2004). Forty years of diffusion of innovations: Utility and value in public health. *Journal of Health Communication, 9* (Suppl 1), 3–11.

Hanson, A., & Levin, B. L. (2010). The complexity of mental health services research data. In B. L. Levin, K. D. Hennessey, & J. Petrila (Eds.), *Mental health services: A public health perspective,* 3rd ed. (pp. 499–510). New York: Oxford University Press.

Healthcare Information and Management Systems Society (HIMSS) (2010). *EHR: Electronic health record.* Website: URL http://www.himss.org/ASP/topics_Ehr.asp.

Howard-Grenville, J. A. (2005). The persistence of flexible organizational routines: The role of agency and organizational context. *Organization Science, 16*(6), 616–636.

Hornik, R. (2004). Some reflections on diffusion theory and the role of Everett Rogers. *Journal of Health Communication, 9,* 143–148.

Hsiao, C-J, Hing, E., Socey, T.C., & Cai, B. (2011). Electronic health record systems and intent to apply for meaningful use incentives among office-based physician practices: United States, 2001–2011. *NCHS Data Brief, 79,* 1–8.

Hutchins, E. (1995). *Cognition in the wild.* Cambridge, MA: MIT Press.

International Organization for Standardization. (1998). *ISO 9241–11. Ergonomic requirements for office work with visual display terminals (VDTs): Part 11: Guidance on usability.* Author. Retrieved from http://www.it.uu.se/edu/course/homepage/acsd/vt09/ISO9241part11.pdf.

International Organization for Standardization. (2001). *ISO/IEC 9126–1 Software engineering: Product quality.* Author.

Jones, K. C. (2009, January 12). Obama wants e-helath records in five years. *InformationWeek.* Retrieved from http://www.informationweek.com/news/healthcare/212800199.

Lambooij, M. S., Engelfriet, P. & Westert, G. P. (2010). Diffusion of innovations in health care: Does the structural context determine its direction? *International Journal of Technology Assessment in Health Care, 26,* 415–420. doi: 10.1017/S0266462310001017.

Leslie, L. K., Hurlburt, M. S., James, S., Landsverk, J., Slymen, D. J., & Zhang, J. (2005). Relationship between entry into child welfare and mental health service use. *Psychiatric Services, 56*(8), 981–987.

Levin, B. L., & Hanson, A. (2011). Mental health informatics. In N. A. Cummings & W. T. O'Donohue WT (Eds.), *Understanding the behavioral healthcare crisis: The promise of integrated care and diagnostic reform* (pp. 59–82). New York: Routledge (Taylor & Francis Group).

Lluch, M. (2011). Healthcare professionals' organisational barriers to health information technologies: A literature review. *International Journal of Medical Informatics, 80*(12), 849–862. doi:10.1016/j.ijmedinf.2011.09.005.

McGinn, C. A., Grenier, S., Duplantie, J., Shaw, N, Sicotte, C., Mathieu, L.... & Gagnon, M. P. (2011). Comparison of user groups' perspectives of barriers and facilitators to implementing electronic health records: a systematic review. *BMC Medicine, 9,* 46. doi: 10.1186/1741–7015-9-46.

Meredith, J. (2010). Electronic patient record evaluation in community mental health. *Informatics in Primary Care, 17*(4), 209–213.

Nielsen, J. (1994). *Usability engineering.* San Diego, CA: Academic Press.

O'Malley, A. S., Grossman, J. M., Cohen, G. R., Kemper, N. M., & Pham, H. H. (2010). Are electronic medical records helpful for care coordination? Experiences of physician practices. *Journal of General Internal Medicine, 25*(3), 177–185.

Peute, L. W., Spithoven, R., Bakker, P. J., & Jaspers M. W. (2008). Usability studies on interactive health information systems: Where do we stand? In S. Kjær Andersen, G. O. Klein, S. Schulz, J. Aarts, & M. C. Mazzoleni (Eds.), *eHealth beyond the horizon: Get IT there: Proceedings of MIE2008: The XXIst International Congress of the European Federation for Medical Informatics* (pp. 327–332). Amsterdam: IOS Press.

Polyani, M. (1966). *The tacit dimension.* London: Routledge.

President's New Freedom Commission. (2003). *Achieving the promise: Transforming mental health care in America: Final report* (DHHS Pub. No. SMA 03–3832). Rockville, MD: The Commission. Retrieved from http://www.mentalhealthcommission.gov/.

Rogers, E.M. (1995). *Diffusion of innovations,* 4th ed. New York: The Free Press.

Rogers, E. M. (2003). *Diffusion of innovations,* 5th ed. New York: The Free Press.

Shaver, E. F. & Braun, C. C. (2008). Assessing devices from the user's perspectives. *Materials Management in Health Care,* September, 30–34.

Shekelle, P., Morton, S., Keeler, E. B., Wang, J. K., Chaudry, B. I., ... Newberry, S. J. (2006). *Costs and benefits of health information technology* (Evidence Report/Technology Assessment, no. 132). Rockville, MD: Agency for Healthcare Research and Quality. Retrieved from http://www.ahrq.gov/downloads/pub/evidence/pdf/hitsyscosts/hitsys.pdf

Tarde, G. (1903). *The laws of imitation* (E. Clews Parsons, Trans.). New York: H. Holt & Co.

Valente, T. W. (1995). *Network models of the diffusion of innovations.* Cresskill, NJ: Hampton Press.

Walker, J. M. (2005). Usability. In J. M. Walker, E. J. Bieber, & F. Richards (Eds.), *Implementing an electronic health record system* (pp. 47–59). New York: Springer.

Wisdom, J., Gabriel, R., Edmundson, E., Bielavitz, S., & Hromco, J. (2008). Challenges substance abuse treatment agencies faced in adoption of computer-based technology to improve assessment. *Journal of Behavioral Health Services & Research, 35*(2), 158–169.

Yen P.-Y. & Bakken, S. (2011). Review of health information technology usability study methodologies. *Journal of the American Medical Informatics Association.* Advance online publication. doi: 10.1136/amiajnl-2010–000020.

In all of the different sectors that have incorporated computer technologies the ethical, legal
and social issues that arise have an impact that affect all stakeholders—from individuals
within the society through to the professionals working in a particular domain. These issues
have not often been clearly seen or anticipated—largely because many of the applications
present new ways of doing things in unfamiliar contexts.

—DUQUENOY, P., GEORGE, C., & KIMPPA, K., 2008, iii

7 Legal and Ethical Issues in Mental Health Informatics

The use of electronic communication technologies has enabled health care professionals to
provide better services for much of the population and has facilitated improved communication between health care professionals and their patients. However, what accompanies
the utilization of these technologies are additional legal and ethical issues and concerns.
It is also important to remember that electronic communication and information technologies includes many types of technologies, such as phone, fax, e-mail, the Internet, still
imaging, and live interactive two-way audio-video communication.

This chapter will address legal and regulatory issues, professional ethics, professional
practice concerns, and conclude with a section on implications for mental health
informatics.

Legislation

Concerns regarding the transmission and utilization of patient information are not new.
The protection of patient privacy and confidentiality abounds throughout federal and state
constitutional privacy rights, federal and state legislation, regulations governing medical
records, credentialing and licensing of health professionals and organizations, and specific
federal and state legislation designed to protect sensitive information. With the development of computerized health data systems in the 1960s, additional privacy, confidentiality, and other legal considerations emerged due to the increasing use of new technologies
(Curran, Stearns, & Kaplan, 1969; Gabrieli, 1973; Gobert, 1976). To address many of these
concerns, the federal government enacted numerous legislative initiatives. In this section,

we will present some of the major and most relevant federal laws regarding confidentiality and privacy in health and mental health care.

The Freedom of Information Act of 1966 (Pub. L. No. 104-231, 5 U.S.C. § 552) has a non-disclosure privacy exemption that exempts federal agency records from public release if individually identifiable medical information is accessible by name or by another personal identifier, such as an employee number or Social Security number. This is deemed "a clearly unwarranted invasion of personal privacy" (§552b(6)). Later amendments of the Act included language addressing the search process through either a manual or a computerized search.

The Privacy Act of 1974 (Pub. L. No. 93-579; 5 U.S.C. § 552a) required that federal agencies utilize fair information practices with regard to the collection, use, or dissemination of "any record" that is contained in "a system of records." It prohibited disclosure of an individual's educational, financial, medical, criminal, and/or employment record without prior written consent, required the de-identification of data (including name, identifying number, symbol, finger or voice prints, or photograph), and provided access to review, copy, and correct records. However, from a public health perspective, the Act applied only to specific institutions, such as federal agencies, federally operated hospitals, and to research or health care institutions operating pursuant to federal contracts (Center for Substance Abuse Treatment, 1994); Gostin, 1995). With the introduction of computer networks, the Computer Matching and Privacy Protection Act of 1988 (Pub. L. No. 100-503) amended the Privacy Act and added procedural requirements for agencies to follow when engaging in computer-matching activities. It also established due process provisions for notice and verification.

However, individuals who seek treatment for mental illnesses or substance use disorders may face discrimination, endure invasion of privacy, or reveal information that may be the basis for public prosecution. Any of these consequences may keep an individual from seeking treatment. Patient confidentiality and privacy in mental health records mirror the restrictions governing medical records. However, additional regulations to protect the identities of persons in alcohol abuse or drug abuse treatment programs began with the Comprehensive Alcohol Abuse and Alcoholism Prevention, Treatment, and Rehabilitation Act of 1970 and the Drug Abuse Prevention, Treatment, and Rehabilitation Act of 1972, which framed substance use as a mental disorder, not a criminal activity.

By 1974, the *Federal Register* (Department of Health, Education, and Public Health Service, 1974) published proposed rules for the confidentiality of alcohol abuse patient records (42 U.S.C. § 290dd-3) and drug abuse patient records (42 U.S.C. § 290ee-3). These rules were authorized by section 408 of the Drug Abuse Prevention, Treatment, and Rehabilitation Act of 1980 (Pub. L. 96-181; 21 U.S.C. 1111). Twelve years later, the Confidentiality Law of 1992 (Pub. L. 102-321; 42 U.S.C. § 290dd-2) consolidated and replaced the two separate but identical laws into a single law dealing with the confidentiality of patients who were seeking treatment for substance abuse. According to the Confidentiality Law, disclosure of patient identifying information by federally assisted programs is permitted only in explicitly delineated circumstances. However, the Confidentiality Law failed to protect information about drug and alcohol abuse entered into medical records in non-federally funded facilities.

The Veterans Omnibus Health Care Act of 1976 (Pub. L. 94-581; 38 U.S.C. § 101) also addressed confidential medical records of treatment relating to the treatment of drug abuse and alcoholism or alcohol abuse. However, it extended protections to persons infected with the human immunodeficiency virus (HIV), or who had sickle cell anemia. Personally identifiable patient information provided or obtained in connection with treatment, education, evaluation, and/or research of certain conditions or diseases was deemed confidential, except with a patient's written consent, or within the Veterans Administration, the Department of Justice, or the Department of Defense.

The Americans with Disabilities Act (ADA) of 1990 (Pub. L. 101-336; 42 U.S.C. 12101 et seq.) provided limited confidentiality of personal health information, applying only to people with a disability as defined by the statute, and to any actions taken by employers based on an individual's disability. Although it prohibited discrimination based on a disability, including HIV or AIDS, it did not directly protect privacy. However, it did provide a remedy for discrimination based on breaches of confidentiality.

The Balanced Budget Act of 1997 (BBA, Pub. L. 105-33) mandated that Medicare reimburse telemedicine care and fund telemedicine demonstration projects. Medicare began accepting claims in January 1999 and reimbursed interactive telemedicine care for Medicare beneficiaries who were in rural health professional shortage areas (HPSAs). In 2000, Congress passed the Benefits Improvement and Protection Act of 2000 (BIPA) (PL 106-554), which replaced the telehealth provisions of the BBA 1997 with an entirely new authority and structure for telehealth reimbursement. Benefits programs affected by BIPA were Medicare, Medicaid, and the State Children's Health Insurance Program (SCHIP).

Although the Health Insurance Portability and Accountability Act (HIPAA) of 1996 (P.L.104-191; 42 U.S.C. 201) was created to make health care delivery more efficient and to increase the number of Americans with health insurance coverage, it also addressed a number of issues arising from legal and ethical concerns in the increased use of technology. Although Title I regulates group health plans and certain individual health insurance policies and amends the Employee Retirement Income Security Act, the Public Health Service Act, and the Internal Revenue Code, Title II has more significance for this chapter.

Title II of HIPAA has two major elements. First, it defines numerous offenses relating to health care and sets civil and criminal penalties for them, and it creates programs to control fraud and abuse within health care systems (42 U.S.C. §1320a-7c, 42 U.S.C. §1395ddd, and 42 U.S.C. §1395b-5), which may affect the illegal use of protected health information (PHI). Second, it establishes the Administrative Simplification (AS) provisions and requires the establishment of national standards for electronic health care transactions and national identifiers for providers, health insurance plans, and employers (45 C.F.R. 160.103, 45 C.F.R. 164.501). The goal of the AS is to increase the efficiency of U.S. health care systems through electronic dissemination (portability) of health care information among covered entities. Covered entities include private and public health plans, billing services, community-based health information systems, and health care providers. It is within Title II that privacy and confidentiality concerns are addressed.

The HIPAA Privacy Rule (45 CFR, parts 160 and 164) regulates the use and disclosure of PHI held by covered entities (US DHHS, 2000). PHI is any information held by a covered entity which concerns health status, provision of health care, or payment for health care that can be linked to an individual, including any part of an individual's medical record or payment history (45 C.F.R. 164.501). It also establishes the requirements for conducting health research.

Historically, confidentiality was defined by state law. However, with the passage and implementation of HIPAA, the federal government established minimum standards for protecting the confidentiality of health and mental health information (McClelland & Thomas, 2002). As part of the Act, federal law preempts state law only when state law would be less protective than the federal law. The confidentiality protections provided would therefore be cumulative, with federal law providing a minimum level of protection (McClelland & Thomas, 2002).

The Health Information Technology for Economic and Clinical Health (HITECH) Act was enacted as part of the American Recovery and Reinvestment Act of 2009. The HITECH Act promotes the adoption and meaningful use of health information technology (HIT) and includes comprehensive safeguards for personal health information. Subtitle A promotes the use of HIT standards, including the use of electronic health records (EHR), enterprise integration, and the creation of the Office of the National Coordinator for Health Information Technology (ONCHIT). The standard for a certified EHR is established, along with the linkage of providers, health plans, and other entities involved in the electronic exchange and use of health information. Enterprise integration enables the electronic exchange and use of health information among all the components of the health care infrastructure and the implementation of application protocols and standards. The director of ONCHIT is responsible for coordinating (1) the department's health information technology policy and programs and the relevant federal agencies; and (2) the HIT Policy Committee and the HIT Standards Committee. A significant component in the success of the use of EHRs is the development of standards and protocols in the protection of patient data.

Subtitle B addresses the role of the National Institute for Standards and Technology (NIST) as well as HIT research and development programs. The NIST has both a regulatory and implementation role, since it tests standards and implementation specifications; addresses issues in the adoption and implementation of these standards, applications, and protocols; and oversees the conformance-testing infrastructure. Subtitle C examines how best to fund the use of health information technology, as well establishing incentives for adoption and implementation.

Subtitle D of the HITECH Act addresses the privacy and security concerns associated with the electronic transmission of health information. In addition, it strengthens the civil and criminal enforcement of the HIPAA rules. Subtitle D also delineates the use of health information technology in the provision of services under Medicaid and Medicare.

As seen in the preceding section, many bills and laws have been passed to enhance the privacy of personal health information. Each piece of legislation has addressed different aspects of personal health information, ranging from disclosure to the actual use of the information. Hence, we can see the importance of legislation in establishing standards and protocols for sharing health information. Further, legislation, at both federal and state levels, is intertwined with the provision of mental health services. Thus, when examining legislation on the provision of health and mental health care, one needs to examine the ethics of care, such as confidentiality.

Confidentiality

Personal health information is maintained by physicians, hospitals, and clinics in their medical databases that document patient treatment or diagnostic services. Personal health information is kept in the records of laboratories that perform tests and in pharmacies. Insurance companies and managed care organizations that accept claims and provide coverage have personal health information transmitted to them, to which they transmit to providers. In addition, universities and pharmaceutical companies receive personal health information to conduct medical and health services research. Further, certain personal health information must be reported to state and local governments, where it is maintained in databases. By law, for example, professionals must report sexually transmitted diseases to public health agencies, child abuse to child welfare agencies, and injuries caused by firearms to law enforcement agencies. Further, most people have little, if any, idea of how many individuals may actually have authorized access to their health records, as seen in this quote from 1996:

> [I]t's hard to keep a secret if more than a couple of people are in on it; in a typical five-day stay at a teaching hospital, as many as 150 people, from nursing staff to X-ray technicians to billing clerks, have legitimate access to a single patient's records. (Gorman, 1996)

Confidentiality, therefore, is a core ethical and legal principle in mental health services delivery (U.S. Department of Health and Human Services, 1999; New Freedom Commission on Mental Health, 2003, 2004; American Mental Health Counselors Association, 2010). The discrimination and stigma experienced by persons with mental and/or substance use disorders often cause barriers to treatment, especially when an individual is divulging not only medical history but events from his or her personal life, items that must require discretion on the part of the health care professional. Hence, communication between a clinical mental health professional and a patient is confidential, including any and all records of treatment in whatever format, including media, paper, audio, video, or electronic.

The principle of confidentiality in mental health is dependent upon three core values (USDHHS, 1999). First, creation of an atmosphere of confidence and trust is essential in a therapeutic relationship. Thus, trust is critical to mental health treatment. Second, confidentiality exists to reduce the possible effects of stigma that might be associated with the treatment of individuals with mental disorders. Third, confidentiality protects individual privacy, which is considered essential in enabling individuals to exercise autonomy in seeking mental health care (USDHHS, 1999).

Certainly, perceptions of privacy may affect an individual's decision to seek mental health care (Beaver & Herold, 2004; Workgroup for Electronic Data Interchange, 2001; USDHHS, 1999; Workgroup for the Computerization of Behavioral Health and Human Services Records, 1998). However, therapists may breach confidentiality without patient consent under a variety of circumstances. These circumstances include during an emergency, during civil commitment, when conforming to child and elder abuse reporting requirements, or when discussing a particular case with supervisors or other clinicians involved in the patient's treatment. In addition, state laws may permit other disclosures without consent to researchers, public health officials, or payers of health care.

Traditionally, confidentiality allowed patients to make full disclosures of information to their health care provider in face-to-face settings to ensure that the provider could properly diagnose illnesses and appropriately treat his or her patients. Providers maintained notes in the patient's file in locked cabinets in a secure location. Access to records, whether by the patient, his or her family, or another provider, required signed authorization and signed receipt whenever documents were delivered. This changed with the passage of HIPAA in 1996.

PROFESSIONAL ETHICS GUIDELINES

Title II of HIPAA requires the health care industry to use electronic media for the transmission of certain patient administrative data. Although HIPAA rules on electronic transactions, code sets, and privacy were established to ensure privacy and confidentiality, numerous health care organizations and associations raised their concerns with the advent of "teleservices." In 1998, the Physicians Insurers Association of America (PIAA) raised numerous ethical issues in its white paper on telemedicine. These ethical issues included the use of e-mail to transmit patient data, clarifying "duty of care," and defining the "standard of care." The PIAA addressed accountability issues regarding jurisdictional differences in liability cases and how they relate to licensure, inclusion of hardware/software vendors and telecommunications carriers in liability cases, and informed consent. The latter was imperative for the protection of participants if a state deemed "tele" consultations as "experimental" in nature.

By 2000, a joint committee of the International Society for Mental Health Online (ISMHO) and the Psychiatric Society for Informatics (PSI) produced and endorsed "Suggested Principles for the Online Provision of Mental Health Services" to address their concerns regarding professional ethics for the online provision of mental health services. The principles addressed informed consent, standard operating procedure, and emergencies. In addition, regulation and legislation at the state and federal levels began to address interstate commerce, benefit designs, payer-payee structures, and liability concerns.

In 2006, the eRisk Working Group for Healthcare published their "Guidelines for Online Communication." The Group comprised the American Medical Association, other national and regional medical societies, and medical malpractice carriers covers more than 70% of insured physicians and state medical licensing boards. The guidelines addressed the special concerns and risks of the technology of online communications and considerations for fee-based online consultations. Areas within the guidelines include informed consent, highly sensitive subject matter, privacy risks, emergency subject matter, doctor-patient relationship (with liability for only online relationships as a concern), licensing jurisdiction (which may subject the provider to increased risk), and the use of or creation of authoritative information. The latter advises health care providers that they are responsible for the web-based and/or e-mail information they provide or make available to their patients (eRisk Working Group for Healthcare's Guidelines for Online Communication, 2006).

A key confidentiality concern in current networked and digital environments is the integrity of health care information (Nass, Levitt, & Gostin, 2009; Vinson, 2011). From a provider perspective, health care data provide analysis on the outcomes and costs of different treatment plans. From a patient perspective, health care data generate "provider report cards" to inform health care users of their treatment options. The possibility that a user could compromise the integrity of such data, be it intentionally, inadvertently, or from sheer negligence, becomes a critically important components in the choice of services delivery.

Licensing, Liability, and Accreditation

Any examination of telemental health services requires a broad understanding of the issues surrounding licensing, liability, and accreditation of professionals, of institutions, and of telecommunication providers to ensure integrity of data, confidentiality, privacy, and treatment. Let us look first at the issue of the transfer of EHRs across state lines and between state and federal governments. The Workgroup on Electronic Data Interchange (1999) provides the following example:

> A Florida resident, insured through their employer in Alabama by a carrier in Connecticut, goes to a California clinic for treatment. Prior to treating the patient, the California clinic would electronically request eligibility information through a local California clearinghouse, which routes the request to another clearinghouse in New York, who then routes it to yet another clearinghouse in Georgia, who finally routes it to the carrier's eligibility contractor in Tennessee. The eligibility contractor's system then generates a response that reverses the path and is delivered back to the clinic, all within 30 seconds of the California clinic generating the initial request. After treating the patient, the clinic would generate an electronic claim that is transmitted to a clearinghouse in Illinois, then sends it to another clearinghouse in Ohio, then routes it to the insurance carrier in Connecticut. After processing the claim, the insurance carrier could then deliver the electronic fund transfer (EFT) and electronic remittance advice (ERA) to a clearinghouse in Indiana that routes it to the clinic's bank in Nebraska who, after balancing with the ERA, deposits the EFT and forwards the ERA on to the clinic for posting.

This example is not even a worst-case scenario. Consider that as these transactions pass through 11 states, none of the transacting agencies or organizations knew the route of any of the transactions. In addition to the number of organizations and states involved in one transaction, add the routing of the electronic data through the local telecommunications carriers. Depending upon bandwidth allocations, routing these transactions through multiple telecommunications carriers could easily add 20 more states to the transaction path. Further, since there is no "tracking" in the provider record of the electronic path that the transaction takes, no covered entity will know which state laws (or how many) are applicable to a single transaction, much less multiple transactions. Finally, because different states have different laws and different levels of protection for this information, it will be difficult to effectively enforce these laws when transferring or using information out of state. Add to the mix payments from federally funded health and welfare programs, and the complexity of issues increases exponentially.

If we look at several of the early state attempts to address this issue, California's Telemedicine Development Act addresses confidentiality in two ways (California, 1996). First, it provides that the state law protect a patient's medical information record transmitted electronically for telemedicine, similar to that of all other medical records. Health and mental health care providers then have certain legal obligations on use, disclosure, confidentiality, retention, maintenance, and access to patient information. Second, providers must inform the patient of his or her rights regarding confidential information and the existing legal protections, and that verbal and written consent be obtained from the patient prior to the use of telemedicine. Arizona (1997) and Texas (1997a, 1997b) also enacted laws requiring confidentiality of all patient medical records generated through care via telemedicine, and guaranteed patient access to his or her medical records resulting from such care. Today, the Arizona Telemedicine Program is recognized as one of the best programs in the United States because telehealth services are seamlessly integrated into routine office practices and systems.

LICENSING

In addition, telemental health has raised new questions regarding licensure and areas of service, as consultations can now easily cross state (and possibly international) borders (National Board of Certified Counselors, 2011; Magenau, 1997; Center for Telemedicine Law, 2003). Since the mission of state agencies involved with the regulation of professional licensing and practice is to protect the health and safety of their citizens, they have a direct interest in interstate telemental health licensure. From the agency's perspective, this is accomplished most effectively by requiring a full license for interstate telemental health practice. An out-of-state professional could be held to the same standard of care and legal responsibility in every state where he or she practices.

State professional health and mental health associations also have a significant interest in interstate telehealth licensure. However, for the private practitioner, the cumulative costs to hold licenses in each state would be prohibitive. In-state health and mental health professionals could lose a significant patient population if barriers to interstate telemental health licensure were reduced. Therefore, health and mental health professional associations would support full licensure requirements for out-of-state health and mental health practitioners. Telecommunication carriers and hardware and software vendors may also need to be licensed (Office for the Advancement of Telehealth, 2001; Wachter, 2002).

There has been a proliferation of state laws and regulations addressing telemental health licensure for mental health professionals. In 2003, 21 states (by law) required a full license for telehealth, 3 states required a full license by regulation or policy, 19 states required full licensure to practice medicine but did not specifically address telehealth (Center for Telehealth, 2003). In 2007, the American Telemedicine Association issued a policy position statement supporting collaborative agreements between the states regarding medical licensure portability at the federal, state, and local levels. In 2010, U.S. Health Resources and Services Administration (HRSA) reported to Congress the state of the portability of telemedicine licensure. It found that 24 states had adopted the Nurse Licensure Compact, and that the 19 states participating in the Physician Licensure Portability Grant Program use multiple models and tools to promote licensure portability, such as online uniform application and centralized credentialing verification (HRSA, 2010). A number of models were in use, ranging from consulting exceptions, endorsement, reciprocity, mutual recognition, registration, and limited, national, or federal licensure (HRSA, 2010).

However, HRSA identified several statutory and regulatory barriers to portability. States may regulate the practice of clinical care under the Tenth Amendment to the U.S. Constitution, so they have the authority to regulate activities that affect the health, safety, and welfare of citizens within their borders. However, states do not have the authority to grant practice privileges in another state or to discipline health care professionals not licensed in their state if patient harm occurs as the result of the provision of health care services by an out-of-state practitioner. In addition, the Commerce Clause of the Constitution limits states' ability to erect barriers against interstate trade (regarding anti-trust laws). Hence, the practice of health care has been held to be interstate trade. The courts have not addressed the potential conflict between the states' power to regulate health care professionals and the prohibition against restraints on interstate commerce.

Effective July 5, 2011, the Centers for Medicare and Medicaid Services (CMS) implemented its final rule on credentialing and privileging by proxy requirements for telehealth practitioners at Medicare hospitals and critical access hospitals (USDHHS, 2011). The final rule permits hospitals to rely on the credentialing and privileging determinations of another hospital or telemedicine entity, rather than make an individualized decision based upon the practitioner's credentials and record. However, states may need to change the regulatory and legislative language of their state statutes and codes to accommodate CMS requirements for credentialing and privileging. For example, mental health professional A is duly credentialed to practice in Alabama. However, for him to participate as a practitioner in New York may require him to undergo additional licensing or credentialing exams. Decisions may be made at the state level as to whether reciprocity of credentialing will be accepted across state lines.

It may be worthwhile for CMS to consider the licensing and credentialing model under the U.S. Health Research and Services Administration (HRSA). The Licensure Portability Grant Program (LPGP) supports state professional licensing boards or national organizations of professional licensing boards that provide services to state professional licensing boards. Funded under the Public Health Service Act (42 USC 254c-18) and the Public Health Service Act Health Care Safety Net Amendments of 2002 (Public law 107-251), LPGP helps state licensing boards with a strong record in implementing cross-border activities to overcome licensure barriers to the provision of telemedicine services across many state lines.

REIMBURSEMENT

These regulations also affect the use of certain technologies in health delivery systems, since use of these technologies may not be eligible for reimbursement in evaluation and management (E & M) services (i.e., patient visits and consultations). Many states require that E & M services be provided in real-time or near real-time (delay counted in seconds or minutes) to qualify as the interactive two-way transfer of health data and information between the patient and practitioner. Therefore, many "store-and-forward" patient visits and consultations are not reimbursable by many federal or state programs unless the transaction involves Hawai'i or Alaska.

In 2000, the Medicare, Medicaid, and SCHIP Benefits Improvement and Protection Act of 2000 (BIPA; United States Congress, 2000) expanded the services that Medicare will reimburse for telehealth. The expansion did include the following mental health services: office and other outpatient consultations; initial inpatient consultations; follow-up inpatient consultations; confirmatory consultations; office and other outpatient services for new and established patients; individual insight oriented, behavior modifying, and/or supportive psychotherapy; and pharmacologic management (CPT codes: 99241 through

99275; 99201 through 99215; 90804 through 90809; and 90862). For more information on implementation, see the Centers for Medicare and Medicaid Services (CMS) concerning implementation policies for the telehealth provisions in BIPA https://www.cms.gov/Regulations-and-Guidance/Regulations-and-Guidance.html.

Currently, Medicare beneficiaries are eligible for telehealth services only if they present from an originating site located in a rural health professional shortage area, in a county outside a Metropolitan Statistical Area, or as a participant in a federal telemedicine demonstration project. Eligible originating sites include the office of a physician or practitioner, hospitals, critical access hospitals, rural health clinics, federally qualified health centers, hospital-based or critical access hospital-based renal dialysis centers (including satellites), skilled nursing facilities, and community mental health centers. Practitioners include physicians, nurse practitioners, physician assistants, nurse midwives, clinical nurse specialists, clinical psychologists, and clinical social workers. However, clinical psychologists and clinical social workers cannot bill for psychotherapy services that include medical evaluation and management services under Medicare. All services delivered must use a real-time interactive audio and video telecommunications system between the physician or practitioner at the distant site and the beneficiary at the originating site. Only federal telehealth demonstration programs, conducted in Alaska or Hawai'i, may use asynchronous "store and forward" technology.

Unlike Medicare, CMS has not formally defined telemedicine for Medicaid. Since the federal government does not mandate reimbursement for telehealth services under Medicaid, states have the option to reimburse selectively for Medicaid services delivered through telehealth. The Code of Federal Regulations (CFR at 42 CFR 430 and 447) offers regulatory guidance to states in implementing Medicaid State plan payment rates consistent with the Social Security Act. Each state specifies what telemedicine/telehealth services, if any, are eligible for Medicaid reimbursement.

A number of issues affect reimbursement. First, the therapy provided must fall under the state's Medicaid covered services. If it falls under optional services, the provider may not receive payment through Medicaid. If the health professional is not on the state's Medicaid list of qualifying providers, again, there is no reimbursement through Medicaid. Finally, there are additional specific requirements that providers must follow when submitting claims for services furnished using telehealth, such as the proper coding, forms, and verifications.

Approximately 12 states allow for some reimbursement for telehealth services, including Medicaid. However, each state has its own coverage and billing requirements, which vary widely. For example, although Virginia's new telemedicine statute allows the use of interactive audio, video, or other electronic media used for the purpose of diagnosis, consultation, or treatment, it does not allow services provided using an audio-only telephone, e-mail message, fax transmission, continuing medical education, or call center services (Silva, 2010). In Maine, the law supplements Medicaid reimbursement for telemedicine services delivered only by interactive video sessions. In New Hampshire, Medicaid covers telemedicine only in selected pilot waiver programs (Macios, 2011).

MODEL LEGISLATION

Although most states have dealt with telehealth and telemental health licensure through regulations, not legislation, there have been attempts to develop model legislation.

The first attempts were in 1996 by the Association of Telemedicine Service Providers (ATSP) and the Federation of State Boards of Medical Licensure. The ATSP compact focused on reducing the barriers to practicing interstate telemedicine by utilizing a limited license, mutual recognition model, while the Federation model proposed a limited licensing mechanism, permitting telemedical consultations only in remote (i.e., rural or frontier) states. The passage of SB600 by Oregon in April 1999, which focused on out-of-state physicians practicing on Oregon patients, was considered a possible model for other licensed professions (Oregon State Legislature, 1999).

The Federation of State Boards of Medical Licensure, currently known as the Federation of State Medical Boards, is a national non-profit organization whose membership includes 70 medical licensing and disciplinary boards in the United States and the U.S. territories. In 1996, it developed "A Model Act to Regulate the Practice of Medicine Across State Lines" (Federation of State Medical Boards, 2002). By 2009, the Federation of State Medical Boards had developed model agreements across 13 states in the Northeastern and Western regions (Maine, Massachusetts, Vermont, Connecticut, Rhode Island, and New Hampshire; and North Dakota, Kansas, Colorado, Minnesota, Iowa, Idaho, and Oregon). Its Federation Credentials Verification Service (FCVS) is a central repository of health professionals' credentials maintained by the Repository. Massachusetts and Wyoming are implementing the laws necessary to allow licensure portability by endorsement.

In addition, the Nurse License Compact, developed by the National Council of State Boards of Nursing, has been adopted by 23 states (HRSA, 2009). The Nurse Compact is a mutual recognition model under which nurses are licensed in one state and practice both in person and virtually in other states.

The Uniform Emergency Volunteer Health Practitioners Act (UEVHPA) was drafted by the National Conference of Commissioners of Uniform State Laws in 2007. During a declared emergency or disaster, UEVHPA allows state governments to give reciprocity to emergency services providers who have licenses in other states so that licensed individuals may provide services without meeting the emergency/disaster state's licensing requirements. Eleven states have enacted the UEVHPA (Colorado, Nevada, Utah, New Mexico, Oklahoma, Arkansas, Louisiana, Tennessee, Kentucky, Indiana, and Illinois) (US DHHS, 2009).

However, work continues on telehealth models. In 2011, California convened a Telehealth Model Statute Work Group to develop a model statute, which revised its 1996 statute and expanded coverage of interactive telemedicine services. For this group, the emphasis was on redefining telemedicine as telehealth and incorporating telehealth into the state workforce law (Center for Connected Health Policy, 2011).

The Ad Hoc Rural Mental Health Provider Work Group (Pion, Keller, & McCombs, 1997) recommended the use of creative applications of telecommunications to reduce barriers to accessing rural mental health services. Furthermore, they recommended sound evaluations of the effectiveness of the information technology strategies. The three most prevalent forms of telehealth are store-and-forward, real-time video, and hybrid systems. A study by the Center for Information Technology Leadership estimated a savings of over $4 billion a year if hybrid systems were adopted nationally across emergency rooms, prisons, nursing home facilities, and physician offices (Pan, Cusack, Hook, et al., 2008). Another study showed that real-time video telehealth was cost-effective for home care and on-call hospital specialists but had mixed results for rural services delivery (Wade, Karnon, Elshaug, et al., 2010).

Professional Practice Concerns

When using health information technology such as telehealth or electronic health records, it is critical that ethical and legal considerations are part of everyday professional practice. Patient confidentiality and autonomy are essential to services delivery, and privacy/confidentiality issues are present on daily basis. Although there are numerous health and behavioral health care settings relevant to a discussion of confidentiality issues, our focus in this chapter will include rural populations and prison/forensic settings.

RURAL POPULATIONS

Approximately 20% of non-metropolitan counties lack mental health services. The vast majority of Mental Health Professional Shortage Areas (MHPSAs, or areas listed by the U.S. government as having a critical need for psychiatrists, psychologists, and other mental health professionals) are rural (Mohatt, Adams, Bradley, & Morris, 2006). To put this into perspective, 95 million people live in 3,781 MHPSAs. To meet the need for mental health services, the HRSA estimates that it would take 6,226 mental health practitioners, or a population to practitioner ratio of 10,000:1 (HRSA, n.d.). One reason for the critical shortage of practitioners in rural areas is that fewer mental health professionals settle in rural areas, since practicing in rural areas is somewhat isolated and lacks the access to services vis-à-vis urban and suburban practitioners (Schank & Skovholt, 2006). Telehealth and telemental health services are seen as a way to combat the isolation and lack of available treatment resources.

Warner et al. (2005) conducted surveys of community-based primary care and mental health clinics in rural New Mexico and Alaska. They found that approximately 50% of providers reported that their patients were reluctant to be open in therapeutic sessions because of stigma, discrimination, and possible breaches of privacy and confidentiality. Rural clinicians also reported that their patients expressed more concern about knowing them in both personal and professional roles.

In a mental health practice, clerical staff know the clients, handle personal health information, process billing claims, process referrals to other health care providers or social services agencies, and transcribe session notes. In a rural community, everyone "knows everyone's business." Therefore, rural mental health professionals should be very sensitive to where services are delivered and take extra care in training their staff in the appropriate confidentiality and privacy protocols and practices to assure compliance with state and federal legislation and ethical practice (Fisher, 2009).

FORENSIC AND CORRECTIONAL FACILITIES

Telemental health treatment in forensic and correctional facilities differs significantly from telemental health treatment in community-based or outpatient clinics (Antonacci et al.,

2008). In correctional and forensic facilities, for example, a corrections officer or orderly may be physically located in the room where the patient will receive telehealth services. Other staff may sit in on the therapeutic session with the mental health professional without the knowledge of the client on the other end of the videoconference. The room itself in which services are delivered may not be soundproofed or may have observation windows. This eliminates the privacy traditionally available in a provider-patient relationship.

Sullivan et al. (2008) described a case in which a patient in a forensic mental health facility hid a recording device in a team meeting room, taping team meetings where patient care was discussed and personal conversations of the staff. In another case, they describe an incident in which the therapist did not verify that the video and audio feeds were terminated before discussing the case with a trainee, who sat in on the session without the knowledge or consent of the patient. Unfortunately, the patient heard a most unflattering and non-professional assessment of his or her condition between the therapist and the trainee.

Finally, in matters involving judicial disposition, they warned against relying only on videoconferenced assessments (Sullivan et al., 2008). Poor video or audio feed may result in misinterpretation of behavior or discussion, which results in an inappropriate or incorrect diagnosis. The consequences of misdiagnosis may have serious consequences for the patient as to facility assignation or release or, from a larger perspective, for community safety (Jones et al., 2006). This is an important consideration for U.S. practitioners, as a clinical interaction conducted by teleconference has the same legal standing as a face-to-face consultation.

CASE STUDY

Lisa is a mental health professional practicing in rural North Dakota. She is meeting with Tom, a client with co-occurring disorders: smoking addiction and depression. She is unfamiliar with initiating a smoking cessation program in concert with behavioral interventions for depression. She arranges for a teleconference call from the local health clinic to David, a colleague who specializes in smoking cessation programs. To prepare Tom for the consultation, Lisa tells him that he will be meeting David over the new videoconference equipment at the clinic. Lisa and Tom arrive at a small conference room next to the waiting area of the clinic. Even with the door to the room closed, they can hear the conversations in the waiting area.

The telesession begins with David introducing himself and starting the clinical interview. The audio reception is problematic, which the audio technician solves partially by turning up the volume, which then masks the conversations in the waiting room. During their conversation, Lisa notices that David appears to be talking to someone but is unsure if perhaps David is just restating what Tom has said or reformulating his thoughts aloud to David and to her. There is the sound of a chair being moved, and Tom asks David if someone is there. David acknowledges that he has a psychology intern sitting in on the session with him, but there is no need to worry. In addition, David mentions that he is storing the session for review. David clicks off the session. As Tom and Lisa leave through the waiting room, Tom feels the people sitting closest to the teleconference room watching him leave the building. Tom then mentions to Lisa his concerns that people in the waiting room have overheard their session.

There are a number of problems regarding privacy and confidentiality with the scenario described above. First, there is a lack of adequate patient informed consent. Lisa should have informed Tom about the protocols surrounding a tele-consultation and explained to him the benefits and the disadvantages of this type of therapy. David should have explained to Tom that he would have an intern sitting in on the session and received Tom's written consent to the presence of a third party, for treatment, for storing the session for later review, and for examination of the videotape by other professionals. In addition, the location of the teleconference next to a busy and public waiting area in a local health clinic may not provide the level of privacy comparable to a traditional face-to-face encounter, especially with technology transmission and receipt problems. Finally, there is a potential loss of trust between Tom as patient and David and Lisa as health care providers.

This example illustrates the difficulty in ensuring privacy and confidentiality in the provision of telehealth services, as clinical encounters are "broadcast" beyond the privacy of a therapist's office or examination room. Whether the technology is e-mail, telephone, e-conferencing, or other electronic media, it is difficult to know who is actually involved in the session or if the session or records are being "examined" by anonymous individuals. Although breaches in confidentiality can be intentional or accidental, any unauthorized viewing of patient information of any kind is unethical and does not meet compliance with current legislation or regulatory policies on privacy and confidentiality.

Implications for Mental Health Informatics

Confidentiality is a matter of both ethical and legal concern. Although health and mental health professions endorse confidentiality and privacy as essential tenets of ethical practice, the legal and judicial systems establish the basic rules that govern confidentiality in practice. Examples that come to mind are the U. S. Supreme Court decision in *Jaffee v. Redmond* that determined psychotherapeutic privilege applies in Federal court, or the *Tarasoff v. Regents of the University of California* decision determined by the California Supreme Court which decided that mental health professionals had an obligation to protect third parties who could be endangered by a client in treatment. Further, the creation of disease-specific registries or web-based access to de-identified health data may bring up additional issues regarding confidentiality, consent and access to data, reducing risks to the privacy of individuals, and minimizing legal challenges to professionals. The U. S. Surgeon General noted:

> It is clear that confidentiality is not absolute. There are other competing values that require its breach in certain circumstances. However, it also seems clear that there are significant gaps in the current legal framework that protects the confidentiality of mental health information. Consideration of an appropriate level of legal protection for mental health information should acknowledge that mental illness continues to be a category of illness that may subject a person receiving a diagnosis to discrimination and other disadvantages. (U.S. Department of Health and Human Services, 1999)

Considering the complexity of ethical and legal issues in a paper-based world, the issues are even more complex in the online services environment. It is critical for any professional, provider, or practitioner working in health and mental health to understand licensure, credentialing, privacy, security, confidentiality, informed consent, and professional liability in this digital age.

References

American Mental Health Counselors Association. (2010). *Code of ethics, 2010 revision.* Retrieved from http://www.amhca.org/assets/content/AMHCA_Code_of_Ethics_11_30_09b1.pdf

American Psychiatric Association Board of Trustees. (1998). Telepsychiatry via videoconferencing: Resource document (APA Document Reference No. 980021). Retrieved from http://www.telepsychiatry.com/apa.pdf.

American Telemedicine Association. (2007). *Licensure portability, position statement and recommendations.* Retrieved from http://media.americantelemed.org/news/Whitepapers/Medical%20Licensure%20Portability%20Position.pdf.

Antonacci, D. J., Bloch, R. M., Saeed, S. A., Yildirim, Y., & Talley, J. (2008). Empirical evidence on the use and effectiveness of telepsychiatry via videoconferencing: Implications for forensic and correctional psychiatry. *Behavioral Sciences and the Law, 26*, 253–269. doi:10.1002/bsl.812.

Arizona. H.B. 2224. (1997). 43rd Leg., 1st Reg. Sess.

Beaver, K., & Herold, R. (2004). *The practical guide to HIPAA privacy and security compliance* (pp. 23–34). Boca Raton, FL: RCR Press LCC.

California. Cal. S.B. 1665 § 2290.5. (1996). California Telemedicine Act.

Center for Connected Health Policy (2011). *Advancing California's leadership in telehealth policy: A telehealth model statute & other policy recommendations.* Sacramento, CA: The Center. Retrieved from http://www.connectedhealthca.org/policy-projects/telehealth-model-sta.

Center for Substance Abuse Treatment. (1994). *Confidentiality of patient records for alcohol and other drug treatment* (Technical Assistance Publication Series, No. 13). Washington, DC: Author. Retrieved from http://kap.samhsa.gov/products/manuals/taps/13.htm.

Center for Telemedicine Law. (2003). *Telemedicine licensure report.* Washington, DC: Center for Telemedicine Law, prepared for the Office for the Advancement of Telehealth, 2003. Retrieved from http://www.hrsa.gov/ruralhealth/about/telehealth/licenserpto3.pdf.

Curran, W. J., Stearns, B., & Kaplan, H. (1969). Privacy, confidentiality and other legal considerations in the establishment of a centralized health-data system. *New England Journal of Medicine, 281*(5), 241–248.

Department of Health, Education, and Public Health Service. (1974, August 22). Confidentiality of alcohol and drug abuse patient records: Proposed rules. *Federal Register, 39*/164(30426–30437), 0097-6326.

Duquenoy, P., George, C., & Kimppa, K. (2008). *Ethical, legal and social issues in medical informatics.* Hershey, PA: IGI Global.

eRisk Working Group for Healthcare's Guidelines for Online Communication (2006). Medem, Inc. Retrieved from http://www.calrhio.org/crweb-files/docs-privacy/20061121/2006%20eRisk%20 Guidelines%20Final.pdf.

Federation of State Medical Boards. (2002). *Report of the Special Committee on License Portability: A policy document of the Federation of State Medical Boards of the United States, Inc.* Retrieved from http://www.fsmb.org/pdf/2002_grpol_License_Portability.pdf.

Fisher, M. A. (2009). Ethics-based training for nonclinical staff in mental health settings. *Professional Psychology: Research and Practice, 40,* 459–466.

Gabrieli, J. D. (1973). Privacy of medical information: Do not bend, fold, or mutilate. *Journal of Clinical Computing, 3*(1), 57–70.

Gobert, J. J. (1976). Accommodating patient rights and computerized mental health systems. *North Carolina Law Review, 54*(2), 153–187.

Gorman, C. (1996, May 6). Who's looking at your files. *Time, 147*(19), 60–62.

Gostin, L. (1995). Health information privacy. *Cornell Law Review, 80,* 451–528.

Health Research and Services Administration (2009). *Program guidance, 2009.* (Licensure Portability Grant Program, HRSA-09-196, Catalog of Federal Domestic Assistance (CFDA) No. 93.211). Washington, DC: The Administration. Retrieved from https://grants.hrsa.gov/webexternal/FundingOppDetails.asp?FundingCycleId=832CBBE5-683C-4F98-B581-0F5808F83BC9&ViewMode=EU&GoBack=&PrintMode=&OnlineAvailabilityFlag=True&pageNumber=1.

Health Resources and Services Administration. (2010). *Health licensing board report to Congress: Requested by: Senate report 111-66.* Retrieved from http://www.hrsa.gov/rural-health/about/telehealth/licenserpt10.pdf

International Society for Mental Health Online & Psychiatric Society for Informatics. (2000). *Suggested principles for the online provision of mental health services.* Retrieved from https://www.ismho.org/suggestions.asp [officially endorsed version].

Jones, R. M., Leonard, S., & Birmingham, L. (2006). Setting up a telepsychiatry service. *The Psychiatrist, 30,* 464–467. doi: 10.1192/pb.30.12.464.

Macios, A. (2011, July 14). Payment for telemedicine gaining momentum. *Medscape Today.* Retrieved from http://www.medscape.com/viewarticle/725115

Magenau, J. L. (1997). Digital diagnosis: Liability concerns and state licensing issues are inhibiting the progress of telemedicine. *Communications and the Law, 19,* 25–43.

McClelland, R., & Thomas, V. (2002). Confidentiality and security of clinical information in mental health practice. *Advances in Psychiatric Treatment, 8,* 291–296.

Mohatt, D. Adams, S. J., Bradley, M. M., & Morris, C. A. (2006). *Mental health and rural America: 1994–2005.* Washington, DC: U.S. Department of Health and Human Services Health Resources and Services Administration, Office of Rural Health Policy. Available http://www.ask.hrsa.gov/detail_materials.cfm?ProdID=3899.

Nass, S. J., Levit, L. A., & Gostin, L. O. (2009). *Beyond the HIPAA privacy rule: Enhancing privacy, improving health through research.* Washington, DC: National Academies Press for the Institute of Medicine. Retrieved from http://www.nap.edu/catalog.php?record_id=12458.

National Board of Certified Counselors. (2011). *The practice of internet counseling.* Retrieved from http://www.nbcc.org/Assets/Ethics/internetCounseling.pdf.

New Freedom Commission on Mental Health. (2003). *Achieving the promise: Transforming mental health care in America. Final report* (DHHS Pub. No. SMA-03-3832). Rockville, MD: The Commission. Retrieved from http://govinfo.library.unt.edu/mentalhealthcommission/reports/FinalReport/downloads/downloads.html.

New Freedom Commission on Mental Health, Subcommittee on Rural Issues. (2004). *Background paper* (DHHS Pub. No. SMA-04-3890). Rockville, MD: The Commission. Retrieved from http://web.archive.org/web/20100527091216/http://www.mentalhealthcommission.gov/papers/Rural.pdf.

Office for the Advancement of Telehealth. (2001). *2001 report to Congress on telemedicine.* Retrieved from ftp://ftp.hrsa.gov/telehealth/report2001.pdf.

Oregon State Legislature. (1999). *Telemedicine Licensure*, Senate Bill 600.

Pan E, Cusack C, Hook J, et al. (2008). The value of provider-to-provider telehealth. *Telemedicine Journal of E- Health, 14*(5), 446–453.

Pion, G. M., Keller, P., & McCombs, H. (1997). *Mental health providers in rural and isolated areas: Final report of the Ad Hoc Rural Mental Health Provider Work Group.* Rockville, MD: Center for Mental Health Services. Retrieved from http://web.archive.org/web/20050301073846/http://www.mentalhealth.org/publications/allpubs/SMA98-3166/.

Physicians Insurers Association of America. (1998). *Telemedicine: A medical liability white paper.* Rockville, MD: Physicians Insurers Association of America.

Schank, J. A., & Skovholt, T. M. (2006). *Ethical practice in small communities.* Washington, DC: American Psychological Association.

Silva, C. (2010, April 19). Telemedicine coverage now mandated in Virginia. *American Medical News.* Retrieved from http://www.ama-assn.org/amednews/2010/04/19/gvsb0419.htm.

Sullivan, D. H., Chapman, M., & Mullen, P. E. (2008). Videoconferencing and forensic mental health in Australia. *Behavioral Sciences and the Law, 26,* 323–331. doi: 10.1002/bsl.815.

Texas H.B. 2033. (1997a). 75th Leg., Reg. Sess.

Texas Revised Civil Statutes Art. 4495b. (1997b). § 3.06(I).

United States Congress. (2000). *Medicare, Medicaid and SCHIP Benefits Improvement and Protection Act of 2000* (Benefits and Improvement Protection Act). PL 106-554, 106th Congress.

U.S. Department of Health and Human Services. (1999). Confidentiality of mental health information: Ethical, legal, and policy issues In *Mental health: A report of the Surgeon General.* Rockville, MD: U.S. Department of Health and Human Services, Substance Abuse and Mental Health Services Administration, Center for Mental Health Services, National Institutes of Health, National Institute of Mental Health, 1999. Retrieved from http://www.surgeongeneral.gov/library/mentalhealth/toc.html#chapter7.

U. S. Department of Health and Human Services (2000, December 28). Standards for privacy of individually identifiable health information. Office of the Assistant Secretary for Planning and Evaluation, DHHS: Final rule. *Federal Register, 65*(250):82462–82829. Retrieved from http://frwebgate.access.gpo.gov/cgi-bin/getdoc.cgi?dbname=2000_register&docid=f:28der2.pdf.

U.S. Department of Health and Human Services. (2011, May 5). 42 CFR Part 482 and 485: Medicare and Medicaid programs: Changes affecting hospital and critical access hospital conditions of participation: Telemedicine credentialing and privileging. *Federal Register, 76*(87), 25550–25565. Retrieved from http://www.gpo.gov/fdsys/pkg/FR-2011-05-05/html/2011-10875.htm.

U.S. Department of Health and Human Services. (2009). *Pandemic and All-Hazards Preparedness Act Public Law 109-417: Telehealth report to Congress.* Washington, DC: USDHHS. Retrieved from http://www.phe.gov/Preparedness/legal/pahpa/Documents/telehealthrtc-091207.pdf.

Vinson, D. D. (2011). No more paper tiger: Promise and peril as HIPAA goes HITECH. *Journal of Healthcare Risk Management, 30*(3), 28–37. doi: 10.1002/jhrm.20058.

Wachter G. (2002). Law and policy in telemedicine: Interstate licensure for tele-nursing. Silver Spring, MD: American Nurses Association.

Wade, V. A., Karnon, J., Elshaug, A. G., et al. (2010). A systematic review of economic analyses of telehealth services using real time video communication. *BMC Health Services Research,* 10, 233. Retrieved from http://www.biomedcentral.com/content/pdf/1472-6963-10-233.pdf.

Warner, T. D., Monaghan-Geernaert, P., Battaglia, J., Brems, C., Johnson, M. E, & Roberts, L. W. (2005). Ethical considerations in rural health care: A pilot study of clinicians in Alaska and New Mexico. *Community Mental Health Journal, 41*(1):21–33. doi: 10.1007/s10597-006-2597-1 Retrieved from http://www.ncbi.nlm.nih.gov/pmc/articles/PMC1599854/pdf/nihms12234.pdf.

Workgroup for the Computerization of Behavioral Health and Human Services Records. (1998). *The Virtual Consumer and Family-Focused Behavioral Health and Human Services Record.* Rockville, MD: Center for Mental Health Services.

Workgroup for Electronic Data Interchange. (1999, August 25). WEDI board submits preliminary recommendations on pending privacy regulations. Retrieved from http://www.wedi.org/public/articles/details~25.shtml.

Workgroup for Electronic Data Interchange. (2001). *SNIP—Security and Privacy Work Group, 2001.* Retrieved from http://www.wedi.org/snip/public/articles/spwg3.1-preemption.pdf.

8   Taking Research to Practice

Health services research examines the utilization, costs, quality, accountability, delivery, organization, financing and outcomes of health care services from both a population- and individual-level perspective to add to the existing knowledge base in mental health (Field, Tranquada, & Feasley, 1995).

The National Research Council (2011) suggests that health services research is the key to improving the delivery of health care in the United States. Not only does health services research document deficiencies in patient and population health and in the provision of health services, it also identifies factors which contribute to these deficiencies. However, it is critical to tie knowledge of services delivery and outcomes to the analytical process, to conduct, interpret, and apply empirical research, thereby incorporating a systemic perspective of applying research to practice.

Translational and implementation research, two additional areas identified in the report, provide the knowledge base to move clinical research to clinical practice and to effectively adapt clinical research to real-world practice settings. Meeting the challenge of translational research draws upon "marketing research, adult learning, and real-time decision support technologies" (National Research Council, 2005, p. 79).

In this chapter, we will examine the challenges in moving research to practice, delineate the differences between evidence-based and best practices, show how informatics plays a key role, and address the role of leadership necessary for implementation.

Translational Research

Translational research, as a term in the literature, is relatively new (NLM, 2011). Although the phrase has been in use since the 1990s, there are many definitions of translational research, which includes a focus on different areas. Translational research, especially in medicine, has a strong clinical research focus. The National Institutes of Health (NIH; Nathan, 1998; *NIH Director's Panel*, 1997) uses a three-part definition for clinical research: (1) patient-oriented research (mechanisms of human disease, therapeutic interventions, clinical trials, or development of new technologies); (2) epidemiologic and behavioral studies; and (3) outcomes research and health services research.

With the growing interest in moving research to practice (bench to bedside), the NIH (2007) suggested the following definition for translational research:

> Translational research includes two areas of translation. One is the process of applying discoveries generated during research in the laboratory, and in preclinical studies, to the development of trials and studies in humans. The second area of translation concerns research aimed at enhancing the adoption of best practices in the community. Cost-effectiveness of prevention and treatment strategies is also an important part of translational science. [http://grants.nih.gov/grants/guide/rfa-files/RFA-RM-07–007.html; Section 2, para. 2]

The first area of translation, from laboratory findings to clinical practice, emphasizes that the way to improve health is through a connected approach of research and practice. The second area of translation, to the community and back, has long been a focus of public health and mental health researchers and practitioners.

Translational research, however, is much more than simply moving research evidence into practice. Translational research should inform decision making at all levels of health care systems, from clinical to organizational to public policy. Further, it should emphasize the testing of effective and efficient interventions to improve clinical practice, enhance patient safety, and sustain changes in practitioner behavior. In addition, translational research should facilitate the rapid and widespread adoption of evidence in decision making and implementation of evidence-based interventions into processes of care, and should effectively measure the impact of these efforts to ensure quality of health care and the reduction of disparities in health care.

Why the emphasis on translational research? Creating a new medication or intervention is only the beginning of a very long process. It is estimated that it takes an average of 17 years for approximately 14% of new clinical discoveries to become day-to-day clinical practice (Balas & Boren, 2000). Basic science work performed in laboratories must be understood in terms of human behavior, physiology, and neurology. These understandings must then be translated into diagnostic procedures, medicines, and interventions in clinical practice. The intervention must be assessed in terms of patient outcomes, which in turn should inform the basic science research that in turn informs human behavior.

As previously mentioned in this text, the costs of mental illnesses are staggering. Mental illnesses are chronic, that is, long-term illnesses. Much like other chronic illnesses, such as diabetes, many mental illnesses can be managed but are not considered "curable." As seen in Figure 8.1, the direct and indirect costs of mental illnesses affect the quality of life and workplace productivity of both individuals and populations (Insel, 2008; Kessler et al., 2008; Mark et al., 2007).

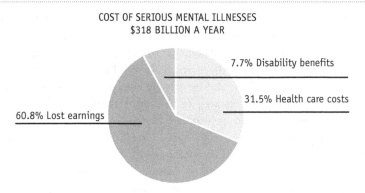

COST OF SERIOUS MENTAL ILLNESSES
$318 BILLION A YEAR

7.7% Disability benefits

31.5% Health care costs

60.8% Lost earnings

FIGURE 8.1 Cost of Serious Mental Illnesses, 2008.
Figure adapted from National Institute of Mental Health Strategic Plan. Retrieved from http://www.nimh.nih.gov/about/strategic-planning-reports/nimh-strategic-plan-2008.pdf. Document in public domain.

As seen from the impact of the direct and indirect costs of mental illnesses, moving research to practice is a priority. In 1997, the NIMH Clinical Treatment and Services Research Workgroup was charged with the "urgent task" of developing tools to bridge the gap from research to practice and to "better enable people with mental illnesses to receive optimal care" (para. 1). The Workgroup emphasized research on efficacy, effectiveness, practice, and service systems to assess the needs and outcomes of potential users of the research (i.e., patients and families, clinicians, public and private purchasers, insurers and MCOs, and policy makers).

In 2000, NIMH funded a number of Translational Research Centers in Behavioral Science (TRCBS). These Centers were intended to support integrated research teams across the fields of basic behavioral and social sciences, including neuroscience, epidemiology, prevention, academic mental health, and mental health services delivery. The TRCBS initiative resulted from the publication of two seminal documents addressing the translation of research to practice in behavioral health. The first document, an Institute of Medicine report, emphasized "the need to understand the entire human organism, not just one part of it, is driving disciplines toward each other as scientists seek better ways to prevent, diagnose, treat, and control" mental illnesses (Pellmar & Eisenberg, 2000, p. 1) to bridge the behavioral, and clinical sciences. The second document, by the National Advisory Mental Health Council Behavioral Science Workgroup (2000), recommended strategies for NIMH to foster translational research; to assist the adoption, development, and dissemination of translational research tools and methods; and to share research findings among clinical and services researchers and other stakeholders.

The "New Perspectives in the Translational Neuroscience of Late Life Mental Disorders Conference" focused on neuropathological mechanisms, biology of aging, and pathophysiology in the study of late life mental disorders (NIMH, 2009). The participants suggested that a better understanding of the biological and pathophysiological models of aging could be linked to risk and protective factors that also change as people age, especially with the onset of later life psychotic disorders.

More recently, the NIMH *Strategic Plan* (2010) stressed the use of translational research to gain a more complete understanding of the many factors (genetic, neurobiological, behavioral, environmental, and experiential) that contribute to mental disorders and to chart the trajectories of mental illnesses across the lifespan. The NIH Roundtable on Opportunities to Advance Research on Neurologic and Psychiatric Emergencies (D'Onfrio, 2010) established the need for translational research to investigate the pathobiology of symptoms and symptom-oriented therapies, to incorporate innovative informatics technologies, and to develop a research infrastructure for the rapid identification, consent, and tracking of research subjects. The Roundtable also emphasized the development of diagnostic strategies and tools necessary to understand key populations and the process of medical decision making, bringing basic science concepts into the clinical arena to enhance the collaboration of practitioners and researchers in the development and successful implementation of research to practice.

The Committee on the Science of Adolescence (2011) suggested that developmental changes during adolescence in the central and peripheral processes of the brain may account for differences in the brain functions between adolescents and adults. Further, specific neurobehavioral changes may account for risk-taking and sensation-seeking behaviors in adolescents. Hence, there are "reciprocal dynamics among the many processes that affect adolescents' behavior and risk-taking" (Committee on the Science of Adolescence, 2011, p. 90).

Thus, translational research in behavioral health focuses on integrating genetics and neuroimaging methods into the study of behavioral disorders. This will build a knowledge base to increase our understanding of the complexity involved in addressing such issues as treatment response variability, clinical courses and outcomes, comorbidity, and research methodologies. Research has suggested that there are biological susceptibilities to mood disorders, which are exacerbated by genetic, vascular, neurochemical, and neurodegenerative factors (Smith et al., 2007; D'Onofrio et al., 2010). However, the data necessary to draw conclusions that lead to applied interventions spans numerous disciplines and technologies, and requires linkages to or development of clinical and cognitive measures to effectively diagnose and prescribe appropriate treatments.

The *NIMH Strategic Plan* acknowledged, "Scientific progress is generally slow and incremental—too slow and incremental for families who need effective treatments today" (p. iii). The report identified four strategic objectives that emphasized (1) basic, translational, and clinical research; (2) longitudinal charting of mental disorders; (3) development of innovative and personalized treatments; and (4) moving research to practice (Figure 8.2). We will see later in this chapter how mental health informatics supports translational and implementation research.

Today, NIMH has a number of translational research programs, such as the Adult Translational Research and Treatment, Developmental Translational Research, and Translational Research on the Development of Novel Interventions for Mental Disorders. Its translational research programs emphasize the impacts of efficacious interventions and innovative delivery strategies, the cost-effectiveness of those strategies, the fidelity/adaptation of implementation, and the identification of client reactions and outcomes to prevention and adherence interventions. An important component that cuts across

1. Promote discovery in the brain and behavioral sciences to fuel research on the causes of mental disorders.

2. Chart mental illness trajectories to determine when, where and how to intervene.

3. Develop new and better interventions that incorporate the diverse needs and circumstances of people with mental illnesses.

4. Strengthen the public health impact of NIMH-supported research.

FIGURE 8.2 NIMH Strategic Objectives.

National Institute of Mental Health (2008). *NIMH strategic plan* (NIH Publication No. 08–6368). Retrieved from http://www.nimh.nih.gov/about/strategic-planning-reports/nimh-strategic-plan-2008.pdf. Document in public domain.

all four objectives is the gathering, sharing, and analysis of data gathered during research, implementation, assessment, and outcomes.

Implementation Research

Dissemination research and implementation research are often confused. Dissemination research is the systematic study of the processes and factors that lead to widespread use of evidence-based interventions by a target population. Much of the dissemination research focuses on adoption of evidence-based interventions. Implementation research has two foci. Not only does it seek to understand the factors associated with integration of evidence-based interventions in particular settings (level 1), it also determines the fidelity of implementation in the real-world setting (level 2). Level 1 translational research examines how best to integrate evidence-based interventions in particular settings and applies to both dissemination and the first goal of implementation research.

The second goal of implementation research is considered level 2 of translational research, which brings research findings to the community, implements them, assesses outcomes, and takes those findings back to researchers. It is the systematic study of how a specific evidence-based intervention is integrated successfully within a specific setting. Factors that are studied in implementation research include adaptation (modification of the intervention), adoption (use of intervention by population and/or implementers), fidelity (adherence to original treatment protocol), generalizability (applicable to additional populations, conditions, and/or settings than the original study), integration (combination of evidence-based and local contextual knowledge into application of intervention), outcomes (impact on functioning, health, quality of life, etc.), scalability (scales to a larger population while retaining effectiveness and efficacy), and sustainability.

Evidence-Based and Best Practices

Much of the literature on translational and implementation research emphasizes the use of evidence-based practices in the treatment of mental illnesses. Derived from the term *evidence-based medicine* (NLM, 1997), evidence-based practice (EBP) is:

> A way of providing health care that is guided by a thoughtful integration of the best available scientific knowledge with clinical expertise. This approach allows the practitioner to critically assess research data, clinical guidelines, and other information resources in order to correctly identify the clinical problem, apply the most high-quality intervention, and re-evaluate the outcome for future improvement. (NLM, 2009, para. 1; http://www.nlm.nih.gov/hsrinfo/evidence_based_practice. html)

Thus, evidence-based practices use the best scientific evidence available to guide clinical decision making for the purposing of attaining the best outcomes. EBPs are reflected in clinical practices guidelines, evidence reports, and evidence summaries.

EBP research uses numerous empirical methodologies, including meta-analyses, randomized controlled trials, non-randomized trials, cross-sectional studies, case control studies, pre-test and post-test studies, time series studies, non-comparative studies, retrospective cohort studies, and prospective cohort studies. Other methodologies include systematic literature reviews, non-systematic or narrative literature reviews, quality improvement research, and case series.

EBPs differ from best practices in that EBPs show evidence of effect with a strong research design (experimental or quasi-experimental), sustained effect (at least one year beyond treatment), and multiple site replication. Best practices often have evidence of effect with a strong research design (experimental or quasi-experimental); however, they may not show sustained effect (at least one year beyond treatment) and/or multiple site replication. For example, the National Registry of Evidence-Based Programs and Practices (NREPP, 2007) uses a "quality of research rating" based upon six criteria: (1) reliability; (2) validity; (3) intervention fidelity; (4) missing data and attrition; (5) potential confounding variables; and (6) appropriateness of analysis.

There are numerous types of evidence. Glasgow and Emmons (2007) examined the strengths and weaknesses of 18 types of evidence. They found that, although process or quality of care information is a very important assessment criterion for policy makers, process information may not translate to improved outcomes. In addition, contextual information, which is often used in the interpretation of results, may also mask what is relevant regarding outcomes, adoption, and implementation (see Table 8.1).

Mercer and Pignotti (2007) also created taxonomy to address quality in research studies. They divided research studies into five broad categories: (1) EBPs; (2) evidence-supported interventions; (3) evidence-informed treatments; (4) belief-based interventions; and (5) potentially harmful treatments. Within these categories, they then subdivided types of studies to more closely examine methodological issues (see Table 8.2).

Let's take a closer look at a specific type of evidence: systematic reviews. Systematic reviews seek to "collate all evidence that fits pre-specified eligibility criteria in order to

TABLE 8.1

Types of Evidence and Associated Strengths and Weaknesses

Evidence type	General strength	Frequent weakness
Theoretical or mechanism data	Helps to understand how and why treatment works	Are concerns about length of assessments
Feasibility/implementation evidence	Helps to understand delivery issues and adaptations	Requires detailed monitoring and tracking information
Contextual information— e.g., constraints, history, resource availability	Helps in judging applicability and interpretation of other results	Is not clear exactly what is relevant
Intended primary outcome evidence	Is optimal for evaluations of a priori hypotheses	Can be limiting and researcher-centric
Unintended or unanticipated outcome results	Is important from systems perspective	May be retrospective and anecdotal
Process or quality-of-care results	Is key concern of policy makers and useful for quality improvement	May not translate to outcomes
"Outcome" or clinical data	Is often important goal of programs	Is only part of the picture
Quality-of-life data and adverse consequences data	Addresses bottom line issues and participant perspective	Requires more questions of participants
Quality improvement data	Encourages refinement and adaptation	Is seen by some as "low quality" or uncontrolled
Marketing and opinion poll data	Is helpful for program design	Can be costly
Surveillance data on trends over time	Presents bottom line, population-based data	Are many potential confounders
Cost and economic data	Is key for decision makers	Can be complex and costly to collect and interpret
Qualitative data	Helps to understand how and why programs work (or do not work)	Are subjectivity, and in some cases, reliability issues
Local data	Assesses applicability	May not be generalizable
Systematic review data	Synthesizes and evaluates "quality" of evidence	Can be overly narrow or restrictive about what is included
Simulation data on project impact	Saves time and can identify important, nonintuitive factors	Can be expensive
Internal validity evidence	Helps determine causality and rule out confounding factors	Can lack relevance, if "decontextualized"

(*continued*)

TABLE 8.1

Types of Evidence and Associated Strengths and Weaknesses (*continued*)

Evidence type	General strength	Frequent weakness
External validity evidence	Is important for translation, decision makers, and practitioners	Can be challenging to collect

From Glasgow, R.E., & Emmons, K. M. (2007). How can we increase translation of research into practice? Types of evidence needed. *Annual Review of Public Health, 28,* 413–433.

TABLE 8.2

Taxonomy of Research

Intervention	Method	Replication	Outcome Evaluation	Manual
Evidence-based	Randomized designs, comparisons to established treatments	Independent replications of results	Blind evaluation	Yes
Evidence-supported	Nonrandomized or within subjects designs	Independent replications of results	Blind evaluation	Yes
Evidence-informed	Case studies, interventions tested on populations other than the targeted group	No independent replications	No evidence of harm or potential for harm	Yes
Belief-based	No published research; based on religious or ideological principles	No independent replications	No evidence of harm or potential for harm	Yes/No
Potentially harmful	Harmful mental or physical effects have been documented	Harmful mental or physical effects have been documented	Harmful mental or physical effects have been documented	Shows potential for harm

Adapted from Mercer, J., & Pignotti, M. (2007). Shortcuts cause errors in systematic research syntheses. *Scientific Review of Mental Health Practice, 5*(2), 59–77.

address a specific research question" (Green et al., 2008, p. 3). Since 1993, the Cochrane Collaborative, which is attributed with creating the term *evidence-based medicine*, is considered the gold standard in its methodology to create a systematic review. Comprising over 15,000 contributors from more than 100 countries, the Collaborative has 51 Cochrane Review Groups (CRGs), which are supported by Methods Groups, Centers, and Fields. The Methods Groups are the primary developers of the *Cochrane Handbook for Systematic Reviews of Interventions* (the *Handbook*) (Higgins & Green, 2011).

A Cochrane systematic review uses explicitly stated methods with the intent to minimize bias and to provide reliable findings. Key characteristics of a systematic review are:

> a clearly stated set of objectives with pre-defined eligibility criteria for studies; an explicit, reproducible methodology; a systematic search that attempts to identify all studies that would meet the eligibility criteria; an assessment of the validity of the findings of the included studies, for example through the assessment of risk of bias; and a systematic presentation, and synthesis, of the characteristics and findings of the included studies. (Green et al., 2008, p. 6)

Since the *Handbook* focuses on the effects of interventions, it is oriented primarily to randomized clinical trials (RCTs).

As with any evidence used to establish the effectiveness and efficacy of an intervention in moving it from research to practice, it is important to be aware of how research studies are constructed, how evidence is constructed, and to critically review any larger review study or meta-analysis. This is important for mental health informatics since health services and translational research competencies position critical thinking, construction of research questions, and study methodologies as key, foundational elements.

Translational Research Informatics

Within the area of translational research is the specialty area of translational research informatics (TRI). A sister domain of clinical research informatics, TRI manages logistics, data integration, and collaboration among translational investigators. To do so, TRI integrates with health information technology, electronic medical record systems, clinical trial management systems, clinical research informatics, statistical analyses, and data mining. A 2010 NIMH workshop, Mental Health and Health IT Research: The Way Forward, examined opportunities to leverage emerging technologies toward improved research and services delivery. Key areas of concern addressed: the effectiveness of technology-supported service delivery models that allow for asynchronous assessment, services delivery, and monitoring; effectiveness of mobile technologies to increase use of mental health services and adherence to treatments; and the use of technologies to improve data capture, real-time assessment, and prediction of risk and acute service need.

In earlier chapters within this text, we discussed the electronic health record (EHR) and data standards. Let's take a moment to consider the key requirements for EHRs that will support translational research needs. One of the first requirements will be reliable and complete data. The EHR documents each action (orders, procedures, observations, medications, supply, and registration) taken to treat a patient. The relationship between these actions leads to a next step in the diagnostic or treatment protocol. However, an EHR is not designed to link patients across disease groups, diagnostic categories, or patient demographics. It is designed to enhance clinical decision making, which limits its use in translational research. Although the notion of "complete data" will be driven by the needs of the different research specialties, standards in data collection and naming as well as in the detection and correction of errors will improve the reliability of data.

The two most significant factors that affect data quality are data collection error and staging error. Data collection errors can be corrected using validation processes that show the source of the errors and allow for correction. Staging errors occur due to incomplete queries or partial data extraction. Both types of errors require staff time to correct; however, the quality of the data is improved in both the provider source system and data warehouses. Standards also will ensure that the data architecture is interoperable across multiple systems and convertible from legacy systems.

A second requirement is searchability. Federated search engines allow the simultaneous search of multiple searchable resources in real-time. A user makes a single query request that is distributed to the search engines in the federation. Then, the federated search aggregates the results from the search engines and presents an integrated display to the user. One example is the Science.gov portal, which federates over 30 research and development sites of the U.S. federal government.

MANAGING DATA DISCOVERY AND RETRIEVAL

There are a number of TRI initiatives investigating data discovery and retrieval. Harris et al. (2009) described an innovative work-flow methodology designed for rapid development and deployment of research using electronic data capture tools. Their program, REDCap (research electronic data capture), uses a metadata-driven methodology to capture and study data from over 208 research projects across 27 institutions. Although the REDCap project is considered to successfully meet the needs for researcher-controlled data services and secure data collection, storage, and export, there are several limitations. The first is a flat-file structure, which works well for collected research data but not so well for data storage or mining. Also, there are no data-naming standards, which can create difficulty in searching and retrieving relevant research information. These are issues currently under consideration for further development of REDCap.

At Stanford University, Lowe et al. (2009) created an integrated standards-based translational research informatics platform. The STRIDE (Stanford Translational Research Integrated Database Environment) consists of three integrated components: (1) a clinical data warehouse; (2) an application development framework for building research data management applications on the STRIDE platform; and (3) and a biospecimen data management system. The data warehouse contains almost 20 years of clinical information on over 1.3 million pediatric and adult patients. Based on the HL7 Reference Information Model (RIM), it uses defined vocabulary domains: SNOMED-CT; RxNorm; ICD-9CM; and CPT. Although STRIDE is cost-effective in terms of time and use for large-scale projects, Lowe and colleagues (2009) are currently researching the use of REDCap to handle small to medium-sized research projects.

Anderson et al. (2011) adapted software from the Informatics for Integrating Biology and the Bedside (i2b2) program to create a federated search of over 5 million de-identified aggregated clinical data sets stored across separate institutional environments. To accomplish this, however, required significant investment in standardizing technical infrastructures, policies, and semantic metadata.

Ohio State University Medical Center IW (Information Warehouse) is a prime example of the transformation of a business system to a networked platform able to support translational research. Its IW integrated a clinical data repository, a research data repository, an application development platform, and a business intelligence environment (Kamal et al, 2010). Similar to other translational research databases and platforms, the IW uses standard terminologics (SNOMED-CT, ICD-9 CM, RxNorm, American Hospital Formulary Service classifications, and CPT).

IDENTIFYING POTENTIAL RESEARCH COHORTS

One of the more practical sides of translational research informatics is the identification of potential research patient cohorts and patient suitability. Weber et al. (2010) describe their use of event stream processing (ESP) to identify individuals who are patients in emergency rooms who may meet eligibility criteria for clinical studies at Stanford. Using the STRIDE platform, ESP handles data analysis from real-time HL7 message streams rather than pulling from data previously entered into a database. In simple terms, ESP analyzes data as it enters a system before it is stored. Complex event processing (CEP) handles more than one message stream at a time. For example, it may monitor laboratory order streams and radiology order streams. In this case, Weber and colleagues (2010) were able to parse ICD-9-coded values in the message streams and to generate an electronic alert by pager and by e-mail to the study coordinator. This first alert contained no protected health information (PHI). If the patient was interested in being a part of the study, a second message was sent that contained PHI to streamline the study enrollment process.

STRIDE also offers researchers the ability to review stored data as well to determine potential patient cohorts, using a series of query tools. In addition, its research cohort data review tool, which meets stringent IRB (Institutional Review Board) and HIPAA (Health Information Portability and Accountability Act) requirements, allows authorized users to access all clinical data captured as part of direct clinical care at the Stanford University Medical Center (Lowe et al., 2009). Unlike STRIDE's query tools, Ohio State's IW uses a question-and-answer approach to build complex queries and to store those queries as query conditions for future searches.

HUMAN SUBJECT PROTECTION

One of the key issues in identifying patient cohorts is human subject protection. To ensure that no harm comes to participants in clinical trials, IRB and HIPAA security protocols are established. With the increase in multi-site health research, especially with the NIH's Clinical and Translational Science Award program, human subject protection is of paramount importance. Whether the study is prospective or retrospective, there are issues with PHI. In a prospective study, researchers query databases to determine potential participants who meet minimum criteria data, followed by a request to enroll in the study. In a retrospective study, researchers use historical data that are still covered by confidentiality and privacy.

Regardless of the type of study, there are steps to be followed in the process. First, the researcher submits the IRB application to the IRB. The IRB reviews and approves the study. The researcher submits the IRB application to the data administrator. The administrator reviews the IRB application and provides the data to the researcher. However, the IRB review system and the data access process are two separate systems. This can cause problems, particularly for multi-site applications.

At the University of Utah's Center for Clinical and Translational Science, a federated data repository combines five of the largest patient data warehouses in the state (state public health system, VA healthcare system, the Utah Population Database, Intermountain Healthcare, and the University's health care system) (He, Hurdle, Botkin, & Narus, 2010). The Federated Utah Research and Translational Health e-Repository (FURTHeR) integrates the IRB review system and the data access process using the HL7 Regulated Clinical Research Information Management (RCRIM) content to increase operability across the systems. RCRIM allows interoperability among legacy databases as well as scalability among systems. Not only does FURTHeR provide stricter and more controlled access to researchers, it also makes ethics review for multi-site studies easier, since the federated hub allows the IRBs to exchange information (He, Hurdle, Botkin, & Narus, 2010).

Getting from There to Here: Effective Translation

The National Institutes of Health's *Roadmap* is of great interest to mental health clinical and services research because there are numerous ways to approach translational research in behavioral health. Wang et al. (2009) suggested that clinical epidemiology plays an important role in moving research to practice and taking questions raised in practice to research. Epidemiology provides data on incidence, and allows us to calculate prevalence and to study clusters of disease. Further, rapid developments in informatics, emphasis on large sample collection for genetic and biomarker studies, and interest in relative and absolute risk factors provide exciting new venues for translational research. For example, Weissman, Brown, and Talati (2011) suggested that community surveys are an excellent resource for translational research: gathering DNA or other biomarkers for the NIMH genetic repository, providing samples for future case-control studies based upon risk factors, and generating hypotheses for population studies on illnesses, such as schizophrenia or substance abuse. Longitudinal cohort studies, although observational in nature, lend themselves to the formulation of hypotheses based upon data in the field, which leads back to human and animal genetic research studies in the lab.

New methodological and computational advances now permit better data analyses in behavioral health research studies. Joint modeling of longitudinal data examines the differential effects of personal characteristics, environmental factors, and/or interventions on the multiple dependent variables. Generalized linear mixed modeling, group-based trajectory modeling, and latent growth curve modeling currently are considered state-of-the-art tools.

Charnigo et al. (2011) suggested that researchers can best analyze the impact of interventions on multiple behavioral outcomes by (1) treating the outcomes as distinct, and (2) employing one or more analytic strategies to assess the impact on all of the outcomes simultaneously where appropriate. By using complementary approaches, that is, "the difference between fitting multiple marginal (or conditional) models within a particular analytic paradigm … and fitting a single joint model within that same analytic paradigm" (p. 195), researchers transcend specific research silos and broaden their opportunities to take research to practice.

Weiss et al. (2011) maintained that effective translation of interventions from research to practice requires reach, effectiveness, adoption, implementation, and maintenance. Using the RE-AIM model (train-the-trainer) for implementation of cognitive behavioral stress management program for economically disadvantaged minority women living with AIDS, Weiss and colleagues suggest that four elements contributed to the successful translation of their intervention: (1) open communication; (2) formative and process assessments of clinical and site outcomes; (3) clear measures of fidelity; and (4) program maintenance. They also suggested that consideration of cultural and subcultural values are essential in successful translation of research to practice (Weiss et al., 2011).

Young and Borland (2011, p. 256) discussed the challenges for researchers and practitioners as one of "practical ontologies." Researchers and practitioners operate as mirror images, as researchers work from specific to universal contexts and practitioners try to incorporate the universal contexts into specific contexts that work in their everyday environments. Creating a translational environment, where practitioners can ask questions that they would like to see answered and researchers can take these questions and answer them, would be a new area for development in informatics.

Thus, recreating the notion of translational research as interlocking loops, as opposed to bi-directional conduits, may be an effective way to re-address how health services research is structured (Callard, Rose, & Wykes, 2011). Callard and colleagues (2011) advocated for embedding service users and other stakeholders into the translational research process. The benefits of this involvement may result in improved recruitment rates within clinical trials, identifying new research hypotheses and questions, and improved implementation of EBPs within the community. More important, such a perspective reinforces the role of participation in translational research (Zerhouni, 2007).

Barriers to real-world implementation are influenced by content, context, and process. Content concerns the development, testing, and interpretation of evidence. A study that works well in a controlled clinical study with a narrowly defined population may not transfer successfully to a community mental health setting if extended to a different population. Context addresses the political, professional, economic, social, organizational attitudes and behavior of local stakeholders, both providers and consumers.

In Chapter 5, we discussed the issues of adoption of health information technology; it is also critical that organizations implement evidence-based practices, practitioners are able to deliver the intervention without adversely affecting how they deliver services, and consumers are satisfied with interventions and improve their quality of life. To do so requires a process that examines behavior change strategies, supervisory/management practices, and engagement, again at the individual, organizational, and system levels. One of the greatest barriers to successful implementation is a mismatch between an intervention/research design, on the one hand, and the realities inherent to the target practice setting on the other hand. A very intensive intervention to a very small, selective group of elderly patients in a residential treatment setting may not generalize to a less intensive interpretation for a population of younger adults in a community mental health center.

To offset these barriers, Glasgow and Emmons (2007) offered two suggestions. First, researchers need to pay greater attention to context and external validity. External validity refers to "inferences about the extent to which a causal relationship holds over variations in persons, settings, treatments, and outcomes" (Shadish, Cook, & Campbell, 2002). Too often, researchers present only internal validity results, which may lack relevance to the setting if they are not contextualized to the needs of the stakeholders. Second, researchers need to create and maintain "partnerships with relevant decision-makers and target audiences" (Glasgow & Emmons, 2007, p. 427) to enhance effective implementation of evidence-based interventions in the community.

Clearly, the science related to the transportability of efficacious programs to real-world settings and the dissemination of these programs on a broad scale lags far behind the research that develops the programs (Fixsen et al., 2005). In the next section of this chapter, we take a closer look at one implementation research project that did not work as planned, and the resulting lessons learned by the investigators.

CASE STUDY

Zayas, McKee, and Jankowski (2004) described the challenges that their research team experienced in implementing a multi-modal psychosocial intervention addressing perinatal depression in community health centers. Their target population was urban, low-income, pregnant minority women ($n = 187$) across three health centers in the south Bronx in New York City. The three components of the intervention included an eight-session cognitive behavioral treatment specifically developed for depression prevention in primary care, four psycho-educational sessions (videotaped and written materials) on infant development and maternal sensitivity, and ongoing social support from a therapist (14 visits). The therapists were female minority graduate students in social work, trained and supervised in cultural sensitivity and in the specific intervention. The interventions were offered twice a month at the health centers or at the participants' homes. Two of the three health centers had formal psychosocial service teams, while the third health center was a family practice site with a part-time social worker. Not only did the health centers have little experience with conducting research, but none of the health centers had experience with implementation studies.

The researchers found that a number of challenges affected the study outcomes. The first challenge was the lack of organizational buy-in by the health centers. The administrators of the three centers voiced concerns over compromises in service delivery. In addition, operational challenges often involved changes in patient scheduling due to a lack of space to conduct the intervention, lack of secure storage for equipment, logistical barriers to videotaping the interventions, and conflicts with normal center operations. These challenges affected the fidelity of the intervention. Since the researchers were unable to video- or audiotape the sessions, their ability to effectively examine the delivery of the intervention by the student therapists was affected.

Participant attrition was also a major problem. Over a third (38%) of the participants did not complete the study. Attrition was attributed to several factors. One was the use of student therapists. Constraints with the academic calendar (and thus the student therapists' availability) affected the continuity of care to participants. Some participants dropped out of the study due to the many changes in their therapists over the four-month time period.

Patient adherence and expected outcomes were identified as other factors affecting implementation. Not only did patients decide what parts of the intervention they would attend or accept, their expectations regarding the help they needed were significantly different from those of the researchers. Many of the participants saw themselves as stressed, not depressed, and opted out of the depression component of the intervention. Surprisingly, for example, the option to have the intervention delivered at home was not as popular as the researchers had expected. Many of the participants liked the social component of coming to the health centers. Other participants had concerns for the safety of the therapists if they came to the participants' homes. Several participants said that their partners opposed home visits.

However, the researchers did learn much from this study in how best to handle client-program mismatch. They offer four recommendations for adapting research design to address stakeholder and service system characteristics (Zayas et al., 2004). First, determine what the target population will accept from an intervention. This would include learning about key issues in participants' lives that can be addressed as part of the intervention and what they see as critical outcomes for them. Second, determine the type of interventions that clinicians are most likely to offer in their settings within the time and operational constraints of their practice. This increases local staff and organization buy-in. Third, determine the site's capacity to accommodate intervention research. If adaptations are necessary to accommodate fiscal or policy needs, it does not mean that the fundamental research design is necessarily compromised. Finally, collect additional data as it emerges. It is impossible to identify all the data that may emerge from a study. Systematically collecting additional ethnographic and anecdotal information for review from all members of the team may indicate emerging challenges to the intervention (Zayas et al., 2004).

Implications for Mental Health Informatics

Translational research is an important component of health and mental health services research design and analysis. It provides the knowledge base to move scientific discoveries from clinical or population studies into clinical applications in real-world settings. The National Institute of Mental Health (NIMH) articulated its challenge as how to "redefine disorders by understanding them as unfolding developmental processes, recognizing that these disease processes can have different consequences at different life stages" (NIMH, 2011, p. 12). Early detection of risk factors leads to early intervention, which leads to more successful outcomes for persons of all ages diagnosed with mental illnesses (Landa, Holman, & Garrett-Mayer, 2007; Cannon et al., 2008).

Certainly understanding the biological, developmental, genetic, psychological, and behavioral markers and relationships is critical in translational research (National Advisory Mental Health Council Workgroup on Neurodevelopment, 2007; National Advisory

Mental Health Council Workgroup, 2010).). However, environmental and experiential components also should be integrated into models of mental illnesses. One question is how to define, classify, and analyze these components in a meaningful way to add to our understanding and the development of effective interventions. Further, an important aspect of this translation is in the implementation of these studies into the community. Here, we are faced with determining factors that affect access to service, quality and cost of services, and how to best disseminate and implement newly discovered effective mental health interventions (National Advisory Mental Health Council, 2011).

There is a continuing need to support the national health information infrastructure, to develop integrated applications in informatics, and to implement standards to facilitate the collection and sharing of clinical information (National Institutes of Health Roadmap Working Group, 2004). Programs, such as the Clinical Research Networks and the National Electronics Clinical Trials and Research network, created inventories of clinical research, providing snapshots of federally and privately sponsored networks. These initiatives led to the NIH Clinical and Translational Science Award program, which has continued to focus attention on the infrastructure tools and the support needed to facilitate multidisciplinary team building within and across academic medical centers, universities, and communities, which has addressed many of the barriers to translational research at a national level (Sung et al., 2003).

Effectively assessing the impact of research is critical. Banzi et al. (2011) suggest four types of information are crucial to understanding impact: (1) program reach on representativeness; (2) implementation and adaptation; (3) outcomes for decision making; and (4) maintenance and institutionalization. If researchers took the time to incorporate this information into their research designs, it would create a unified conceptual framework when reviewing the results of research studies, thus providing a valuable baseline for future assessment.

Finally, we suggest that the levels of translational research (T1 and T2) be integrated as a continuum to enhance the transition from discovery to clinical application to practice. From a public mental health perspective, that would create a more seamless process and natural linkages in translational research. Whether we are advancing knowledge, building capacity, informing decision making, enhancing health benefits, or addressing broad socioeconomic benefits, moving research to practice benefits all of us involved in health and mental health services research and services delivery.

References

Anderson, N., Abend, A., Mandel, A., Geraghty, E., Gabriel, D., Wynden, R., ... & Tarczy-Hornoch, P. (2011). Implementation of a deidentified federated data network for population-based cohort discovery. *Journal of the American Medical Informatics Association.* Advance online publication. doi: 10.1136/amiajnl-2011-000133.

Balas, E. A., & Boren, S. A. (2000). *Yearbook of medical informatics: Managing clinical knowledge for health care improvement.* Stuttgart, Germany: Schattauer Verlagsgesellschaft mbH.

Banzi, R, Moja, L, Pistotti, V, Facchini, A, & Liberati, A. (2011). Conceptual frameworks and empirical approaches used to assess the impact of health research: an overview of reviews. *Health Research Policy and Systems, 9*, 26. doi:10.1186/1478-4505-9-26.

Callard, F., Rose, D., Wykes, T. (2011). Close to the bench as well as at the bedside: Involving service users in all phases of translational research. *Health Expectations*. Advance online publication. doi: 10.1111/j.1369–7625.2011.00681.x.

Cannon, T. D., Cadenhead, K., Cornblatt, B., Woods, S.W., Addington, J., Walker, E., Seidman, L.J., Perkins, D., Tsuang, M., McGlashan, T., & Heinssen, R. (2008). Prediction of psychosis in high risk youth: A multi-site longitudinal study in North America. *Archives of General Psychiatry, 65*(1), 28–37.

Charnigo, R., Kryscio, R., Bardo, M. T., Lynam, D., & Zimmerman, R. S. (2011). Joint modeling of longitudinal data in multiple behavior change. *Evaluation and the Health Professions, 34*(2), 181–200.

Clinical Treatment and Services Research Workgroup (1997). *Bridging science and service: A Report by the National Advisory Mental Health Council's Clinical Treatment and Services Research Workgroup.* Rockville, MD: National Institute of Mental Health. Retrieved from http://web.archive.org/web/20010303185256/http://www.nimh.nih.gov/research/bridge.htm.

Committee on the Science of Adolescence; Board on Children, Youth, and Families; Institute of Medicine and National Research Council. (2011). *The science of adolescent risk-taking: Workshop report.* Washington, DC: National Academies Press. Retrieved from http://www.nap.edu/catalog.php?record_id=12961.

D'Onofrio, G., Jauch, E., Jagoda, A., Allen, M. H., Anglin, D., Barsan, W. G., ... & Zatzick, D. (2010). NIH Roundtable on Opportunities to Advance Research on Neurologic and Psychiatric Emergencies. *Annals of Emergency Medicine, 56*(5):551–564. doi: 10.1016/j.annemergmed.2010.06.562.

Field, M. J., Tranquada, R. E., & Feasley, J. C. (1995). *Health services research: Work force and educational issues.* Washington, DC: National Academy Press. Retrieved from http://www.nap.edu/catalog.php?record_id=5020.

Fixsen, D. L., Naoom, S. F., Blase, K. A., Friedman, R. M., & Wallace, F. (2005). *Implementation research: A synthesis of the literature* (FMHI Publication #231). Tampa, FL: University of South Florida, Louis de la Parte Florida Mental Health Institute, the National Implementation Research Network. Retrieved from http://cfs.cbcs.usf.edu/_docs/publications/NIRN_Monograph_Full.pdf.

Glasgow, R.E., & Emmons, K. M. (2007). How can we increase translation of research into practice? Types of evidence needed. *Annual Review of Public Health, 28,* 413–433.

Green, S., Higgins, J. P. T., Alderson, P., Clarke, M., Mulrow, C. D., & Oxman, A. D. (2008). Introduction. In J. P. T. Higgins & S. Green (Eds.), *Cochrane handbook for systematic reviews of interventions* (pp. 1.1–1.2). Chichester, UK: John Wiley & Sons.

Harris, P. A., Taylor, R., Thielke, R., Payne, J., Gonzalez, N., & Conde, J. G. (2009). Research electronic data capture (REDCap): A metadata-driven methodology and workflow process for providing translational research informatics support. *Journal of Biomedical Informatics; 42*(2), 377–381. doi: 10.1016/j.jbi.2008.08.010.

He, S., Hurdle, J. F., Botkin, J. R., & Narus, S. P. (2010). Integrating a federated healthcare data query platform with electronic IRB information systems. *AMIA Annual Symposium Proceedings, 13,* 291–295. Retrieved from http://www.ncbi.nlm.nih.gov/pmc/articles/PMC3041360.

Higgins, J. P. T. & Green, S. (2011). *Cochrane handbook for systematic reviews of interventions 5.1.0.* Chichester, UK: John Wiley & Sons. Retrieved from http://www.cochrane-handbook.org/.

Insel, T. R. (2008). Assessing the economic cost of serious mental illness. *American Journal of Psychiatry, 165*(6), 663–665.

Kamal, J., Liu, J., Ostrander, M., Santangelo, J., Dyta, R., Rogers, P., & Mekhjian, H. S. (2010). Information warehouse: A comprehensive informatics platform for business, clinical, and research applications. *AMIA Annual Symposium Proceedings, 13,* 2010:452–456. Retrieved from http://www.ncbi.nlm.nih.gov/pmc/articles/PMC3041278/?tool=pubmed.

Kessler, R. C., Heering, S., Lakoma, M. D., Petukhova, M., Rupp, A. E., Schoenbaum, M., Wang, P.S., & Zaslavsky, A. M. (2008). Individual and societal effects of mental disorders on earnings in the United States: Results from the National Comorbidity Survey Replication. *American Journal of Psychiatry, 165*(6), 703–711.

Landa, R. J., Holman, K. C., & Garrett-Mayer, E. (2007). Social and communication development in toddlers with early and later diagnosis of autism spectrum disorders. *Archives of General Psychiatry, 64*(7):853–864.

Lowe, H. J., Ferris, T. A., Hernandez, P. M., & Weber, S. C. (2009). STRIDE: An integrated standards-based translational research informatics platform. *AMIA Annual Symposium Proceedings,* 391–395. Retrieved from http://www.ncbi.nlm.nih.gov/pmc/articles/PMC2815452.

Mark, T. L., Levit, K. R., Coffey, R. M., McKusick, D. R., Harwood, H. J., King, E. C., Bouchery, E., Genuardi, J. S., Vandivort- Warren, R., Buck, J. A., & Ryan, K. (2007). *National expenditures for mental health services and substance abuse treatment.* Rockville, MD: United States Department of Health and Human Services, Substance Abuse and Mental Health Services Administration.

Mercer, J., & Pignotti, M. (2007). Shortcuts cause errors in systematic research syntheses. *Scientific Review of Mental Health Practice, 5*(2), 59–77.

Nathan, D. G (1998). Clinical research: perceptions, reality, and proposed solutions. National Institutes of Health Director's Panel on Clinical Research. *JAMA, 208*(16), 1427–1431.

National Advisory Mental Health Council Behavioral Science Workgroup. (2000). *Translating behavioral science into action* (NIH Publication No. 00–4699). Retrieved from http://web.archive.org/web/20010209155349/http://www.nimh.nih.gov/council/bswreport.pdf.

National Advisory Mental Health Council Workgroup. (2010). *From discovery to cure: Accelerating the development of new and personalized interventions for mental illnesses.* Rockville, MD: National Institute of Mental Health. Retrieved from http://www.nimh.nih.gov/about/advisory-boards-and-groups/namhc/reports/fromdiscoverytocure.pdf.

National Advisory Mental Health Council Workgroup on Neurodevelopment. (2007). *Transformative neurodevelopmental research in mental illness.* Retrieved from http://www.nimh.nih.gov/about/advisory-boards-and-groups/namhc/neurodevelopment_workgroup_report.pdf.

National Institute of Mental Health. (2011, May 06). *Harnessing advanced health technologies to drive mental health improvement.* Rockville, MD: NIMH. Retrieved from http://www.nimh.nih.gov/research-funding/grants/concept-clearances/2011/harnessing-advanced-health-technologies-to-drive-mental-health-improvement.shtml.

National Institute of Mental Health. (2009). *Meeting summary: New perspectives in the translational neuroscience of late life mental disorders.* Rockville, MD: NIMH, Division of Adult Translational Research and Treatment Development. Retrieved from http://www.nimh.nih.gov/research-funding/scientific-meetings/2009/new-perspectives-in-the-translational-neuroscience-of-late-life-mental-disorders.shtml.

National Institute of Mental Health. (2008). *NIMH strategic plan* (NIH Publication No. 08–6368). Rockville, MD: National Institute of Mental Health. Retrieved from http://www.nimh.nih.gov/about/strategic-planning-reports/nimh-strategic-plan-2008.pdf.

National Institutes of Health. (2007). *Institutional clinical and translational science award* (U54) RFA-RM-07–007. Retrieved from http://grants.nih.gov/grants/guide/rfa-files/RFA-RM-07–007.html.

National Institutes of Health Roadmap Working Group (2004). *NIH roadmap: Reengineering the Clinical Research Enterprise Regional Translational Research Centers interim report.* Rockville, MD: NIH. Retrieved from https://commonfund.nih.gov/clinicalresearch/rtrc/pdf/rtrc_interimreport.pdf.

National Library of Medicine. (1997). *Evidence-based medicine.* MeSH. Retrieved from http://www.ncbi.nlm.nih.gov/mesh/68019317.

National Library of Medicine. (2009). *Evidence-based practice.* MeSH. Retrieved from http://www.ncbi.nlm.nih.gov/mesh/68055317.

National Library of Medicine. (2011). *Translational research.* MeSH. Retrieved from http://www.ncbi.nlm.nih.gov/mesh/68057170.

National Registry of Evidence-based Programs and Practices. (2007). *NREPP review criteria.* Washington, DC: Substance Abuse and Mental Health Services Administration. Retrieved from http://web.archive.org/web/20080719121619/http://nrepp.samhsa.gov/review-criteria.htm.

National Research Council. (2005). *Advancing the nation's health needs.* Washington, DC: National Academies Press. Retrieved from http://grants.nih.gov/training/nas_report_2005.pdf.

National Research Council. (2011). *Research training in the biomedical, behavioral, and clinical research sciences.* Washington, DC: National Academies Press. Retrieved from http://www.nap.edu/catalog.php?record_id=12983.

NIH Director's Panel. (1997). *The NIH Director's Panel on Clinical Research report to the Advisory Committee to the NIH Director.* Rockville, MD: National Institutes of Health. Retrieved from http://web.archive.org/web/20070310065147/http://www.nih.gov/news/crp/97report/.

Pellmar, T., & Eisenberg, L. (2000). *Bridging disciplines in the brain, behavioral, and clinical sciences.* Washington, DC: National Academies Press. Retrieved from http://books.nap.edu/catalog/9942.html.

Shadish, W. R., Cook, T. D., & Campbell, D. T. (2002). *Experimental and quasi-experimental design for generalized causal inference.* Boston, MA: Houghton Mifflin.

Smith, G. S., Gunning-Dixon, F. M., Lotrich, F. E., Taylor, W. T., and Evans, D. D. (2007). Translational research in late-life mood disorders: Implications for future intervention and prevention research. *Neuropsychopharmacology, 32,* 1857–1875. doi:10.1038/sj.npp.1301333.

Sung, N.S., Crowley, W. F. Jr., Genel, M., Salber, P., Sandy, L., Sherwood, L. M., Johnson, S. B., … & Rimoin, D. (2003). Central challenges facing the national clinical research enterprise. *JAMA, 289*(10), 1278–1287.

Wang, P. S., Heinssen, R., Oliveri, M., Wagner, A., & Goodman, W. (2009). Bridging bench and practice: Translational research for schizophrenia and other psychotic disorders. *Neuropsychopharmacology, 34*(1):204–212.

Warren, R., Buck, J. A., & Ryan, K. (2007). *National expenditures for mental health services and substance abuse treatment.* Rockville, MD: United States Department of Health and Human Services, Substance Abuse and Mental Health.

Weber, S., Lowe, H. J., Malunjkar, S., & Quinn, J. (2010). Implementing a real-time complex event stream processing system to help identify potential participants in clinical and translational research studies. *AMIA Annual Symposium Proceedings, 13*, 472–476.

Weiss, S. M., Jones D. L., Lopez, M., Villar-Loubet, O., Chitalu, N. (2011). The many faces of translational research: A tale of two studies. *Translational Behavioral Medicine, 1*(2), 327–330. doi: 10.1007/s13142–011–0044–0.

Weissman, M. M., Brown, A. S., & Talati, A. (2011). Translational epidemiology in psychiatry: Linking population to clinical and basic sciences. *Archives of General Psychiatry, 68*(6), 600–608.

Young, D., & Borland, R. (2011). Conceptual challenges in the translation of research into practice: it's not just a matter of "communication." *Translational Behavioral Medicine, 1*(2), 256–269. doi: 10.1007/s13142–011–0035–1.

Zayas, L. H., McKee, M. D., & Jankowski, K. R. (2004). Adapting psychosocial intervention research to urban primary care environments: A case example. *Annals of Family Medicine, 2*(5):504–508.

Zerhouni, E. A. (2007). Translational research: Moving discovery to practice. *Clinical Pharmacology and Therapeutics, 81*, 126–128.

Part 3 Competencies and Strategies

All health professionals should be educated to deliver patient-centered care as members
of an interdisciplinary team, emphasizing evidence-based practice, quality improvement
approaches, and informatics.

—BOARD ON HEALTH CARE SERVICES, 2003, p. 3

9 Research, Professional, and Educational Competencies

The range of data used in mental health services, research, and practice is very broad. To successfully work with data, information, and systems requires a series of literacies and competencies. Further, given the way in which behavioral health services research and practice are defined, how can one be best prepared in data-intensive information and computing environments? In this chapter, we will look at the skills and competencies that are necessary to conduct mental health and substance abuse services research in an increasingly complex and changing online environment.

Working with Data, Data Types, and Data Reports

Working with data requires a number of skills and competencies. Differences in academic disciplines affect how faculty and students conduct research. Individuals in the physical sciences and engineering often use search strategies based upon specific problem-solving processes, while individuals in the humanities or social sciences are more likely to use search strategies based upon a topical interest that is extensively researched (Palmer, 2005). Järvelin and Wilson (2003) stated "Conceptual models may and should map reality, guide research and systematize knowledge, for example, by integration and by proposing systems of hypotheses" (para. 9). Therefore, understanding diverse analytical models of task-based information seeking is key to understanding the research process.

By suggesting that researchers have explicit or implicit cognitive models of the domain of interest at the particular point in time when they are conducting research, Ingwersen (1992; 1996) supports Järvelin and Wilson's (2003) contention that individuals interpret the same objective task differently, particularly for what is perceived to be a complex task. How the user perceives the task is the basis for the actual performance of the task, the interpretation of his or her information needs, and the decision making to ensure satisfaction, or successful completion of the task. These tasks range from simple computational tasks to decision-making tasks, which increase with the complexity of the information and process needed to complete the tasks.

Further, the style of learning also affects the process. Some users are "big picture" learners, with a broad, divergent learning style (Heinström, 2006). These individuals typically start their research process through an overall understanding of a topic, addressing several aspects of the information needs at the same time, relating new information, and determining causal relations between variables. Other users may use a convergent, rational, problem-focused style, concentrating on one item at a time (Heinström, 2006). These individuals often generate precise searches, mastering one component of a topic before moving on to the next. For these users, the broad or big conceptual picture emerges later in the search. Thus, learning styles have implications for the development of effective research competencies.

LITERACIES

Traditionally, *literacy* is defined as the ability to read, write, and think critically. At a global level, *literacy* is defined as "the ability to identify, understand, interpret, create, communicate, compute, and use printed and written materials associated with varying contexts. Literacy involves a continuum of learning, enabling individuals to achieve their goals, to develop their knowledge and potential, and to participate fully in their community and wider society" (UNESCO, 2005, p. 21).

In 2003, the National Assessment of Adult Literacy (NAAL) examined three types of literacy: (1) prose literacy; (2) document literacy; and (3) quantitative literacy (Kutner et al., 2007). Prose literacy deals with whole works, such as articles and book chapters, while document literacy deals with parts of texts, such as maps and tables. Surveying over 19,000 adults, the NAAL found that only 13% of adults surveyed had proficient skills in all three areas of literacy. Approximately 40% of adults had below basic or basic prose literacy, a third of the adults had below basic or basic document literacy, and a little over half of adults surveyed had basic or basic quantitative literacy (Kutner et al., 2007).

Information Literacy

In academic settings, an important component of research skills revolves around information literacy. Information literacy focuses on the user's (1) ability to recognize when information is needed; (2) ability to locate the needed information; (3) ability to evaluate the suitability of retrieved information; and (4) ability to effectively and appropriately use the needed information (Association of College and Research Libraries, 2000). However, today's researchers need to have a range of skills: (1) determining the nature and extent of the information needed; (2) using information effectively to accomplish a specific purpose; (3) solving problem scenarios; and (4) answering data-based questions. To do so requires proficiency in a number of competency standards, from theoretical and philosophical concepts to mastering methodologies. Compounding requisite skill sets is the inevitable need to judge the reliability and validity of information as well as the evaluation of current and emergent technologies in the research process.

Shapiro and Hughes (1996) suggested that there are additional literacies necessary to succeed as a researcher. These include literacies in the context of information in academia (such as the import of discipline and scholarly publications). Social-structural literacy, research literacy, and publishing literacy address how information is socially situated and produced, how tools are used to conduct research, and the processes of publication and production of research results. Tool and resource literacy is the ability to use print and electronic resources and software and to understand their form, format, and access issues. Finally, there are emerging technology literacy and critical literacy, which address the adaptation, adoption, and evaluation of information technology in terms of their intellectual and social capital and their benefits and costs (Shapiro & Hughes, 1996).

Technology Literacy

The intensive computational and technology skills sets necessary to work with data today require additional approaches to literacy. Bloom's taxonomy of learning domains, a standard in education, addresses how individuals learn. The three domains are (1) cognitive (mental skills or knowledge); (2) affective (feelings or attitudes); and (3) psychomotor (manual or physical ability or skills) ([1956] 1984). When working with technology, all three domains play a critical part in identifying elements of competencies. For example, in the cognitive domain, Bloom suggests that there are six attendant processes or behaviors: (1) knowledge; (2) comprehension; (3) application; (4) analysis; (5) synthesis; and (6) evaluation (1984, 1956), which play a critical role in how we learn.

Using Bloom's processes, Vitolo and Coulston (2002) created a "competency taxonomy" to address the analytical and model-based reasoning processes used by researchers (see Table 9.1). They mapped the six levels of the educational objectives of Bloom's taxonomy ([1956] 1984) to the five fundamental units of information systems (Shelly, Cashman, & Rosenblatt, 1998). Devised to express educational objectives ("intended behaviors which the student shall display at the end of some period of education"; Bloom, 1984, p. 16), Vitolo and Coulston tied Bloom's taxonomy to larger information literacy competencies, for example, "intended behaviors *in the context of information literacy* which the student shall display at the end of some period of education" (Vitolo and Coulston, p. 46).

In the context of mental health informatics, understanding these elements framed across knowledge, skills, and attitudes allows us to work from and across macro-, meso-, and micro-levels of how information and processes intersect.

This method of looking at skills and competencies makes sense in a statistically intensive, computing-intensive, and quickly evolving field such as mental health services research and services delivery. The evolution of the national health information infrastructure will require clinicians and academicians to address multi-institutional standards and the dynamic nature of health and mental health information, since public health and mental health data are large, interconnected databases of statistics, surveillance, and survey data, with high-resolution images, textual data sets, and complicated decision-making algorithms.

TABLE 9.1

The "Information Literacy Competency" Taxonomy

	Knowledge	Comprehension	Application	Analysis	Synthesis	Evaluation
Hardware	What are the hardware components of a system?	What do the components of a hardware system do?	When would the hardware suit my needs?	How does this piece of hardware work?	How would I build this hardware?	What improves hardware design?
Software	What are the software components of a system?	What is the role of software is in a system?	When would the software fit the situation?	How does this software work?	How would I build this software?	What conditions produce quality software?
Data	Where can I get data?	What does this data mean?	When would I use this data?	How is this data interpreted?	How do I appropriately gather the data?	What factors increase the value and reliability of data?
Procedure	What actions can be taken?	What is the purpose of an action?	When would an action occur?	What are the steps of the action?	How would I define the steps of the action?	Which aspects of an action are necessary and which are sufficient?
People	Who are the stakeholders?	What are the roles and relationships of individuals in a situation?	When should an individual become involved?	How is the person responding?	How can the individuals have their responses changed?	What significance does an individual have to the progress of a system?

Reprinted with permission of publisher. Vitolo, T. M. & Coulston, C. (2002). Taxonomy of information literacy competencies. *Journal of Information Technology Education, 1*(1), 43–51. Retrieved from http://jite.org/documents/Vol1/v1n1p043–052.pdf.

Statistical (Quantitative) Literacy

Another important element of research competency is quantitative literacy or numeracy. Numeracy is the ability to work effectively with numbers and other mathematical concepts and theories. Statistical literacy has "the ability to read and interpret summary statistics in the everyday media: in graphs; tables; statements; surveys; and studies" (Bidgood, Hunt, & Jolliffe, 2010, p. 135).

Schield (2008) notes that approximately 40% of college graduates are in a non-quantitative major. These students need to understand percentages and ratios, which are common mathematical constructs in policy making, politics, journalism, and law. Lutsky (2008) suggested that students and researchers more effectively incorporate quantitative reasoning into their work. For the student, this would create a more comfortable and productive environment for students in support of their work.

Just as with the other forms of literacy, the context (how it will be used), content (necessary knowledge), and cognitive/affective processes (such as adaptive reasoning, which links content and context, and procedural fluency) are key components of quantitative literacy (Ginsburg, Manly, & Schmitt, 2006) and create research competencies.

Health Services Research Competencies

As an example, health services research is an integrative, interdisciplinary field, utilizing basic and applied research to examine the "use, costs, quality, accountability, delivery, organization, financing and outcomes of health care services" for both populations and individuals (Field, Tranquada, & Feasley, 1995, p. 3). These actions would thereby "increase knowledge and understanding of the structure, processes, and effects of health services for individuals and populations" (p. 3). The inclusion of knowledge and understanding as an outcome for health services research ties new knowledge to the analytical process: to conduct, interpret, and apply empirical research, thereby incorporating a systemic perspective of "moving" research to practice.

To determine competencies for health services researchers, we need to understand who works in health services research. From a discipline-based perspective, the list is very broad: "biostatistics, clinical sciences, economics, epidemiology, political science, psychology, sociology, and statistics …. actuarial science, anthropology, decision theory, demography, engineering, ethics, finance, gerontology, geography, health education, history, law, marketing, medical informatics, nutrition, operations research, and pharmacy" (Thaul, Lohr, & Tranquada, 1994). However, since health services research is inter- and transdisciplinary, the question becomes: What competencies best apply? Let's start with a look at interdisciplinary competencies.

INTERDISCIPLINARY RESEARCH COMPETENCIES

Interdisciplinary research is seen as the standard rather than the exception, since health services and health policy research are inextricably entwined within and across multiple disciplines. The National Institutes of Health's *Roadmap* (n.d.) describes interdisciplinary research as an area that "integrates the analytical strengths of two or more often disparate scientific disciplines to solve a given biological problem"; by doing so, it eliminates "traditional gaps in terminology, approach, and methodology" (para. 10). Using theoretical frameworks from multiple disciplines, interdisciplinary research seamlessly integrates study designs, methodologies, perspectives, and skills of those disciplines throughout the research process (Aboelela et al., 2007). This definition was the foundation of an interdisciplinary competencies document created to allow an individual researcher to move successfully from discipline-based work to successful participation in interdisciplinary work. Aboelela et al. (2007) also identified three key characteristics of interdisciplinary research: "the qualitative mode of research (and its theoretical underpinnings), existence of a continuum of synthesis among disciplines, and the desired outcome of the interdisciplinary research" (p. 329). In their systematic review of the literature, only 11 papers provided an explicit definition of interdisciplinarity and only 5 papers provided a conceptual framework.

Gebbie et al. (2008) observed that knowledge alone is not a sufficient measure of ability; a combination of knowledge, skills, and attitude comprises competency. In their Delphi study, 27 scholars from medicine, health sciences, public health, environmental sciences, natural sciences, and social sciences participated. The group developed 17 interdisciplinary research competencies grouped across three domains: (1) conduct research (5 competencies); (2) communicate (7 competencies); and (3) interact with others (5 competencies). The competencies are defined broadly to best work across disciplines.

Under the conduct of research, for example, a scholar who has completed doctoral work should be able to "use theories and methods of multiple disciplines in developing integrated theoretical and research frameworks" and to "integrate concepts and methods from multiple disciplines in designing interdisciplinary research protocols" (p. 69). In addition, he or she should be able to use a multidisciplinary lens when examining hypotheses, to work collaboratively to obtain funding with scholars from other disciplines, and to disseminate the results of interdisciplinary research across and within disciplines.

Since these competencies are non-discipline-specific, they can be used as preliminary competencies in pre- and post-doctoral training programs, as well as in the development of research agendas and enhancing academic/scholarly careers. Gebbie and colleagues (2008) also caution that there should be a periodic review conducted every two to three years due to the rapidly evolving nature of interdisciplinary research. However, in these competencies, there is no explicit mention of technology or informatics as part of research competencies. Rather, it is implied through words (methods, training) and domains (communicate).

PUBLIC HEALTH COMPETENCIES: TWO PERSPECTIVES

Since the interdisciplinary research competencies above primarily addressed scholars, in this section we will examine research competencies for public health professionals.

The *Core Competencies for Public Health Practitioners* were developed by the Council on Linkages Between Academia and Public Health Practice (Council on Linkages, 2001). The *Competencies* served dual purposes: addressing the competencies needed by public health organizations as well as academic and practice organizations. The competencies cover the following domains: (1) Analytic/Assessment Skills; (2) Policy Development/ Program Planning Skills; (3) Communication Skills; (4) Cultural Competency Skills;

(5) Community Dimensions of Practice Skills; (6) Public Health Sciences Skills; (7) Financial Planning and Management Skills; and (8) Leadership and Systems Thinking Skills. Competencies were listed under each domain, broken out by tiers: non-management entry-level public health professionals (tier 1); individuals with program management and/ or supervisory responsibilities (Tier 2); and senior managers and/or leaders of public health organizations (Tier 3).

In 2002, informatics competencies were created for public health professionals as a complement to the *Core Competencies*. The Public Health Informatics Competencies Working Group defined public health informatics competency as "a public health worker's observable or measurable performance, skill, or knowledge related to the systematic application of information and computer science and technology to public health," (O'Carroll, 2002, p. 7). Using the tiered workforce model created by the Council on Linkages, the Working Group addressed three classes of competencies: (1) the use of information per se; (2) the use of IT to increase one's personal and professional effectiveness; and (3) the management of IT projects to improve the effectiveness of public health from a systemic perspective (O'Carroll, 2002). Not only did the Working Group consider that these competencies should be applicable to the developing world, they clearly stated that clinical informatics competencies were not in the scope of its document.

The Working Group added a competency to the Council on Linkages' list of core competencies (see Table 9.2). To the first class of "the use of information per se," it added "the systematic management of public health information as a key strategic resource of a public health organization" (O'Carroll, 2002, p. 11).

Linked to each domain are specific competencies. Some domains are limited to a single competency, others are linked to more than one. To review research competencies, one would need to closely examine each domain. For example, under Class 1 in the domain of Analytic/Assessment Skills, competency 1 requires an understanding of quantitative and qualitative data, which ties into the need for literacy in understanding text and numbers. In addition, understanding qualitative and quantitative data are found in several other areas, such as Policy Development & Program Planning (Class 1 domain), in the interpretation, analysis, and decision making in health planning, Information and Knowledge Development (Class 2 domain) to support decision making, and in Research (Class 3 domain), in the monitoring and application of research findings to improve public health practice. To do so requires the public health professional to have an integrative literacy, that is, to comprehend how numbers substantiate an understanding of a policy or population in policy development or in resource allocation (Lutsky, 2008).

The rapid evolution of information technology as a discipline resulted in another review of informatics competencies for public health professionals in 2009. Input was requested from members of the Centers for Disease Control and Prevention (CDC) Public Health Information Network, American Medical Informatics Association, and major public health professional associations. However, unlike the 2002 competencies, which were created for public health professionals working with informatics, this set of competencies was developed specifically for public health informaticians (PHIs). PHIs are defined as "persons with a core identity and expertise in informatics" (Centers for Disease Control and Prevention, CDC, 2009, p. 4) and whose roles are "more expert in informatics than a

TABLE 9.2

2002 Public Health Informatics Competencies for Public Health Professionals

Class 1. Effective Use of INFORMATION Domains/Competencies		Class 2: Effective Use of INFORMATION TECHNOLOGY Domains/Competencies		Class 3: Effective Management of IT PROJECTS Domains/Competencies	
Analytic/Assessment Skills	1–8	Digital literacy	1	System development	1–3
Policy Development & Program Planning Skills	9–10	Electronic communications	2	Cross-disciplinary communication	4
Communication Skills	11–13	Selection and use of IT tools	3	Databases	5
Community Dimensions of Practice Skills	14	On-line information utilization	4	Standards	6
Public Health Sciences Skills	15–19	Data and system protection	5–6	Confidentiality & security systems	7
Financial Planning and Management Skills	20–21	Distance learning	7	Project management	8
Leadership and Systems Thinking Skills	23–24	Strategic use of IT to promote health	8	Human resources management	9
		Information and knowledge development	9	Procurement	10
				Accountability	11
				Research	12

Adapted from http://www.nwcphp.org/resources/informatics/phI_print.pdf [Public domain document].

highly functional public health professional who assists with informatics-related challenges or supports personal productivity with IT" (p. 6). Competency in public health informatics was defined as a "public health worker's observable or measurable performance, knowledge, skills, and abilities to organize information and use it for public health purposes, leveraging technology within the public health setting" (p. 19). Thirteen specific competencies provide the foundation "to understand how information systems can improve the practice and science of public health while contributing to the evidence-based practice of public health informatics" (CDC, 2009, p. 11). As with the 2002 document, there is still the need for the PHI to understand qualitative and quantitative data, as shown in Table 9.3, cells I-2f and I-3a.

There were several significant differences between the 2002 and the 2009 reports. First, the 2009 Work Group created a new domain to add to the Council of Linkages original eight domains. The additional domain focused completely on public health informatics competencies. Second, the Work Group created a working definition for the term public health informatician (PHI). Third, the Work group did not specifically map the competencies to the 2001 Council on Linkages eight domains. Instead of mapping the competencies, the Work Group created a list of competencies, further sub-divided into two levels (e.g., A.1.a.). Fourth, the Work Group created a two-tier personnel model, broken out as PHIs and senior PHIs. A PHI may be a project or program manager responsible for operations and maintenance, or a researcher responsible for developing information systems or methodologies. A senior PHI may be a policy adviser or administrator at the highest levels within an agency or organization responsible for strategic planning or implementation of IT projects or systems. Fifth, the language used in the competencies differs significantly from the competencies for a more traditional IT professional. Since a PHI works within the broad discipline of public health, he or she is uniquely qualified to understand how IT can improve the practice and science of public health. Finally, as with all competencies, this set may be influenced by competencies within other disciplines that influence public health as well as the broader research agenda on public health. Hence, these competencies should be viewed as an evolving document.

TABLE 9.3

Competencies for Public Health Informaticians

A. Supports development of strategic direction
    for public health informatics within the
    enterprise.
B. Participates in development of knowledge
    management tools for the enterprise.
C. Uses informatics standards.
D. Ensures that knowledge, information, and
    data needs of project or program users and
    stakeholders are met.
E. Supports information system development,
    procurement, and implementation that
    meet public health program needs.
    F1. Manages IT operations related to
        project or program (for public health
        agencies with internal IT operations).
    F2. Monitors IT operations managed by
        external organizations.
G. Communicates with cross-disciplinary
    leaders and team members.
H. Evaluates information systems and
    applications.

(continued)

TABLE 9.3

Competencies for Public Health Informaticians (*continued*)

I. Participates in applied public health informatics research for new insights and innovative solutions to health problems.

I-2. Supports applied informatics research to determine how IT can change and improve public health practice

I-2f. *Assists in analysis and synthesis of data*

J. Contributes to development of public health information systems that are interoperable with other relevant information systems.

I-3. Supports development of new insights into potential uses of public health informatics for programs

I-3a. *Assesses uses and value of different types of data to answer public health questions*

K. Supports use of informatics to integrate clinical health, environmental risk, and population health.

L. Implements solutions that ensure confidentiality, security, and integrity while maximizing availability of information for public health.

M. Conducts education and training in public health informatics.

Adapted from http://www.cdc.gov/informaticscompetencies/downloads/PHI_Competencies.pdf, p. 16. [Public domain document].

HEALTH SERVICES RESEARCH COMPETENCIES

So far, we have examined research competencies from an interdisciplinary perspective and from a dual perspective in a specific discipline. Since the "social and behavioral sciences deal with the most complex and the least predictable phenomena that affect the nation's health" (National Research Council, 2005, p. 36), by blurring the demarcations between health services research, health care management, and health policy, health services research is broadened as to discipline, foci, and competencies (Field, Tranquada, & Feasley, 1995), particularly in the use of informatics and clinical decision making. As the interdisciplinary research competencies were directed also toward graduates of doctoral programs, let us review the development of health services research competencies created for doctoral programs.

Health services research as a field has grown dramatically over the past half century. Unlike biomedical research, health services research addresses observational and quasi-experimental studies, comparative effectiveness studies, economic evaluations, financing and organizational decision making across a variety of settings using mixed methodologies. Knowledge and technology transfer is critical, as is the dissemination of applied research and knowledge translation. As shown in the previous examples, the process of creating a competencies document is critical to obtaining consensus. Forrest et al. (2009) conducted a review of the literature and a textual analysis of accreditation documents submitted to the Council on Education for Public Health to develop an initial draft of core competencies for health services research doctoral programs. The 2005 Consensus Conference defined competency as "knowledge or skill-based assets that doctoral trainees in [Health Services Research] HSR should acquire during their training; they are the common outcomes across all training programs. Core competencies help to define professional role expectations and are likely to be broader in scope than individual program competencies" (Forrest et al., 2009, para. 7). Participants created 14 broad knowledge- and skills-based competencies common to all health services professionals (see Table 9.4).

TABLE 9.4

2005 Consensus Conference Health Services Research Doctoral Core Competencies

#	Core Competency	Associated Learning Objective Content Areas
1	Demonstrate *breadth of HSR theoretical and conceptual knowledge* by applying alternative models from a range of relevant disciplines.	Biomedicine, Economics, Epidemiology, Informatics, Management Sciences, Political Science, Psychology, Sociology, Statistics
2	Apply *in-depth disciplinary knowledge and skills* relevant to health services research.	Variable depending on the discipline or interdisciplinary area of specialization
3	Apply knowledge of the structures, performance, quality, policy, and environmental context of health and health care to *formulate solutions for health policy problems.*	Access and Use, Financing of Health Care, Health, Health Economics, Health Policy, Organization of Health Care, Quality of Care
4	*Pose innovative and important health service research questions*, informed by systematic reviews of the literature, stakeholder needs, and relevant theoretical and conceptual models	Scientific Method and Theory, Literature Review, Proposal Development
5	*Select appropriate interventional, observational, or qualitative study designs* to address specific health services research questions.	Study Design for Interventions, Observational Study Design, Qualitative Research

(continued)

TABLE 9.4

2005 Consensus Conference Health Services Research Doctoral Core Competencies
(*continued*)

#	Core Competency	Associated Learning Objective Content Areas
6	Know how to *collect primary health and health care data* obtained by survey, qualitative, or mixed methods.	Survey Research, Qualitative Research, Primary Data Acquisition and Quality Control
7	Know how to *assemble secondary data* from existing public and private sources.	Health Informatics, HSR Data Sources, Secondary Data Acquisition and Quality Control
8	*Use conceptual models and operational measures* to specify study constructs for a health services research question and develop variables that reliably and validly measure these constructs.	Measurement Theory and Methods, Variable Construction
9	*Implement research protocols* with standardized procedures that ensure reproducibility of the science.	Research Management
10	*Ensure the ethical and responsible conduct of research* in the design, implementation, and dissemination of health services research.	Research Ethics
11	*Work collaboratively in multi-disciplinary teams.*	Teamwork
12	*Use appropriate analytical methods* to clarify associations between variables and to delineate causal inferences.	Advanced HSR Analytic Methods, Advanced Statistics, Economic Evaluation, Decision Sciences
13	*Effectively communicate the findings and implications of HSR* through multiple modalities to technical and lay audiences.	Proposal Development, Dissemination
14	*Understand the importance of collaborating with stakeholders*, such as policy makers, organizations, and communities to plan, conduct, and translate health services research into policy and practice.	Community Participatory Research, Translating research into practice and policy

Forrest, C. B., Martin, D. P., Holve. E., & Millman. A. (2009). Health services research doctoral core competencies. *BMC Health Services Research, 25*(9), 107. doi: 10.1186/1472–6963-9-107 [OPEN ACCESS] http://www.biomedcentral.com/1472–6963/9/107/table/T1.

Three years later, in 2008, a second consensus conference was convened. Health Services Research Competencies Conference (Martin, 2008) examined 38 health services research doctoral programs to update expected competencies for future professionals. Researchers used a number of methods to gather information: a review of the literature; text analyses of institutional accreditation self-studies submitted to the Council on Education for Public Health; and a consensus conference of health services research educators from U.S. educational institutions. After reviewing the data, the Conference determined that there were 11 core competencies (see Table 9.5). Four of these 11 competencies (Conceptual models and operational methods, #4; Data collection and management methods, #6; Data analysis, #8; and Knowledge transfer, #11) appear particularly relevant, especially with the increased emphasis on informatics as a key competency for health services research.

As one can see from Table 9.5, these are broad competencies that cross multiple disciplines. The emphasis is on creating competencies that can be adopted and adapted by academic programs and professional organizations to establish program evaluation, professional development, and to further the translation of research to practice, particularly in mental health.

BEHAVIORAL HEALTH COMPETENCIES

In 1995, a national consensus-building project was started to bring together numerous stakeholders to review and develop standards and competencies for services delivered to at-risk populations. Numerous professional groups also participated, including psychology, psychiatry, nursing, social work, counseling, and psychosocial rehabilitation. From the Behavioral Health Standards and Competencies Initiative, a series of competencies and guidelines were developed addressing the needs of adults and older adults with serious mental illnesses and/ or co-occurring disorders, as well as for specific racial and ethnic populations. Competency was defined as "attitudes, values, knowledge, and skills that staff need to deliver high quality services" (Adult Panel of the Managed Care Initiative, 1998, p. 3). This is a very different tenor for competencies than a focus only on research. It is important to note that several of the service competencies have applications to the translation of research to practice. Three of the competencies addressed the need to demonstrate "current knowledge of issues related to mental illness," "best practices of intervention," and "methods of evaluation" (p. 5).

In the summary report created on competencies for working with persons with co-occurring disorders, a section entitled "Provider Competencies for Dual Diagnosis Treatment in Managed Care Systems" addressed familiarity with an "integrated conceptual framework" for treatment, "principles of public sector managed care, and its implications for horizontal and vertical service integration and flexibility," "knowledge of basic utilization management guidelines for mental health, substance abuse, and comorbid disorders," as well as an "integrated longitudinal assessment" and methodologies (Co-Occurring Mental and Substance Disorders Panel, 1998, pp. 42–53) across the domains of attitudes, values, knowledge, and skills. Considering the interdisciplinary nature of services delivery in the public sector and the added complexities in treating comorbid disorders, the Panel advocated review and revision as "new concepts, new program models, and new research are emerging regularly" (p. 4). In addition, the Co-Occurring Mental and Substance Disorders Panel also created recommendations for curriculum, with a focus on clinical services.

TABLE 9.5

Health Services Research (HSR) Doctoral Level Core Competencies

Label	Competency
1. **Foundational knowledge**	Acquire knowledge of the context of health and health care systems, institutions, actors, and environment
2. **Theoretical knowledge**	Apply or develop theoretical and conceptual models relevant to health services research
3. **Relevant & important HSR question development**	Pose relevant and important research questions, evaluate them, and formulate solutions to health problems, practice and policy
4. **Conceptual models and operational methods**	Use or develop a conceptual model to specify study constructs for a health services research question and develop variables that reliably and validly measure these constructs
5. **Study designs**	Describe the strengths and weaknesses of study designs to appropriately address specific health services research questions
6. **Data collection and management methods**	Sample and collect primary health and health care data and/or assemble and manage existing data from public and private sources
7. **Research conduct management**	Execute and document procedures that ensure the reproducibility of the science, the responsible use of resources, the ethical treatment of research subjects
8. **Data analysis**	Demonstrate proficiency in the appropriate application of analytical techniques to evaluate HSR questions
9. **Professional development**	Work collaboratively in teams within disciplines, across disciplines, and/or with stakeholders
10. **Communication**	Effectively communicate the process, findings, and implications of health services research through multiple modalities with stakeholders
11. **Knowledge transfer**	Knowledge translation to policy and practice

Adapted from Table 4. Health Services Research (HSR) Doctoral Level Core Competencies. Retrieved from http://www.ahrq.gov/fund/training/hsrcompo8tab4.htm.

In 2001, the Annapolis Coalition convened a national conference to determine the effectiveness and relevance of the education of mental health and substance abuse treatment professionals. Over the next three years, the Coalition enlisted the support of experts to create position papers and recommendations for review at the next conference. In 2004, the Coalition made a number of recommendations. The Coalition defined the behavioral health workforce as providers within the formal behavioral health system, the general and specialty health care system and human service system, and persons with mental health and substance use disorders and their families. The latter group was included due to the emphasis on self-care and peer support. The Coalition recommended the identification and assessment of competencies in behavioral health, achieving "reliability and validity through the use of established methods of competency development" (Hoge et al., 2005, pp. 654). The Coalition further delineated competencies as core (common to a discipline or organization), job family competencies, and tiered-level competencies (direct care, supervisory, program administration). In addition, the Coalition recommended that organizational competencies be determined at the team, organization, and system level. All of these competencies again lead to improving the translation of research to practice.

TRANSLATIONAL RESEARCH COMPETENCIES

Translational research is an important component of health services research design and analysis. It provides the knowledge base to move scientific discoveries from clinical or population studies into clinical applications in real-world settings. However, an important aspect of this translational approach is the implementation of these studies in the community (2001).

Funded by the National Center for Research Resources within the National Institutes of Health, the Clinical and Translational Science Awards (CTSAs) program used the parameters from the *NIH Roadmap for Medical Research* (Zerhouni, 2003) to create competencies for moving research to practice. Based upon input from 15 working groups, three themes were developed: (1) "new pathways to discovery," which addresses technologies and approaches necessary to meet contemporary research challenges; (2) "research teams for the future," which looks at new ways of combining skills and disciplines; and (3) "re-engineering the clinical research enterprise," which seeks to create new partnerships among patient, community, and academic communities. This is achieved with new clinical protocols, innovative use of information technologies to provide and document care, and enhancements to workforce development.

There are 14 domains of 91 core competencies addressing clinical and translational research (Clinical and Translational Science Awards, 2009). The transition from research to practice requires an emphasis on clinical skills that can be placed within a translational framework. Hence, similar to the other competencies discussed in this chapter, each domain has specific competencies (Table 9.6).

TABLE 9.6

Clinical and Translational Research Questions

1. Clinical and translational research questions (7)	6. Statistical approaches (10)	11. Translational teamwork (7)
2. Literature critique (7)	7. Biomedical informatics (9)	12. Leadership (5)
3. Study design (9)	8. Responsible conduct of research (ethics: 9; conduct: 8)	13. Cross disciplinary training (4)
4. Research implementation (4)	9. Scientific communication (5)	14. Community Engagement (5)
5. Sources of error (7)	10. Cultural diversity (5)	

Adapted from Core Competencies in Clinical and Translational Research. http://www.ctsaweb.org/uploadedfiles/Core%20Competencies_Posting_July%2009.pdf.

Helfland et al. (2011) made the case for incorporating a patient-centered comparative effectiveness research (CER) perspective into clinical and translational research. They argue that the NIH should "accelerate the development and refinement of methods for CER by linking a program of methods research to the broader portfolio of large, prospective clinical and health system studies it supports" (p. 188).

COMPARATIVE EFFECTIVENESS RESEARCH

CER examines cost efficacy and cost effectiveness in a given population. The purpose of CER is to improve health outcomes by developing and disseminating evidence-based information. To determine which interventions are most effective for which patients under specific circumstances, CER compares the benefits and harms of different interventions in "real world" settings (National Research Council, 2011). This is a necessary complement since clinical research does not address issues such as generalizability, cost, or implementation practice.

In 2008, the Institute of Medicine Roundtable on Value & Science Driven Health Care examined the infrastructure necessary to implement and coordinate CER in U.S. health care (Olsen, Grossman, & McGinnis, 2011). One of the goals of the Roundtable was to have 90% of clinical decision making supported by evidence-based practice. Additional goals addressed bridging technology and practice, keeping pace with health information technology, and creating a trained workforce. To do so will require creating hardware, analytic tools and methods, workforce training, effective workflow processes, and strategic implementation. Participants emphasized a need for multidisciplinary training so researchers have knowledge and skills in numerous methodologies for use in clinical trials, observational studies, and syntheses.

In 2009, the IOM indicated its national priority areas for CER: health care delivery systems; racial and ethnic disparities; functional limitations and disabilities; psychiatric disorders; alcoholism, drug dependency, and overdose; birth and developmental disorders; neurologic disorders; geriatrics; women's health; emergency and critical care medicine; and complementary and alternative medicine. There were also a number of other physical disorders included as national priorities for CER (Committee on Comparative Effectiveness Research Prioritization, 2009).

The IOM also recommended 14 research priorities by types of intervention (Committee on Comparative Effectiveness Research Prioritization, 2009). Of those 14, systems of care, standard of care, behavioral treatment, treatment pathways, and prevention are important from a behavioral health perspective. Four recommendations were made for research study methodologies: (1) randomized trials; (2) prospective observational studies; (3) database research; and (4) systematic reviews.

The final list of 100 priority topics was divided into quartiles (Committee on Comparative Effectiveness Research, 2009). We are most interested in the list from an integrative CER/behavioral health perspective. Health care delivery services, wraparound home, community-based services, and residential treatment for treating children with serious emotional disturbances were in the first quartile. In addition, health care delivery systems also include the use of the electronic health record, provider and patient decision support tools, informed consent, medication adherence, and disease management.

This mirrors federal and consortia initiatives found in *Healthy People*, the National Quality Forum, and the Cochrane Collaborative.

Autism spectrum disorders, early childhood interventions (0 to 3 years of age), transition support services, different residential settings for adults with functional limitations, major depressive disorders in adults and adolescents, and coordinated long-term and end-of-life care for the elderly were listed in the next (2nd quartile). Increasing health care professionals' use of electronic health reports (EHR) and evidence-based practice (EBP); disease prevention, acute and chronic disease care, and rehabilitation services; and management strategies following suicide attempts were found in the third quartile. Care coordination for children with special needs, alternative behavioral interventions for children and adults, integrating primary and specialty psychiatric care to reduce early mortality and comorbidity among people with persistent and serious mental illnesses, and co-location of primary and specialty care on improving outcomes for persons with mental and physical disabilities or functioning were relevant for behavioral health and were listed in the fourth quartile (Committee on Comparative Effectives Research, 2009). It is important to note that (1) there are elements across quartiles that address behavioral health concerns; and (2) quartile rank does not indicate a lesser emphasis on a population or disorder. The quartiles were a way of classifying "like" or similar priority areas together. This list clearly shows the interdisciplinary and complex nature of comparative effectiveness research in health services.

In 2011, the Workgroup on Education, Training, and Workforce Development approached competencies based upon classes of individuals who worked "within" the CER workforce or "outside" the workforce. Those individuals who were within the CER workforce actually conduct CER (investigators, technical staff, and knowledge translators). Those individuals "outside" the workforce work in translational areas ranging from knowledge discovery to health outcomes (empirical investigators, patient and clinician participants, and stakeholders).

Based upon these classes, the Workgroup defined competencies as "the knowledge and skills that workers need to perform their work well. Competencies are ideally stated in behavioral terms and framed as something that is measureable" (p. 5). The Workgroup created 27 competencies and categorized them in five domains:

1. Asks relevant research questions;
2. Recognizes or designs ideal CER studies;
3. Executes or uses CER studies;
4. Uses appropriate statistical analyses for CER; and
5. Communicates and disseminates study results to allow for implementation of the results of research (p. [7–8]).

To evaluate an individual, each of the areas is subdivided into functional and applied task-oriented competencies. For example, under competency 1, "Asks relevant research questions," one of the *foundational* tasks is "Seeks and identifies strong evidence for decision-making." This can be measured in terms of an individual's skills at finding relevant CER studies in the literature to use in his or her clinical decision making. In addition, there are two *applied* tasks: "Phrases questions about health care delivery as key questions for comparative effectiveness research" and "Phrases questions about prevention, screening and diagnosis, in addition to treatment, appropriately as comparative effectiveness question" (p.7). By creating large conceptual domains, then subdividing the domains into theoretical and applied skills, levels of competencies can be concretized and evaluated.

Implications for Mental Health Informatics

The National Research Council (2011) sees health services research as key to documenting deficiencies in patient and population health, in the provision of health services, and in identifying factors that contribute to these deficiencies. Translational and implementation research, two additional areas identified in the report, provide the knowledge base to move clinical research to clinical practice and to effectively adapt clinical research to real-world practice settings. Meeting the challenge of translational research draws upon "marketing research, adult learning, and real-time decision support technologies" (National Research Council, 2005, p. 79).

Integrating data and technology can provide real benefits to both the researcher and the community. It could foster interaction among the various governance boards or departments within a municipality in the quality and depth of their own data needs and requirements. It would be economical over the long run and, more important, would show the true inter- and multidisciplinary nature of local problems and issues. In addition, the rapid and continuous change in how we use health information "will result in the translation and implementation processes being continual and not one-time or infrequent events." This may require "fundamental re-thinking of information flow and how it supports all aspects of health services" (National Research Council, 2011, p. 103).

As with the implementation of any research competencies, it is critical that they show rigor and applicability to the field. Edgar, Mayer, and Scharff (2009) describe their study in which they examined the validity and reliability of the Core Competencies for Public Health Professionals, as promulgated by the Council on Linkages Between Academia and Public Health (COL). Using principal component analysis, correlation, reliability analysis, and known-groups comparisons, they recommended a 65-item, eight-factor framework that corresponds with the eight COL domains. More studies, such as these, continue to support the evidence- and practice bases for competencies in health services research.

References

Aboelela, S. W., Larson, E., Bakken, S., Carrasquillo, O., Formicola, A., Glied, S. A., Haas, J., & Gebbie, K. M. (2007). Defining interdisciplinary research: Conclusions from a critical review of the literature. *Health Services Research, 42*(1 Pt 1), 329–346. Retrieved from http://www.ncbi.nlm.nih.gov/pmc/articles/PMC1955232/?tool=pubmed.

Adult Panel of the Managed Care Initiative. (1998). *Competencies for direct service staff who work with adults with serious mental illness in public health/managed care systems.* University of Pennsylvania Health System, Center for Mental Health Policy and Services Research. Retrieved from http://www.med.upenn.edu/cmhpsr/documents/AdultCompetenciesSet1. PDF.

Association of College and Research Libraries. (2000). *Information literacy competency standards for higher education*. Chicago, IL: ACRL. Retrieved from http://www.ala.org/acrl/standards/informationliteracycompetency.

Bidgood, P., Hunt, N., & Jolliffe, F. (2010). Assessing statistical literacy: Take CARE. In M. Schield (Ed.), *Assessment methods in statistical education* (pp. 133–152). New York: Wiley.

Bloom, B. S. (1984). *Taxonomy of educational objectives. Handbook 1: Cognitive domain*. New York: Longman.

Board on Health Care Services, Institute of Medicine. (2003). *Health professions education: A bridge to quality*. Washington, DC: National Academies Press. Retrieved from http://www.nap.edu/catalog/10681.html.

Centers for Disease Control and Prevention. (2009). *Competencies for public health informaticians 2009*. Atlanta, GA: CDC. Retrieved from http://www.cdc.gov/informaticscompetencies/downloads/PHI_Competencies.pdf.Clinical and Translational Science Awards. (2009). *Core competencies in clinical and translational research: Draft*. Retrieved from http://www.ctsaweb.org/uploadedfiles/Core%20Competencies_Posting_July%202009.pdf.

Committee on Comparative Effectiveness Research Prioritization. (2009). *Initial national priorities for comparative effectiveness research June 30 2009*. Washington, DC: National Academies Press. Retrieved from http://www.nap.edu/catalog.php?record_id=12648.

Co-Occurring Mental and Substance Disorders Panel. (1998). *Co-occurring psychiatric and substance disorders in managed care systems: Standards of care, practice guidelines, workforce competencies, and training curricula*. University of Pennsylvania Center for Mental Health Services Managed Care Initiative. Retrieved from http://www.med.upenn.edu/cmhpsr/documents/Coocurring_MH_DA_Panel_Report.pdf.

Council on Linkages Between Academia and Public Health Practice (2001). *Core competencies for public health practitioners*. Washington, DC: Public Health Foundation.

Edgar, M., Mayer, J. P., & Scharff, D. P. (2009). Construct validity of the core competencies for public health professionals. *Journal of Public Health Management Practice, 15*(4), E7-E16.

Field, M. J., Tranquada, R. E., & Feasley, J. C. (1995). *Health services research: Work force and educational issues*. Washington, DC: National Academy Press. Retrieved from http://www.nap.edu/catalog.php?record_id=5020.

Forrest, C. B., Martin, D. P., Holve. E., & Millman. A. (2009). Health services research doctoral core competencies. *BMC Health Services Research, 25*(9), 107. doi: 10.1186/1472-6963-9-107.

Gebbie, K. M., Meier, B. M., Bakken, S., Carrasquillo, O., Formicola, A., Aboelela, S. W., Glied, S., & Larson, E. (2008). Training for interdisciplinary health research: Defining the required competencies. *Journal of Allied Health, 37*(2), 65–70.

Ginsburg, L., Manly, M., & Schmitt, M. J. (2006). *The components of numeracy* [NCSALL Occasional Paper]. Cambridge, MA: National Center for Study of Adult Literacy and Learning. Retrieved from http://www.ncsall.net/fileadmin/resources/research/op_numeracy.pdf.

Heinström, J. (2006). Broad exploration or precise specificity: Two basic information seeking patterns among students. *Journal of the American Society for Information Science and Technology, 57*(11), 1440–1450.

Helfand, M, Tunis, S., Whitlock, E. P., Pauker, S. G., Basu, A., Chilingerian, J., … & Kent D. M. (2011). A CTSA agenda to advance methods for comparative effectiveness research. *Clinical & Translational Science, 4* (3), 188–198. doi: 10.1111/j.1752-8062.2011.00282.x.

Hoge, M. A., Morris, J. A., Daniels, A. S., Huey, L. Y., Stuart, G. W., Adams, N., ... & Dodge, J. M. (2005). Report of recommendations: The Annapolis Coalition Conference on Behavioral Health Work Force Competencies. *Administration and Policy in Mental Health, 32*(5), 651–663. doi: 10.1007/s10488-005-3267-x.

Ingwersen, P. (1992). *Information retrieval interaction*. London: Taylor Graham. Retrieved November 2006 from http://comminfo.rutgers.edu/~muresan/614_IR/2004_Fall/Resources/OnlineBooks/Ingwersen_IRI/Ingwersen_IRI.pdf.

Ingwersen, P. (1996). Cognitive perspectives of information retrieval interaction: Elements of a cognitive IR theory. *Journal of Documentation, 52*(1), 3–50.

Järvelin, K., & Wilson, T. D. (2003). On conceptual models for information seeking and retrieval research. *Information Research: An International Electronic Journal, 9*(1), Article No.163. Retrieved November 2006 from http://informationr.net/ir/9-1/paper163.html.

Kutner, M. Greenberg, E., Jin, Y., Boyle, B., Hsu, Y-C, & Dunleavy, E. (2007). *Literacy in everyday life: Results from the 2003 National Assessment of Adult Literacy* (NCES Number: 2007480). Washington, DC: National Center for Education Statistics.

Lutsky, N. (2008). Arguing with numbers: A rationale and suggestions for teaching quantitative reasoning through argument and writing. In B. L. Madison & L. A. Steen (Eds.), *Calculation vs. context: Quantitative literacy and its implications for teacher education* (pp. 59–74). Washington, DC: Mathematical Association of America.

Martin, D. (2008). *Health services research core competencies: Final report*. Rockville, MD: Agency for Healthcare Research and Quality. Retrieved from http://www.ahrq.gov/fund/training/hsrcompo8.htm

National Institutes of Health. (n.d.). "NIH Roadmap for Medical Research" released. Retrieved from http://www.cossa.org/NIH/nihroadmap.htm.

National Research Council. (2005). *Advancing the nation's health needs*. Washington, DC: National Academies Press. Retrieved from http://grants.nih.gov/training/nas_report_2005.pdf.

National Research Council. (2011). *Research training in the biomedical, behavioral, and clinical research sciences*. Washington, DC: National Academies Press. Retrieved from http://www.nap.edu/catalog.php?record_id=12983.

O'Carroll, P. W. (2002). *Public Health Informatics Competency Working Group: Informatics competencies for public health professionals*. Seattle, WA: Northwest Center for Public Health Practice; 2002.

Olsen, L., Grossman, C., & McGinnis, J. M. (2011). *Learning what works: Infrastructure required for comparative effectiveness research: Workshop summary*. Washington, DC: National Academies Press. Retrieved from http://www.nap.edu/openbook.php?record_id=12214.

Palmer, C. L. (2005). Scholarly work and the shaping of digital access. *Journal of the American Society for Information Science and Technology, 56*(11), 1140–1153.

Schield, M. (2008). Quantitative literacy and school mathematics: Percentages and fractions. In B. L. Madison & L. A. Steen (Eds.), *Calculation vs. context: Quantitative literacy and its implications for teacher education* (pp. 87–107). Washington, DC: Mathematical Association of America.Shapiro, J. J., & Hughes, S. K. (1996). Information literacy as a liberal art: Enlightenment proposals fora new curriculum. *Educom Review 31*(2)[HTML]. Retrieved from http://www.educause.edu/pub/er/review/reviewarticles/31231.html

Shelly, G. B., Cashman, T. J., & Rosenblatt, H. J. (1998). *Systems analysis and design,* 3rd ed. Cambridge, MA: Course Technology.

Thaul, S., Lohr, K., & Tranquada, R. E. (1994). *Health services research: Opportunities for an expanding field of inquiry: An interim statement.* Washington, DC: National Academies Press, Institute of Medicine. Retrieved from http://http://www.nap.edu/openbook.php?record_id=9242.

UNESCO. (2005). *Aspects of literacy assessment: Topics and issues from the UNESCO Expert Meeting, 10–12 June, 2003.* Paris: UNESCO.

Vitolo, T. M., & Coulston, C. (2002). Taxonomy of information literacy competencies. *Journal of Information Technology Education, 1*(1), 43–51. Retrieved from 01/12/02 from http://jite.org/documents/Vol1/v1n1p043–052.pdf.

Workgroup on Education, Training, and Workforce Development for the Clinical and Translational Science Awards Consortium Key Function Committee for Comparative Effectiveness Research. (2011). *Competencies and workforce development for comparative effectiveness research.* Retrieved from http://www.ctsaweb.org/uploadedfiles/Text_CER_6_23_11.pdf.

Zerhouni, E. (2003). The NIH Roadmap. *Science, 302,* 63–72. Retrieved from http://www.sciencemag.org/site/feature/plus/nihroadmap.pdf.

A graphic representation of data abstracted from the banks of every computer in the human system. Unthinkable complexity. Lines of light ranged in the nonspace of the mind, clusters and constellations of data. Like city lights, receding.

—WILLIAM GIBSON, 1984, p. 69

10 Types of Data

In *A Mapmaker's Dream*, Fra Mauro, a fictional sixteenth-century Viennese cartographer, attempts to create a *mappa mundi*, a perfect map of the world without ever leaving his monk's cell (Cowan, 2007). Similarly, today's online environment allows a researcher to create a *mappa mundi* from his or her desktop by (re)-constructing the world based upon many types of information from a multitude of resources, including online, print, spatial, numeric, and media. This requires researchers to have expertise in a variety of data applications and databases, as well as how to map and navigate their way across often "uncharted seas" of information. This chapter will examine the types of data used in mental health services and research from an informatics perspective, the types of databases most commonly used in research, and the types of research studies that may be encountered. The chapter then examines how data establishes future research priorities, and concludes with implications for mental health informatics.

Types of Data

There are many types of data used in mental health informatics. There is primary data, which is "raw" or original data. Numeric and spatial data sets, electronic health information, and interviews are primary data. Secondary data are analyses run on primary data, which are often formatted or preselected into tables, charts, figures, spreadsheets, coded data, or maps. A report, which synthesizes raw data into a list of neighborhood strengths and weaknesses, is an example of secondary data. The Centers for Disease Control and Prevention's (CDC's) Web-Based Injury Statistics Query and Reporting System (WISQARS™)

TABLE 10.1

Primary, Secondary, and Tertiary Data Flow Chart

Primary data	Secondary data			Intent Self Harm	Tertiary data
WISQARS™ http://wisqars.cdc.gov	Hospitalizations and	Type of Cost Mechanism			2009 *Community Health Scan* Report http://www.flhsa.org/Community%20Health%20Scan.pdf
		# Hospitalized	—	250222	
		Medical Cost	Average	$8183	
			Total	$2,047,479,000	
	All Mechanisms of Injury	Work Loss Cost	Average	$14,102	
			Total	$3,528,529,000	
		Combined Cost	Total	$22,284	
			Total	$5,576,008,000	

Secondary data section of table adapted from NonFatal Injuries, Hospitalizations, Both Sexes, All Ages, United States, 2005; Estimated Number of Nonfatal Injuries and Estimated Lifetime Costs Classified by Mechanism and Intent; Costs Expressed in Year 2005 United States Prices [http://wisqars.cdc.gov:8080/costT/].

mortality and morbidity database is an example of secondary data. For example, a summary report (secondary data) that can be created from the WISQARS™ site may then be further examined to generate a formal report in the Centers for Disease Control and Prevention's (CDC) publication entitled *Morbidity and Mortality Weekly* (*MMWR*) comparing nonfatal self-inflicted injuries among adults 65 years of age and older in the United States (CDC, 2005). Tertiary data are the synthesis of the numeric, health, spatial data, and secondary data, which is then re-purposed into specific contexts within mental health informatics. An example would be a 2009 *Community Health Scan* report by the Finger Lakes Health Systems Agency (2009, p. 89), which included the *MMWR* article (mentioned above) in its section on unintentional injury.

As one can see in Table 10.1, primary data generates secondary data, which are then used in the creation of a report (modeled after *Health, United States*) to contrast national trends to local health district trends in the Finger Lakes District in rural New York. This type of comparative analysis provides a solid foundation for planning and priority setting, especially when determining long- and short-range implications of a current situation. Examining demographics, health determinants, mortality, and disease to plan for services utilization and improved health outcomes requires a 360-degree scan of a community or region through the use of quantitative data in the form of statistics.

Working with Data

Statistics is the study of the collection, organization, analysis, and interpretation of data (Dodge & Marriott, 2003). Statistical data are the result of numerous methods, including surveillance studies, surveys, interviews, and empirical studies, to gather information on a population, a process, a procedure, or a system. Data collected by numerous federal, regional, state, and local authorities are critical in the decision-making process in mental health services delivery. They are also used in program evaluation and outcomes assessment. Statistical data are in demand when examining impacts, effects, and consequences. Understanding how statistical data are used and transformed to other formats is critical to using data effectively in research, teaching, and daily life.

The most commonly used sources of quantitative data in mental health informatics are statistical data, such as epidemiologic data and geographic data. Literature reviews, systematic reviews, meta-analyses, published empirical studies, and grey literature are also frequently used. As with all data, there are frameworks for the conceptualization and notation of data in mental health informatics.

EPIDEMIOLOGIC DATA

Epidemiology may be defined as the study of the factors that determine the frequency and distribution of disease in populations. The focus of epidemiologic studies changes over time. Current sociocultural values can influence definitions and perceptions of disease (especially mental and addictive disorders). In addition, improvements in diagnostic instrumentation can lead to earlier detection of disease. However, the underlying and constant premise of epidemiology is that disease does not occur at random, but rather in patterns that can be studied to determine the underlying causal factors of the disease.

Epidemiologic methods determine the extent of disease in the community. By examining the natural history and progression of disease, we can identify associations and potential disease etiology (causes) as well as the risk factors for a disease. Epidemiologic methods aid in the evaluation of new preventive and therapeutic measures and innovative modes of health care delivery. Finally, these methods help to provide a foundation for developing public health policy and regulatory decisions relating to societal and environmental problems that affect a population's health.

So what is the relationship between epidemiology and clinical practice? By using population data, clinicians are better able to define diagnoses based upon data from large groups of patients. Prognosis of a disease is based upon the experiences of large groups of patients with the same disease, the same stage of disease, and the same treatments. Large treatment studies, such as clinical trials, provide a foundation for selecting evidence-based practices, based upon data that are rigorous and studies that may be replicated and generalized. Studying the frequency and distribution of diseases in large populations allows us to more readily discern the early development of a disease in a community, to better determine threshold levels between sub-clinical and clinical disease presentation in a community, and to assess the co-occurrence of multiple diseases.

In reviewing epidemiologic data, it is important to understand how data is collected. Counts, proportions, ratios, and rates are measures that convey information about the occurrence of disease. *Counts* are the simplest and most frequently performed measure in epidemiology. They refer to the number of cases of a disease being studied. Counts are useful for the allocation of health resources but have limited usefulness for epidemiologic purposes without knowing the size of the source population. *Proportions* tell us the fraction of the population that is affected. They are linked to probability theory (i.e., risk of developing disease). *Rates*, in epidemiology, contain the following elements: disease frequency; the unit size of the population; and the time period during which an event occurs. For example, a crude annual death rate of 8.64 per 1,000 means that about 9 persons in 1,000 died, about 864 persons per 100,000 died, and the risk of dying was about 0.9%.

Incidence of a disease is the number of new cases of a disease that occurs during a specific period of time for a specified population (incidence rate). *Prevalence* of a disease is the number of existing cases of a disease in proportion to the total population. Prevalence may also examine the proportion of a specific population with a disease at a designated point in time (point prevalence) or during a specified period in time (period prevalence). Prevalence rates help health care providers to plan services and assists in the identification of at-risk populations currently with a disease.

Descriptive epidemiology characterizes the amount and distribution of disease (patterns and frequency) within a population. It is used to identify problems in health and patterns of disease that exist in a specific population. In comparison, *analytic epidemiology* examines the determinants (or the risks) of health outcomes. Since descriptive studies generally precede analytic studies designed to investigate determinants of disease, descriptive studies often help to generate research hypotheses. Figure 10.1 illustrates the normal progression of epidemiologic studies.

Epidemiologic data may be in the form of survey data, such as the CDC's Behavioral Risk Factor Surveillance System, which collects data on the prevalence of personal health behaviors among adults associated with premature morbidity and mortality. It is also

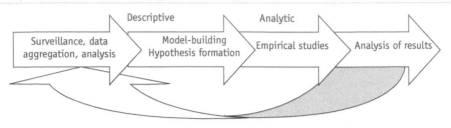

FIGURE 10.1 Flowchart from Descriptive to Analytic Epidemiology.

collected through the CDC's WISQARS™, which collects national incidence data on fatal and non-fatal injury. Epidemiologic data is also used to generate visual representations of disease outbreaks, disease surveillance, and community assessments. The CDC's Epi Info™ 7 software allows users to create questionnaires and data entry forms for data collection, create databases, conduct analyses, generate reports, and to create maps using ESRI (Environmental Systems Research Institute) geographic information system software.

GEOGRAPHIC DATA

A geographic information system (GIS) integrates hardware, software, and data for capturing, managing, analyzing, and displaying all forms of geographically referenced information. It manipulates numeric and spatial data into a visual display, such as a map, charts, or graphs. Geographic data is composed of variables that represent real world phenomena, such as climate regions, topographic features, buildings, city infrastructures, or cable networks. The data representing different aspects of the phenomena are arranged in separate layers, which allow users to reconfigure visual displays of places, over time, and with different boundaries (including zip codes, census tracts, and school districts; see Figure 10.2).

GIS and maps are an area of expanding use in social and behavioral health. A GIS allows one to map places, times, and attributes over time in order to see changes and patterns in services, distribution, and density of populations, and surveillance of disease outbreaks. Further, it also allows one to anticipate future conditions or evaluate the consequences of a policy or intervention.

Another way to conceptualize how a GIS works is to study the variety of applications utilizing six questions most often asked by individuals in government as well as in the private sector, based upon "what" and "how" in reference to a particular location and time (Hanson & Levin, 2010; see Table 10.2).

The first question asks what exists at a particular location (e.g., a neighborhood, a county, or a state). That place can be described in a variety of ways as mentioned above (e.g., place, postal code, geographical coordinates, a local Cartesian coordinate system, or census block). The second question links two locations, such as the particular characteristics between point A and point B. The third question asks if there is a place where certain conditions are satisfied. This is a "true" or "not true" question. For example, do the schedules of local community-based day treatment programs match up to local bus routes and schedules? This is an important question if individuals coming for treatment are completely dependent upon the bus for transportation. The fourth question looks for

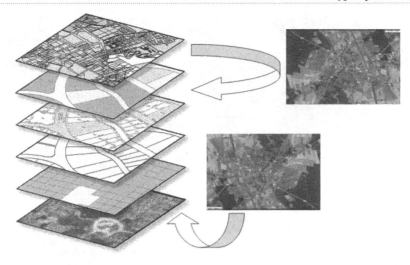

FIGURE 10.2 GIS Layers.

the results of the two moments in time. For example, did a decision to close a unit within a community mental health center in 2008 adversely affect services utilization for center clients in 2011? Question five determines patterns, such as clusters of mental or physical illnesses, services utilization, or increases or decreases in drop-outs. Question six attempts to determine what will happen if something is changed or an innovation implemented (Hanson, 2001, p. 58).

A GIS has two characteristics that allow it to answer these types of questions. The first characteristic is the ability to apply spatial operators to the data (Hanchette, 2003). One example would be to retrieve all instances of adults in the United States who face functional limitations due to a disability (see Figure 10.3). In this case, we would use the Behavioral Risk Factor Surveillance System (BRFSS) as our primary data set and generate a map by selecting the year and the category (disability) from the CDC BRFSS site. The primary GIS data are mapped for both states and metropolitan/micropolitan statistical areas (MMSAs).

The second characteristic is its ability to link data sets together, an essential feature since organizations and agencies collect data for their own objectives without regard to other potential users outside the organization. One example of a local analysis level is the

TABLE 10.2

Who, What, Why, When, and How Questions in a GIS
What is at … ?
How do I get from …. to ….. ?
Where does this condition hold true [or not true]?
What has changed since …. ?
What are the pattern(s)?
What if … ?

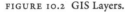

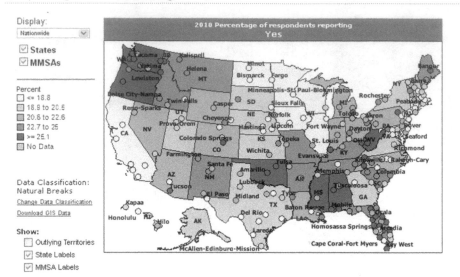

FIGURE 10.3 U.S. Adults Who Are Limited in Any Activities Because of Physical, Mental, or Emotional Problems.

Centers for Disease Control and Prevention (2011). 2010: Adults who are limited in any activities because of physical, mental, or emotional problems. *Behavioral Risk Factor Surveillance System Survey Data*. Atlanta, Georgia: U.S. Department of Health and Human Services, Centers for Disease Control and Prevention. Generated from http://apps.nccd.cdc.gov/gisbrfss/default.aspx.

Community Information Database developed by the Juvenile Welfare Board Children's Services Council of Pinellas (JWB) in Pinellas County, Florida. The JWB was established in 1946 and is one of the largest funding sources for human services in Pinellas County. The JWB also writes state and federal grant proposals to obtain money to provide funding for services to selected populations within their community. In the early 1990s, the JWB created its Community Information Database (CID) to track a number of demographic, health, and socioeconomic status indicators to create a more focused picture of a population, allow decision and policy makers to direct services to areas of greatest need, and to personalize the benefits to area residents (Hall & Gehant, 1994). Today, the JWB offers a "Map of the Month" organized by zip code or census tract, a series of reports specific to Pinellas County, and links to national reports on child health and safety, poverty, homelessness, education, juvenile justice, and risk behaviors (http://www.aboutpinellaskids.org/).

Another example of a local analysis level is the use of GIS data and disaster preparedness for Lee County, Florida (Faris et al., 2005). The Human Services Vulnerability Index and its GIS Map Project were designed as an annual updated disaster preparedness tool for access by all disaster response agencies. It was innovative because it envisioned human services delivery as an additional component to the traditional physical infrastructure planning. Developed in the aftermath of Hurricane Charley in 2004, data is provided on a number of vulnerability indicators, including income, adult poverty, transportation, employment, service wages, physical, disabled over 65 or under 15, transience, length of tenure (English not primary language), and population density. Along with these indicators, basic data sets can be overlaid with data specific to health and mental health. This kind of data is critical to creating management plans, not just for disasters, but also for community growth and development to ensure access to behavioral health services.

Types of Databases

Consider the volume of data generated to substantiate and inform research and practice. Next, consider the volume of academic and research published every day, whether in an academic or research database, a library catalog, or as conference abstracts and presentations posted on a website. Searching for relevant mental health services research requires us to search across numerous resources, all of which have specialty content, multiple formats, and different access procedures. The most commonly used databases in academic, research settings, and practice settings are bibliographic databases and non-bibliographic databases.

BIBLIOGRAPHIC DATABASES

Traditionally, bibliographic databases are comprised of indexing and/or abstracting services (I&A), table of contents services (TOC), and citation databases. Each of these services and/or resources fulfills different functions. Further, all of them may be necessary when conducting a search of the literature to find pertinent materials.

INDEXING AND/OR ABSTRACTING SERVICES

What exactly is an indexing and abstracting service (I&A)? An I&A service provides bibliographic citations, subject headings, and abstracts of the literature of a discipline or subject area. Although many online I&A databases started as print resources, today almost all I&A have converted to an online presence. *Index Medicus*, for example, which started as a print resource in 1879, evolved into the free online PubMed database offered by the National Library of Medicine (National Library of Medicine, 2004) and provides additional search support through the use of its online medical subject headings (MeSH) and concept-to-term mapping.

I&A services vary widely in their structure. Most I&A services are selectively indexed, which means that they do not index every article in every issue of a journal. In addition, since many I&As are discipline-based, one may need to search other discipline-based databases to find certain journal titles or subject areas. Even I&A aggregator databases, which offer a selection of articles across disciplines, are not comprehensive. Therefore, in order to run a comprehensive literature review, one must search in other databases, such as a table of contents service or a citation database, or conduct hand searches of the print literature.

The use and construct of indices and abstracts are important from information-seeking and retrieval perspectives. An index is an alphabetically arranged list of headings, which may consist of personal or corporate names, geographical places, and subjects. Index terms may be pulled directly from the text (e.g., "system of care") or from a controlled vocabulary (e.g., "children's mental health services") that creates linkages across synonymous terms and phrases, indicates broader and narrower terms, and provides related terms. This mapping of terms and phrases ensures that the user of the index is able to retrieve relevant materials, even if he or she is unfamiliar with the vocabulary of a specific discipline.

In Figure 10.4, you can see where the term "controlled vocabulary" resides as you move down the category of "Information Science." The terms indented under controlled vocabulary are narrower terms that are subsets of the term "controlled vocabulary."

Many I&A services, such as PubMed or PsycINFO, use a controlled vocabulary. For PubMed, it is MeSH (Medical Subject Headings). For PsycINFO, it is the *Thesaurus of Psychological Index Terms* (National Library of Medicine, 2010; Tuleya, 2007). Both services have a search feature that allows the user to type in a term or phrase, and then the service "maps" it to possible matches. Professional indexers read and assign subject headings to all items indexed in these services or use machine-assisted indexing, in which computer algorithms are applied to the text of a document and prepares preliminary matches to controlled headings, which are then reviewed by the professional indexers.

Controlled vocabularies and thesauri often include a definition of a term or phrase. In PubMed, the phrase "controlled vocabulary" appears with its definition, the year it was added to the list, and the source of its definition. The "authority record" for that term or phrase may also list synonymous terms. For example, if one searches for the term "thesaurus" in MeSH, one retrieves the same record as the search for "controlled vocabulary" [http://www.ncbi.nlm.nih.gov/mesh?term=thesaurus]. The MeSH redirects the user to the preferred term, which is "vocabulary, controlled" (see Figure 10.5).

An abstract should be a "brief, objective representation of the contents of a primary document or an oral presentation" (NISO, 1996, p. 1) that allows the user to identify quickly the basic content and relevance of the document and decide if it is worth the time

    All MeSH Categories

      Information Science Category

       Information Science

        Information Services

         Documentation

          Vocabulary, Controlled

            Current Procedural Terminology

            Diagnostic and Statistical Manual of Mental Disorders

            Healthcare Common Procedure Coding System

            International Classification of Diseases

            Logical Observation Identifiers Names and Codes

            Subject Headings

              Medical Subject Headings

            Systematized Nomenclature of Medicine

            Unified Medical Language System

FIGURE 10.4 Controlled Vocabulary in the MeSH (*Me*dical *S*ubject *H*eadings).

National Library of Medicine (2011). Vocabulary, Controlled. *MeSH*. Retrieved http://www.ncbi.nlm.nih.gov/mesh?term=thesuarus.

Vocabulary, Controlled

A specified list of terms with a fixed and unalterable meaning, and from which a

selection is made when CATALOGING; ABSTRACTING AND INDEXING; or

searching BOOKS; JOURNALS AS TOPIC; and other documents. The control is

intended to avoid the scattering of related subjects under different headings (SUBJECT

HEADINGS). The list may be altered or extended only by the publisher or issuing

agency. (From Harrod's Librarians' Glossary, 7th ed, p163)

Year introduced: 1996

PubMed search builder options

Subheadings:

☐ history

☐   Restrict to MeSH Major Topic.

☐   Do not include MeSH terms found below this term in the MeSH hierarchy.

Entry Terms:

- Controlled Vocabulary

- Controlled Vocabularies

- Vocabularies, Controlled

- Thesaurus

- Thesauri

- Controlled Thesaurus

- Controlled Thesauri

- Thesauri, Controlled

Thesaurus, Controlled

FIGURE 10.5 MeSH Definition for Term "Controlled Vocabulary".
National Library of Medicine (2011). Vocabulary, Controlled. *MeSH*. Retrieved http://www.ncbi.nlm.nih.gov/mesh?term=thesaurus.

to read the full article. As with many items that deal with information, there are also standards for writing the various types of abstracts, such as the ANSI/NISO Z39.14 *Guidelines for Abstracts* (NISO, 1996).

Professional abstractors write abstracts for the indexed item, or the vendor may choose to use author-written abstracts. Some journals may require a specific format for an abstract. However, abstracts are generally classed in the following categories: critical, indicative, informative (structured), or slanted. A critical abstract contains evaluative comments on the material presented in a document or the style of a presentation. Critical abstracts are generally written by professional abstractors who are also subject specialists. An indicative abstract is generally written for documents that do not contain methodology or results; it provides a description of the document, but it does not paraphrase the document.

In these cases, the abstract reflects theoretical approaches used, arguments presented, and/or background information of the document. An informative abstract, or structured abstract, is generally used for scientific and empirical documents. It is a condensed version of the document and reflects the tenor and content of the document. Often an informative document will follow the IMRaD (introduction, methods, results, and discussion) structure, which is the standard scientific reporting format. However, in some cases, the results and discussion may be placed first, depending upon the preference of the abstracting resource or journal. A slanted abstract is written from a particular point of view.

TABLE OF CONTENTS SERVICES

Unlike the selective indexing that occurs in many I&A services, a Table of Contents (TOC) service provides its users with a reproduction of the table of contents of a complete journal issue. Many TOC services also offer access to the abstracts of the articles in the issue. A TOC service is available through databases, such as *Current Contents Connect*, which provides access to *complete* tables of contents, with bibliographic information and abstracts from selected scholarly journals across a variety of disciplines, or from journal vendor sites, such as Springer's *Journal of Behavioral Services and Research* (Figure 10.6.). TOC services are an excellent resource for professionals and practitioners to remain current with the literature in targeted journals.

Bottom of Form

Current Contents Connect provides coverage of over 8,500 global, peer-reviewed research journals and 9,000 relevant, evaluated websites and documents (Thomson Reuters, 2008). It is classed by edition and by discipline. There are seven editions: (1) Agriculture, Biology, & Environmental Sciences (ABES; 1,170 titles); (2) Social & Behavioral Sciences (SBS; 1,890 titles); (3) Clinical Medicine (CM; 1,380 titles); (4) Life Sciences (LS; 1,400 titles); (5) Physical, Chemical, & Earth Sciences (PCES; 1,270 titles); (6) Engineering, Computing, & Technology (ECT; 1,240 titles); and (7) Arts & Humanities (AH; 1,150 titles) (Thomson Reuters, 2008). Each edition is broken out by disciplines. For example,

ALERTS FOR THIS JOURNAL

Get the table of contents of every new issue published in The Journal of Behavioral Health services &Research.

Your E-Mail Address

SUBMIT

Please send me information on new Springer publications in Public Health.

FIGURE 10.6 *Journal of Behavioral Services and Research*, Current Awareness Service http://www.springer.com/public+health/journal/11414 Used with permission.

the *Journal of Behavioral Services and Research* is in the "Public Health & Health Care Science" discipline, which is one of the 66 disciplines in the "Social & Behavioral Sciences" edition.

CITATION DATABASES

The strength of a citation database is the ability to search who is citing whom and who is citing what. The best-known citation databases are the Thomson/ISI citation databases, that is, *Web of Science, Web of Knowledge,* or the *Social Science, Science,* and *Arts & Humanities Citation Indexes*. Comprised of three major content areas (arts and humanities, social sciences, and science), the Thomson Reuters citation databases index numerous scholarly journals. Each indexed article in the citation databases includes the article's cited reference list (i.e., bibliography), which allows the user to search the databases for articles that cite a known author or work.

The *Social Sciences Citation Index* (1900 to present) indexes 2,697 journals across 55 social science disciplines and selected items from 3,500 of the world's leading scientific and technical journals (Thomson Reuters, 2011). The *Science Citation Index* (1900 to present) indexes 8,300 major journals across 150 disciplines. The *Arts & Humanities Citation Index* (1975 to present) fully indexes over 2,300 arts and humanities journals and selected items over 250 scientific and social sciences journals (Thomson Reuters, 2011). In addition, the citation indexes also index 110 conference proceedings, which make them a good resource for ephemeral, or grey literature.

A user may view the bibliography from a specific record, view citing records, and related records, which map across shared citations, and search across topic (subject), title, author, editor, group author, publication name, doi, the year published, and/or an author's institutional address. In addition, using the *Web of Science* Citation Mapping tool, users may see the other researchers whom Author A has cited, as well as those authors who have cited Author A.

Since the citation indexes and *Current Contents Connect* are part of the Thomson Reuters information suite, users may also link out from the Indexes to *Current Contents* to view a journal issue to see if there are other titles of interest in that journal. For example, linking to the table of contents for the journal issue from a book review on family involvement in treating schizophrenia in the *Journal of Behavioral Health Services & Research* provides access to articles addressing other issues for children with mental illnesses and coping mechanisms for their families.

NON-BIBLIOGRAPHIC DATABASES

In addition to journal literature, there are thousands of non-bibliographic databases used in mental health and substance abuse services research. Although many non-bibliographic databases are numeric or spatial databases, many have some sort of associated text with them, in the form of data dictionaries and chart books. These databases include (open source and proprietary access) general statistics databases, federal and state demographic and population-based databases, and surveillance and epidemiology databases. Data may be available in raw format or pre-defined queries, and/or across micro-, meso-, and macro-levels.

Data may be accessed using an interactive web interface (such as the Centers for Disease Control and Prevention's WISQARS™ mortality and morbidity database) or through specialized software (such as the CDC's EpiInfo and EpiMap module), which can output to commercial software packages (such as Access or SQL Server, or as HTML format).

There are many issues involved in dealing with numeric and spatial databases. Although there may be information on a topic in a numeric database, the actual available data attached to that topic may be nonexistent. The lack of data may be due to proprietary or licensing restrictions, or simply that the available data is not as descriptive as the user may need. Data may not be updated as frequently as the user may wish, as in the case of national suicide data, which has a two-year lag time. There are also the structural issues of interoperability and portability. Interoperability allows computers and users to share and access data and operations through networks. Portability, a component of interoperability, is the ability to transport data between databases and application source code between computer platforms and operating systems.

Data interoperability is also affected by interface design. Standard specifications for data and for operations directed to data are necessary to communicate with one another and to exchange and use information, including content, format, and semantics. Data also may be stored in now obsolete formats or on outdated legacy systems, which require data to be reformatted to current supported applications and platforms, if at all possible. There are also the issues regarding semantic interoperability, which assures that the content is understood in the same way in both systems, as well as by the individuals interacting with the systems. In addition, aggregating data across data sets may be problematic, especially with geospatial data (Gotway & Young, 2002).

A number of different data sets may incorporate geospatial data, such as socioeconomic data, epidemiologic data sets, or textual data sets, in multiple formats, such as vector, raster, or tabular data. All geospatial data must be geocoded (linked to geographic coordinates), most often to a Cartesian coordinate system. To geocode the data, the data is described using attributes of the data, such as its physical, environmental, social, or economic characteristics, the geographic features of the extent of the area (neighborhood, census block, etc.), and linkage to a unique identifier. The unique identifier ensures that the user can retrieve all of the descriptive and geographic data associated with that one point or aggregation of points.

As with bibliographic databases, controlled vocabulary (taxonomy) is essential in spatial and numeric data. In geospatial data, there are issues with ontology development, which formally describes objects and the relations between objects (Hanson, 2008). The grammar of an ontology is used to query data, to disambiguate queries, and for query term expansion. This affects the relevance and ranking of retrieved data and the creation of spatial indexes to increase relevance and precision across multiple databases, particularly in federated searching. It also ensures the successful mapping between a spatial ontology and a geographic conceptual schema (Hanson, 2008).

Types of Research Studies in Databases

In addition to the use of statistical and spatial data, there are data that are found in the published and unpublished literature. Whether the study methodology used qualitative, quantitative, or mixed methods, there are important issues and concerns regarding the publication of research findings. All published empirical studies are not created equal. In addition, the reporting of published empirical studies is certainly not standard. The lack of standards often results in incomplete and inconsistent reporting. Incomplete or inconsistent reporting may result in selecting only certain results or eliminating negative results when conducting systematic reviews and meta-analyses. Although there is a national standard for scientific and technical reports (NISO, 2005), different disciplines, professional societies, and publishers often have their own standards or guidelines tailored to meet their users' needs.

EPIDEMIOLOGICAL STUDIES

Epidemiological studies are often grounded in observational research. Observational research comprises several study designs and many topic areas. While randomized controlled trials (RCTs) provide essential information regarding the effects of an intervention or treatment, observational studies provide a better snapshot of what may be found in daily clinical practice, such as rare or late adverse effects not noted in an RCT. In addition, observational studies often examine risk factors, which cannot be randomly controlled. Meta-analyses of observational studies present particular challenges due to inherent biases, differences in study designs, and sources of variability in results across studies. Therefore, it is important to have a clear understanding of the advantages and limitations of statistical syntheses of observational data.

Reviews of observational epidemiological studies found a number of problems with missing data in the reporting of the research, such as the rationale behind the choice of potential confounding variables, eligibility criteria, and methods to identify cases and controls (von Elm et al., 2008). Two initiatives emerged from the discipline's concern to strengthen observational studies in epidemiology: the Meta-Analysis of Observational Studies in Epidemiology (MOOSE) and the STROBE initiative (Strengthening the Reporting of Observational Studies in Epidemiology).

Spearheaded by the Centers for Disease Control and Prevention (CDC) in 2000, the MOOSE group defined an observational study as an etiologic or effectiveness study using data from an existing database, a cross-sectional study, a case series, a case-control design, a design with historical controls, or a cohort design (Stroup et al., 2000). The group decided not to address "pooled analyses," that is, individual-level data from different studies. The proposed 35-item checklist contains specifications for reporting of meta-analyses of observational studies in epidemiology, including background (6 items), search strategy (10 items), methods (8 items), results (4 items), discussion (3 items), and conclusion (4 items). The checklist applies across all six types of studies (see Table 10.3).

The STROBE Statement, however, focuses on three observational study designs in epidemiology: (1) cohort; (2) case-control; and (3) cross-sectional studies (von Elm et al., 2008). The STROBE Statement is a checklist of 22 items considered essential for good reporting of observational studies. The checklist addresses the title/abstract (1 item), introduction (2 items), methods (9 items), results (5 items), discussion (4 items), and other information (1 item: funding). Eighteen items are common across all three designs. Four items (#6, #12, #14, and #15) are design specific, with different versions for all or part of the item

TABLE 10.3

Observational Studies in Epidemiology as Defined by the MOOSE and STROBE Groups

Moose	Strobe
existing database	—
cross-sectional study	cross-sectional study
case series	—
case-control design	case-control
design with historical controls	—
cohort design	cohort design

depending upon the type of study (see von Elm et al., 2008). Further, some items require separate information for cases and controls in case-control studies, or exposed and unexposed groups in cohort and cross-sectional studies (von Elm et al., 2008). In addition to the Statement, there is an Explanation and Elaboration paper, which includes examples of good reporting from the literature (Vandenbroucke et al., 2007).

Neither is meant to be prescriptive in establishing how studies will be established or conducted or in the writing of the study. Neither the checklist nor the Statement addresses style or format of the manuscript (e.g., APA Style). The intent is to provide a checklist of all the items to be included to effectively and accurately report observational studies. Further, neither is a tool to judge the quality of the research performed. There are other tools available to address quality issues in research (see Sanderson et al., 2007). However, both provide a minimum list of data that need to be addressed in the reporting of observational studies.

CLINICAL TRIALS

During the early 1990s, there was much concern over the inconsistency in the reporting of clinical trials. Two groups, working independently of each other, convened in 1993 to identify a minimum list of requirements for the reporting of clinical trials in the literature. The Standardized Reporting of Trials (SORT) statement (The Standards of Reporting Trials Group, 1994) and the Asilomar Working Group on Recommendations for Reporting of Clinical Trials in the Biomedical Literature (1994) were the outcomes of that meeting. The CONSORT (Consolidated Standards of Reporting Trials) statement was the integration of these two guidelines (Begg et al., 1996). Published in 1996, the CONSORT statement was revised most recently in 2010.

Unlike the *Cochrane Handbook for Systematic Reviews of Interventions* (Green et al., 2008) which addresses the methodology for conducting a systematic review, the CONSORT statement was developed to improve the reporting of clinical trials. Its 25-item checklist specifically addresses information that should be in the title, abstract, introduction, methods, results, discussion, and other information, such as the registration number and name of trial registry, where the full trial protocol is accessed, and sources of funding, other support, and the role of the funders (Schulz, Altman, & Moher, 2010). The checklist is accompanied by a flow chart that addresses the phases of a parallel, randomized trial of two groups (enrollment, intervention allocation, follow-up, and data analysis) (Schulz, Altman,

& Moher, 2010). There are additional explanations and elaborations on key points, as well as CONSORT design (cluster randomized trials, non-inferiority and equivalence trials, pragmatic trials), intervention (non-pharmacological treatments, herbal interventions, and acupuncture extensions), and data extensions (harms-related issues and reporting trials in abstracts; http://www.consort-statement.org/consort-statement/).

META-ANALYSES AND SYSTEMATIC REVIEWS

Meta-analyses and systematic reviews are very common in health care. They are used as current awareness tools to help researchers and practitioners keep up to date in their field, to develop clinical practice guidelines, to appraise new technologies and interventions, and to select and justify new areas of research.

According to the Cochrane Collaborative, a systematic review is a review of a clearly formulated question that uses systematic and explicit methods to (1) identify, select, and critically appraise relevant research, and 2) to collect and analyze data from the studies that are included in the review. Statistical methods (meta-analysis) may or may not be used to analyze and summarize the results of the included studies. Meta-analysis specifically refers to the use of statistical techniques in a systematic review to integrate the results of included studies.

If there are issues in the reporting of clinical trials, consider the issues in the reporting of meta-analyses. However rigorous a systematic review may be, there are a number of pitfalls of which researchers should be aware. Not only may a systematic review data be overly narrow or restrictive in its review of the evidence (Glasgow & Emmons, 2007), it may fail to adequately address the study quality of the RCT. For example, the review may not address patient allocation to the control and treatment groups or how (or if) the study was "blinded." Understanding allocation and blinding is critical to ensure that the clinician, the patient, the researcher, and the analyst do not have any knowledge of who was assigned to what group until after the study and the analyses have been completed (Morissette et al., 2011). Other factors include attrition bias (i.e., who dropped out of the study and the reasons that they dropped); publication bias (which emphasizes the publication of only positive outcomes; Trespidi, Barbui, & Cipriani, 2011; Golder, Loke, & Bland, 2010), and selective reporting (which is defined as the selection of a subset of the original variables recorded for inclusion in publication of trials; Williamson & Gamble, 2005). A major factor that affects comparative effectiveness research is the reporting of outcomes of interest to the researcher but which have little if any value in clinical decision making. Yet another factor that can confound a systematic review is the decision to use statistical criteria rather than clinical criteria in the creation of a meta-analysis or systematic review (Deeks, 2002).

Heterogeneity is an issue in meta-analyses and systematic reviews. There are three types of heterogeneity: (1) clinical diversity; (2) methodological diversity; and (3) statistical heterogeneity (Green et al., 2008). Clinical diversity (a.k.a. clinical heterogeneity) addresses variability in the participants, interventions, and outcomes. Methodological diversity (a.k.a. methodological heterogeneity) examines variability in study design and risk of bias. Statistical heterogeneity is the variability in the intervention effects being evaluated and is a consequence of clinical and/or methodological diversity among the studies. If the observed intervention effects differ so much from each other than one might expect due to random error (chance) alone, that is evidence of statistical heterogeneity. In systematic reviews and meta-analyses, there are a number of reasons that statistical heterogeneity may arise. These include the inappropriate analysis of subgroups, which may result in a small number of results or the use of summary data, both of which affect the power of statistical methods (such as meta-regression or sensitivity analyses). However, if one is looking for new research areas, examining the sources of heterogeneity in clinical studies may be a promising venue.

Considering all of the problems that may emerge in meta-analyses and systematic reviews, guidelines were established to address many of the issues. In 1999, the QUOROM Statement (Quality of Reporting of Meta-Analyses) was published, which focused on the reporting of meta-analyses of RCTs (Moher et al., 1999). To accommodate the inclusion of systematic reviews, the QUOROM Statement was renamed PRISMA (Preferred Reporting Items for Systematic reviews and Meta-Analyses), and adopted the definitions used by the Cochrane Collaboration (Moher et al., 2009).

The PRISMA Statement consists of a 27-item checklist to help authors improve the reporting of systematic reviews and meta-analyses. The 27 items listed address elements across title, abstract, introduction, methods, results, discussion, and funding. Although the PRISMA Statement focuses on RCTs, Moher et al. (2009) suggest that it may also be used for reporting evaluations of interventions. Similar to the CONSORT Statement, the PRISMA Statement also has a flow chart to assist researchers, as well as a supporting Explanation and Elaboration document (Liberati et al., 2009).

DIAGNOSTIC TESTS

In addition to standards for the reporting of empirical studies, meta-analyses, and systematic reviews, similar efforts were being made on behalf of standardizing diagnostic accuracy studies. Diagnostic accuracy refers to the internal and external validity of a diagnostic test. If all evaluations of diagnostic tests were conducted rigorously before use in clinical practice, unwanted clinical consequences and unnecessary testing would be avoided, limiting health care costs and improving patient outcomes.

STARD (Standards for the Reporting of Diagnostic Accuracy Studies) was an outgrowth of a 1996 meeting of the Cochrane Diagnostic and Screening Test Methods Working Group to correct the low methodological quality and sub-standard reporting of diagnostic test evaluations. The meeting produced the STARD Statement, a 25-item checklist addressing five areas of diagnostic accuracy studies: (1) title/abstract/keywords; (2) introduction; (3) methods (participants, test methods, and statistical methods); (4) results (participants, test results, and estimates); and (5) discussion (Bossuyt et al., 2003). Wherever possible, the STARD group based the decision to include an item using evidence derived from narrative articles explaining theoretical principles, papers on statistical modeling, and empirical evidence derived from diagnostic studies. The evidence linked the item to biased estimates (internal validity) or to variation in measures of diagnostic accuracy (external validity) (Bossuyt et al., 2003). Similar to CONSORT and PRISMA, STARD also provides a flow chart and a separate background document that explains the meaning and rationale of each item.

In 2006, the International Committee of Medical Journal Editors included the use of the STARD statement in their Uniform Requirements for Manuscripts Submitted to

Biomedical journals (Smidt et al., 2007). For example, the *Journal of Medical Screening* recommends the use of STARD or of CONSORT to potential authors (http://jms.rsm-journals.com/content/15/1/51.full).

GREY LITERATURE

Grey literature is considered unpublished literature, that is, study reports that have not been formally published or widely distributed. Grey literature comprises ephemeral materials (such as conference abstracts and presentations), state and federal agency reports, and local organization and association reports. Grey literature is most widely used in finding the cutting-edge studies in technology. Let's take a look at the use of grey literature in the appraisal of health technology assessments, especially for rapidly evolving technologies.

In 2006, Dundar et al. (2006) reviewed the seven technology assessment review groups (TARs) for the British National Institute for Health and Clinical Excellence (NICE) to determine how data from conference abstracts and presentations were used as part of NICE health technology appraisal (HTA) process. All seven of the TARs reported that they preferred data in a full publication to data presented only as an abstract or as a presentation. However, five of the seven TARs included studies only available as conference abstracts and/or presentations in their meta-analyses on health technologies. Those five groups reported that they would use the same assessment tools for abstracts and conference presentations as they did for full publications, and would manage the data from these sources in the same way as data in fully published reports. There was inconsistency across the TARs in the policy and practice of searching for and including studies available as conference abstracts/presentations, as well as the level of detail reported in TARs regarding the use of abstracts/presentations. Comparison of the abstracts and/or conference presentations with a formal published study showed data discrepancies in the reporting of results and differences in significance of effect in outcome measures.

Dundar et al. (2006) made a number of recommendations. The first recommendation addressed search strategies and methodologies. TARs should state explicitly their search strategies for identifying conference abstracts and/or presentations, their methods for assessing these for inclusion, and how the data were used and their effect on the results. Second, since incomplete reporting in conference abstracts and presentations limits assessment of the methodological quality of trials, the TARs should obtain further study details by contacting the researchers for more complete information. Third, if there are data discrepancies by including the abstracts and/or conference presentations, the TARs should discuss the effect of including these sources as data, highlight the discrepancies, and carry out sensitivity analyses with and without abstracts and/or conference presentation data included in the analyses (Dundar et al., 2006).

Martin et al. (2005) suggested that the inclusion of grey literature to reduce publication bias may actually affect the results of a systematic review. With the advent of online databases, many researchers favor using these databases as opposed to conducting hand searches of the literature. However, these types of searches often miss a large proportion of relevant RCTs (Adams et al., 1994; Crumley et al., 2005; Hopewell et al., 2007). In their review of the literature, Hopewell et al. (2007) determined that hand searching resulted in more thorough searches for RCTs. Hand searchers identified approximately 92% to 100% of the total number of reports on RCTs; online searchers of Embase, Medline, and PsycINFO identified 49% to 67%.

Therefore, it is critical to understand the parameters of the actual search strategy in determining the breadth and depth of the review, particularly if the majority of trials are published in English language journals, or if there are trials reported in abstracts, letters, conference presentations, or in languages other than English.

Since grey literature is difficult to find, reviewers who plan to use conference abstracts and/or presentations need to create effective search protocols, allocate additional search time, and implement protocols to handle any methodological impacts that these data may have on meta-analyses and literature reviews. Similar to the CONSORT standard created for reporting clinical trials, standards for using grey literature in health and health technology assessments would be a first step in ensuring access to rapidly evolving technologies.

In 2006, the Grey Literature International Steering Committee (GLISC, 2006) adapted the Uniform Requirements for Manuscripts Submitted to Biomedical Journals (URM) of the International Committee of Medical Journal Editors as a guideline for the production of scientific and technical reports. However, while the URM advises potential authors to review its list of guidelines for reporting research methods and findings, the GLISC does not explicitly advise potential authors to review research reporting guidelines.

QUALITY IMPROVEMENT REPORTS

Although there are numerous standards for reporting research studies, there are also standards for reporting other types of research, such as quality improvement. In 1999, the Institute of Medicine reported that over 90,000 people died each year from medical errors (Kohn, Corrigan, & Donaldson, 2000). That year, a new structure was proposed for quality improvement reports (Moss & Thomson, 1999). They suggested the standard scientific form for writing papers, the IMRaD (introduction, methods, results, and discussion). However, the IMRaD structure is not appropriate to use when discussing quality improvement research. In a quality improvement report (QIR), the first methods section would be followed by a second section describing the implementation of change. This may be followed by a third methods section when the measurements are repeated to assess progress, with a second results section describing the improvements (Moss & Thomson, 1999).

Another fundamental difference between QIRs and clinical research is the emphasis that clinical research places on generalizable results. A QIR specifically examines whether the appropriate treatment was provided to patients in a practice setting, monitors the implementation, and evaluates outcomes in the local setting. However, Moss and Thomson (1999) suggested "a well written and structured quality improvement report may include generalizable methods and strategies for change from which others undertaking similar audits would benefit" (p. 76).

The structure for QIRs was initially published in the journal *Quality in Health Care* in 1999. The QIR had eight steps: (1) provide a brief description of context (including relevant details of staff and function of department, team, unit, patient group); (2) provide an outline of the problem to be solved; (3) identify the key measures for improvement;

(4) describe the process of gathering information; (5) provide analysis and interpretation of data; (6) describe the strategy for change; (7) determine if the change led to improved patient outcomes; and (8) discuss what was learned and how that will be use in the future.

In 2005, the journal published SQUIRE (Standards for Quality Improvement Reporting Excellence) guidelines. The SQUIRE Guidelines do not supersede the original QIR structure. Instead, SQUIRE is viewed as an ongoing project that ensures transparency, consensus, updates, and evaluation to improve efficacy, enhance critical scrutiny, clarify thinking, and broaden dissemination of established improvements (Davidoff et al., 2008).

Davidoff and Batalden (2005) suggested that the earlier QIR structure worked well for reporting on smaller improvement projects, which would be the equivalent of clinical case reports. In those types of reports, the primary focus is on a specific problem (clinical or delivery system) rather than on quality improvement methods. Thus, SQUIRE would be appropriate for publications that intend to demonstrate the efficacy of quality improvement methods. Therefore, SQUIRE reorganized and expanded the 8 steps to 16 in its attempt to parallel the construction of a QIR to that of the IMRaD model. With the expansion to 16 items, additional information is available on "prior information available on the problem area; failures, risks or harms encountered; assessment of the project's limitations; evaluation of the project's internal and external validity; and specific plans for assessing maintenance of the improvement" (Davidoff & Batalden, 2005, p. 322).

Establishing Future Research Priorities

Does one create policy from research? Federal legislation emphasizes accountability, incorporation of evidence-based practice, a national health information infrastructure, and continued emphasis on quality of care as well as patient and community outcomes. Meta-analyses and systematic reviews are conducted across mental health services research and practice. They are used to investigate cost-effectiveness (Goodyer et al., 2011), diagnostic questions (Jayaram & Hosalli, 2005), policy making (Coffman, et al., 2009), and allocation of resources (Schuurman, Leight, & Berube, 2008). From a policy perspective, these reviews serve two purposes: to determine the effectiveness of different health care interventions and to provide relevant evidence to inform real-world health care decision making. Further, these reviews not only provide a synthesis of the evidence, but they also identify the gaps in evidence. Decision-making in practice and in policy has become a more complex process than ever before. However, a major question remains: How is priority setting determined in policy decision making?

One issue is which methodology will be used to determine priorities. With the current federal emphasis on comparative effectiveness research, cost-effectiveness analyses are essential. Cost effectiveness research assesses the value of medical treatments using information from diagnostic tests. Generally, cost effectiveness is measured using Cost/QALY (quality of life years), net health benefits (gain in QALYs minus opportunity cost of spending in QALYs), and net monetary benefit (dollar value of improved health minus costs). Value of information (VOI) analysis essentially estimates the potential gains from conducting research to fill a gap, and then ranks research gaps on the basis of expected gains. VOI is particularly useful in framing complex decision-making problems characterized by large uncertainties and high stakes. Thus, VOI can help prioritize research investments, evaluate study designs, and estimate optimal sample size.

Myers and colleagues (2011) specifically examined the use of modeling and value-of-information analysis to set research priorities. In their literature review, they determined that approximately 40% of the articles ($n = 209$) did not specify what method was used to identify research gaps, and only six articles cited a previously published systematic review as a source. In their survey of United States and international institutions, agencies, and organizations involved in research activities, the majority of organizations (26 of 31) described a well-defined priority-setting process. However, only the United Kingdom's National Institute for Clinical Excellence (NICE) explicitly recommended the use of decision-analytical methods and the value of information-based approaches in their decision-making framework about technology adaptation and recommendations for further research (Myers et al., 2011).

Although Myers and colleagues recommend the use of VOI to substantiate decision making, they acknowledge that the complexity and cost of running a full VOI model may prevent many decision makers from using this methodology to set priorities. However, for selected studies, a minimal modeling framework could be applied to VOI analysis. Metzer et al. (2011) suggest that minimal modeling VOI approaches can be readily applied in selected analyses and can provide evidence of the wide variation in the value of research for studies.

For example, the Clinical Antipsychotic Trials of Intervention Effectiveness (CATIE) trial of atypical antipsychotics, which examined the relative effectiveness of second-generation (atypical) antipsychotic drugs with a first-generation antipsychotic in a double-blind study, utilized a minimal modeling VOI approach (Meltzer, Basu, & Meltzer, 2009). A minimal modeling approach is useful when an intervention affects only quality of life so that effects on survival do not need to be modeled in long-term trials that measure comprehensive outcomes, or for adaptive clinical trials when a decision must be made on funding and/ or continuing the trial. However, a minimal modeling approach is not recommended for chronic disease interventions that rely on intermediate outcomes (Metzer et al., 2011).

How are research gaps determined from meta-analyses, systematic reviews, or modeling studies? Robinson, Saldanha, and McKoy (2011) surveyed federal AHRQ Evidence-based Practice Centers (EPCs; $n = 12$) and international organizations ($n = 37$) that conduct systematic reviews, cost-effectiveness analyses, or technology. They found that 33% of the EPCs and 8.1% of the international organizations used variations of the PICO framework (population, intervention, comparison, outcomes), which was the most common across the organizations. Further, they determined that "there is no widespread use or endorsement of a specific formal process or framework for identifying research gaps using systematic reviews" (Robinson et al., 2011, p. ES-5).

They decided to put forth a proposed framework incorporating the three commonly used evidence grading systems: (1) the international Grading of Recommendations Assessment, Development and Evaluation (GRADE) group; (2) the United States Preventive Services Task Force (USPSTF); and (3) the Strength of Evidence (SOE) used by EPCs. The framework identifies the reason(s) that the research gap exists and characterizes the research gap using the PICOS (population, intervention, comparison, outcomes, and setting) elements.

Robinson et al. (2011) also provided a classification for the reasons that the research gap(s) exist: insufficient or imprecise information; biased information; inconsistent or unknown consistency results; or not the right information. Finally, they provided special considerations for diagnostic tests, clinical assessments, screening tests, as well as providing free text for specific research questions, such as: What are the optimal glucose thresholds for medication used in women with gestational diabetes? (Robinson et al., 2011, p. F-3).

As one can read from the issues raised in this chapter, data, methodology, and measures used to assess and compare the quality of health care, provision of care, and health care organizations address numerous structures, processes, or outcomes. To meet federal requirements for accountability in care and to identify existing areas for improvement or to address emerging areas of concern requires careful and clear documentation of change.

Implications for Mental Health Informatics

The enduring question in mental health services, research, and policy is: How do we know that a change is an improvement? The answer is by measurement (Langley et al., 1996). All data collected, whether in research or in practice, intend to answer a specific research question. It is imperative that researchers and practitioners have a clear understanding of the types of data used, how studies are designed, how the data is interpreted, and how outcomes are improved. To do so, mental health services professionals and practitioners need foundational guidelines which allow them to understand how research is conducted and evaluated, the different formats by which data may be presented, the types of resources used to locate research, and to write and read studies that can be examined critically and comparatively.

In the policy-making arena, research serves many functions. Research provides an information base for decision makers. It can be translated into practical measures and action strategies. Evidence, derived from data, is considered the foundation for solving problems in today's society as well as in the future. However, research either explicitly or implicitly embodies a set of values by preferring certain methodologies or frameworks and dispreferring others. These preferences can be seen by the theoretical and empirical constructs used in the research and by its methodology.

One cannot be conversant in all methodologies or theories for all types of research using a variety of data and analytical tools. Therefore, there is a need for guidelines to address specific issues in specific types of research. However, when generating consensus in any group, there is the problem of getting everyone on board to apply the guidelines. This is particularly important as the field of health and mental health become increasingly interdisciplinary and translational in terminology and methodologies across education, practice, and research.

References

Begg, C., Cho, M., Eastwood, S., Horton, R., Moher, D., Olkin, I., ... & Stroup, D. F. (1996). Improving the quality of reporting of randomized controlled trials. The CONSORT statement. *JAMA, 276*, 637–639.

Bossuyt, P. M., Reitsma, J.B., Bruns, D.E., Gatsonis, C.A., Glasziou, P.P., Irwig, L.M, ... & de Vet, H.C.W. (2003). Towards complete and accurate reporting of studies of diagnostic accuracy: The STARD initiative. *Clinical Chemistry, 49*, 1–6. doi: 10.1373/49.1.1

Coffman, J. M., Hong, M. K., Aubry, W. M., Luft, H. S., & Yelin, E. (2009). Translating medical effectiveness research into policy: Lessons from the California Health Benefits Review Program. *Milbank Quarterly, 87*(4), 863–902.

Cowan, J. (2007). *A mapmaker's dream: The meditations of Fra Mauro, cartographer to the Court of Venice.* Boston, MA: Shambhala Publication.

Davidoff, F., Batalden, P., Stevens, D., Ogrinc, G., Mooney, S., & SQUIRE Development Group. (2008). Publication guidelines for improvement studies in health care: Evolution of the SQUIRE Project. *Annals of Internal Medicine, 149*(9), 670–676.

Davidoff, F., & Batalden, P. (2005). Toward stronger evidence on quality improvement. Draft publication guidelines: the beginning of a consensus project. *Quality & Safety in Health Care, 14*, 319–325. doi:10.1136/qshc.2005.014787.

Deeks, J. J. (2002). Issues in the selection of a summary statistic for meta-analysis of clinical trials with binary outcomes. *Statistics in Medicine, 21*(11), 1575–1600. doi: 10.1002/sim.1188.

Dodge, Y., & Marriott, F. H. C. (2003). *The Oxford dictionary of statistical terms,* 6th ed. New York: Oxford University Press.

Dundar, Y., Dodd, S., Dickson, R., Walley, T., Haycox, A., & Williamson, P. R. (2006). Comparison of conference abstracts and presentations with full-text articles in the health technology assessments of rapidly evolving technologies. *Health Technology Assessment, 10*(5), iii–iv, ix–145. Retrieved from http://www.hta.ac.uk/fullmono/mon1005.pdf.

Faris, R., Bizelli, J., Hoyt, A., & Sullivan, C. (2005). Disaster preparedness for human services: A GIS vulnerability index. In *2005 ESRI international user conference proceedings.* Retrieved from http://proceedings.esri.com/library/userconf/proc05/papers/pap1841.pdf.

Finger Lakes Health Systems Agency. (2009). *Community health scan.* Rochester, NY: Finger Lakes Health Systems Agency. Retrieved from http://www.flhsa.org/Community%20Health%20Scan.pdf.

Gibson, W. (1984). *Neuromancer,* p. 69. New York: Ace Books.

Glasgow, R. E., & Emmons, K. M. (2007). How can we increase translation of research into practice? Types of evidence needed. *Annual Review of Public Health, 28*, 413–433. doi: 10.1146/annurev.publhealth.28.021406.144145.

Goodyer, I. M., Tsancheva, S., Byford, S., Dubicka, B., Hill, J., Kelvin, R., ... & Fonagy, P. (2011). Improving mood with psychoanalytic and cognitive therapies (IMPACT): A pragmatic effectiveness superiority trial to investigate whether specialised psychological treatment reduces the risk for relapse in adolescents with moderate to severe unipolar depression: Study protocol for a randomised controlled trial. *Trials, 12,*175. doi: 10.1186/1745–6215–12–175.

Gotway, C. A., & Young, L. J. (2002). Combining incompatible spatial data. *Journal of the American Statistical Association, 97*(458), 632–648.

Grey Literature International Steering Committee (2006). *Guidelines for the production of scientific and technical reports: How to write and distribute grey literature, Version 1.1.* Retrieved from http://www.glisc.info/#4.1.

Hall, J. A., & Gehant, P. K. (1994). Developing a community information database. In Liberton, C. (Ed)., *Proceedings from a system of care for children's mental health.* Tampa: Florida Mental Health Institute, University of South Florida.

Hanchette C. L. (2003). Geographic information systems. In P.W. O'Carroll, W. A. Yasnoff, M. E. Ward, et al. (Eds.), *Public health informatics and information systems,* (pp.431–466). New York: Springer, 2003.

Hanson, A. (2008). Accessibility: Critical GIS, ontologies, and semantics. In J. Abresch, A. Hanson, S. J. Heron, & P. Reehling (Eds.), *Integrating geographic information systems into library services: A guide for academic libraries* (pp. 151–174). Hershey, PA: IGI Global.

Hanson, A. (2001). Community assessments using map and geographic data. *Behavioral and Social Sciences Librarian, 19*(2), 49–62. doi: 10.1300/J103v19n02_04.

Hanson, A. R. M., & Levin, B. L. (2010). Navigating the worlds of information. In B. L. Levin & M.A. Becker (Eds.). *A public health perspective of women's mental health* (pp. 373–390). New York: Springer. doi:10.1007/978-1-4419-1526-9_20.

Hopewell, S., Clarke, M., Lefebvre, C., Scherer, R. (2007). Handsearching versus electronic searching to identify reports of randomized trials. *Cochrane Database of Systematic Reviews, 18*(2), MR000001. doi: 10.1002/14651858.MR000001.pub2.

Jayaram, M. B., & Hosalli, P. (2005). Risperidone versus olanzapine for schizophrenia. *Cochrane Database of Systematic Reviews, 18*(2): CD005237.

Kohn, L. T., Corrigan, J. M., & Donaldson, M. S. (2000). *To err is human: Building a safer health system.* Washington, DC: Institute of Medicine.

Langley, G. J., Nolan, K. M., Nolan, T. W., Norman, C. L., Provost, L. P. (1996). *The improvement guide.* San Francisco: Josey-Bass.

Liberati, A., Altman, D. G., Tetzlaff, J., Mulrow, C., Gøtzsche, P. C., et al. (2009). The PRISMA Statement for Reporting Systematic Reviews and Meta-Analyses of Studies That Evaluate Health Care Interventions: Explanation and elaboration. *PLoS Med 6*(7): e1000100. doi:10.1371/journal.pmed.1000100.

Meltzer, D. O., Basu, A., & Meltzer, H. Y. (2009). Comparative effectiveness research for antipsychotic medications: How much is enough? *Health Affairs, 28*(5), w794–w808. doi: 10.1377/hlthaff.28.5.w794.

Meltzer, D. O., Hoomans, T., Chung, J. W., & Basu, A. (2011). *Minimal modeling approaches to value of information analysis for health research* (Methods Future Research Needs Report, no. 6; AHRQ Publication No. 11-EHC062-EF) Rockville, MD: AHRQ. Retrieved from http://www.effectivehealthcare.ahrq.gov/ehc/products/197/719/MethodsFRN6_06–28–2011.pdf.

Moher, D., Cook, D. J., Eastwood, S., Olkin, I. Rennie, D., et al. (1999). Improving the quality of reporting of meta-analysis of randomized controlled trials: The QUOROM statement. *Lancet, 354,* 1896–1900.

Moher, D., Liberati, A., Tetzlaff, J., & Altman, D.G., for the PRISMA Group. (2009). Preferred Reporting Items for Systematic Reviews and Meta-Analyses: The PRISMA Statement. *PLoS Med, 6*(7): e1000097. doi:10.1371/journal.pmed.1000097.

Morissette, K., Tricco, A. C., Horsley, T., Chen, M. H., & Moher, D. (2011). Blinded versus unblinded assessments of risk of bias in studies included in a systematic review. *Cochrane Database of Systematic Reviews, 7*(9), MR000025. doi: 10.1002/14651858.MR000025.pub2.

Moss, F., & Thomson, R. (1999). A new structure for quality improvement reports. *Quality in Health Care, 8,* 76.

Myers, E., Sanders, G. D., Ravi, D., Matchar, D., Havrilesky, L., Samsa, G., Powers, B., McBroom, A., Musty, M., & Gray, R. (2011). *Evaluating the potential use of modeling and value-of-information analysis for future research prioritization within the evidence-based practice center program* (Report No.: 11-EHC030-EF). Rockville (MD): Agency for Healthcare Research and Quality (US); AHRQ Methods for Effective Health Care. Retrieved from http://www.ncbi.nlm.nih.gov/books/NBK62134/.

National Information Standards Organization. (1996). *ANSI/NISO Z39.14: Guidelines for Abstracts*. Bethesda, MD: NISO Press. Retrieved from http://www.niso.org/kst/reports/standards?step=2&gid=None&project_key%3Austring%3Aiso-8859-1=5944461cb4a1e365ad1688ec6f6c199c9d90ee71.

National Information Standards Organization. (2005). *ANSI/NISO Z39.18–2005: Scientific and technical reports: Preparation, presentation, and preservation*. Bethesda, MD: NISO Press. Retrieved from http://www.dtic.mil/dtic/pdf/customer/STINFOdata/ANSIZ_39182005.pdf.

National Library of Medicine. (2010). MeSH. Retrieved August 11, 2011, from http://www.nlm.nih.gov/mesh.

National Library of Medicine. (2011). Vocabulary, Controlled. MeSH. Retrieved http://www.ncbi.nlm.nih.gov/mesh?term=thesuarus.

Robinson, K. A., Saldanha, I. J., & McKoy, N. A. (2011). *Frameworks for determining research gaps during systematic reviews.* (Methods future research needs report, no. 2; AHRQ Publication No. 11-EHC043-EF). Rockville, MD: AHRQ. Retrieved from http://www.effectivehealthcare.ahrq.gov/ehc/products/201/735/FRN2_Frameworks_20110726.pdf.

Sanderson, S., Tatt, I. D., & Higgins, J. P. (2007). Tools for assessing quality and susceptibility to bias in observational studies in epidemiology: A systematic review and annotated bibliography. *International Journal of Epidemiology, 36,* 666–676. doi: 10.1093/ije/dym018.

Schulz, K. F., Altman, D. G., & Moher, D., for the CONSORT Group. (2010). CONSORT 2010 Statement: Updated guidelines for reporting parallel group randomised trials. *PLOS Medicine, 7*(3), e1000251. doi:10.1371/journal.pmed.1000251.

Schuurman, N., Leight, M., & Berube, M. (2008). A web-based graphical user interface for evidence-based decision making for health care allocations in rural areas. International *Journal of Health Geography, 7,* 49. doi: 10.1186/1476-072X-7-49.

Smidt, N., Overbeke, J., De Vet, H. C. W., & Bossuyt, P. M. (2007). Endorsement of the STARD statement by biomedical journals: Survey of instructions for authors. *Clinical Chemistry, 53*(11), 1983–1985. doi: 10.1373/clinchem.2007.090167.

The Standards of Reporting Trials Group. (1994). A proposal for structured reporting of randomized controlled trials. *JAMA, 272,* 1926–1931.

Stroup, D. F., Berlin, J. A., Morton, S. C., Olkin, I., Williamson, G. D., Rennie, D., Moher, D., … & Thacker, S. B. for the Meta-analysis of Observational Studies in Epidemiology (MOOSE) Group. (2000). Meta-analysis of observational studies in epidemiology: A proposal for reporting. *JAMA, 283*(15), 2008–2012. doi:10.1001/jama.283.15.2008.

Thomson Reuters. (2008). Currrent Contents Connect. Retrieved from http://wokinfo.com/media/pdf/CCCFactsheet_1-08.pdf.

Thomson Reuters. (2011). Web of Knowledge. Retrieved from wokinfo.com/products_tools/multidisciplinary/webofscience/.

Trespidi, C., Barbui, C, & Cipriani, A. (2011). Why it is important to include unpublished data in systematic reviews? *Epidemiology and Psychiatric Sciences, 20*(2):133–135.

Tuleya, L. G. (Ed.). (2007). *Thesaurus of psychological index terms,* 11th ed. Washington, DC: American Psychological Association.

Vandenbroucke, J. P., von Elm, E., Altman, D. G., Gøtzsche, P. C., Mulrow, C. D., Pocock, S. J., ... & Egger, M. for the STROBE Initiative. (2007). Strengthening the Reporting of Observational Studies in Epidemiology (STROBE): Explanation and elaboration. *Epidemiology, 18*(6), 805–835. doi: 10.1097/EDE.0b013e3181577511.

von Elm, E., Altman, D. G., Egger, M., Pocock, S. J., Gøtzsche, P. C., & Vandenbroucke, J. P., for the STROBE Initiative. (2008). The Strengthening the Reporting of Observational Studies in Epidemiology (STROBE) statement: Guidelines for reporting observational studies. *Journal of Clinical Epidemiology, 61*(4), 344–349. doi: 10.1016/j.jclinepi.2007.11.008.

Williamson, P. R., & Gamble, C. (2005). Identification and impact of outcome selection bias in meta-analysis. *Statistics in Medicine, 24*(10), 1547–1561. doi: 10.1002/sim.2025.

Working Group on Recommendations for Reporting of Clinical Trials in the Biomedical Literature. (1994). Call for comments on a proposal to improve reporting of clinical trials in the biomedical literature. *Annals of Internal Medicine, 121*, 894–895.

It is about common formats for integration and combination of data drawn from diverse sources.... It is also about language for recording how the data relates to real world objects. That allows a person, or a machine, to start off in one database, and then move through an unending set of databases which are connected not by wires but by being about the same thing.

—WC3, 2011, November, 2

I I   Information Retrieval, Interfaces, and Strategies

Over the past several decades, major federal reports have repeatedly prioritized two areas of critical importance for improving the health and mental health of Americans: (1) reducing the time it takes to move research to practice; and (2) the development of a national health information system for surveillance of health and mental health data. As practice and research generate data that finds its way into numerous databases, the data are repurposed into different formats, structures, and outputs. Mental health data are collected and disseminated by a variety of organizations, including federal, state, county, and local public agencies. In addition, academia creates and disseminates hundreds of thousands of publications a year in mental health through technical reports, academic and research publications, and online venues. This plethora of information makes it difficult to determine where these resources are housed and the constraints that limit the resources and data. From an informatics perspective, how one accesses information, strategizes searches, and recognizes the limitations of information is a never-ending quest, full of numerous caveats. Information seeking and information-seeking behaviors are key to mental health services research, practice, and education.

This chapter presents how best to navigate the systematized body of knowledge that constitutes mental health. The chapter contents examine (1) the importance of developing organized information systems for mental health; (2) the intellectual foundation of organizing information, including an overview of information-seeking behaviors; (3) current and emerging technologies which affect how one finds and retrieves information; and (4) the implications that emerging technologies and information seeking behaviors have on mental health research, education, services delivery, and policy.

Background

A number of federal reports have supported the use of communication and information technology to improve mental health services and research (U.S. Department of Health and Human Services, 1991, 1999, 2000; and The President's New Freedom Commission, 2003). These reports also suggested the development of a public health infrastructure by increasing efforts to collect, track, and disseminate national health and mental health data in order to build and maintain data, databases, and surveillance systems.

In addition, with the increased federal emphasis on comparative effectiveness research, quality of care, and patient outcomes, open access to the research literature and data has increased in importance. For example, since 2005, all National Institutes of Health (NIH)– funded research must be made available in an open access venue. NIH requires that these papers are accessible to the public on PubMed Central no later than 12 months after publication. PubMed Central is the free full-text archive of biomedical and life sciences journal literature at the U.S. National Institutes of Health's National Library of Medicine (NIH/NLM). PubMed Central is just one of the many systems available to access the research literature, and in some cases, actual data. However, there are numerous ways that information is organized to enhance access to digital and print repositories (Svenonius, 2000). Understanding how information is organized is often the first step toward understanding the efficacy of various search engines.

Organizing Information

Numerous cataloging codes and practices have been created to describe new resources (a.k.a. "works"), to provide networked access to resources, and to respond more effectively to an increasingly broad range of user expectations and information needs. Issues surrounding the quality and relevance of metadata (bibliographic access) become more critical in online venues, especially with non-textual data. One of the paradigms of access was proposed by Charles Ammi Cutter (1904). His constructs of m*eans and objects* enable the finding of information more easily in an early database: the library catalog. Cutter's *objects* were to (1) enable a person to find a book of which either the author, title, or subject is known; (2) show what the library has by a given author, on a given subject, or in a given kind of literature; and (3) assist in the choice of a book as to its edition (bibliographically) or to its character (literary or topical). His *means*, or method of doing so, provides numerous access points, including author-entry with necessary references; title-entry or title-reference; subject-entry, cross-references, and classed subject-table; form-entry; and edition and imprint, with notes when necessary (Cutter, 1904). These principles are still the foundation of best cataloging practice, including the notion of specificity, the consideration of the user as the principal basis for subject heading decisions, the practice of standardizing terminology, the use of cross-references to show preferred terms and hierarchical relationships, and solving the problem of the order of elements. To bring the terminology of the nineteenth century into the twenty-first century, replace "resource" for "book," prefix it with any number of adjectives (e.g., print, digital), and call it metadata.

Metadata, like Cutter's means, tell "who, what, where, when, why, and how" about every facet of a piece of data or service. When properly constructed, metadata answer a wide range of questions about information resources, including what data or texts are available, how to evaluate quality and suitability for use, and how to access, transfer, and process them. To ensure consistency for access and retrieval, metadata are standardized to provide a common set of terms, definitions, and organization.

With databases, libraries, and other information repositories now available as remote, online resources, users still search for works by a specific author, title, or subject. In many instances, title and subject searches may be based upon keywords in the title, notes, abstracts, and subject headings. Databases and catalogs still show what they contain as to authors, titles, and subjects. Users incorporate this information in their decisions to select, retrieve, and read the work. The increasing access points provided in databases and catalogs also increases the possibility of retrieving relevant information on a specific topic or author, as well as retrieving associated works by the author(s).

In the development of databases, there are many issues to consider. In addition to the issues of relevance, specificity, and recall, a sustainable system must also incorporate the three R's: reliability, redundancy, and replication of results. These "three R's" can be seen in the development of the functional requirements for the bibliographic record (FRBR) relationship model for works, expressions, manifestations, and items, which is one of the current international standards used in the information field (Tillett, 2003).

First, however, a schema must be created, supported by syntax rules and constraints. Schemas typically restrict element and attribute names and their allowable containment hierarchies. The constraints in a schema may also include data type assignments that affect how information is formatted and processed. For example, date elements would be formatted in a specific way, such as MM/DD/YYYY or MM/DD/YY. Most databases and catalogs use three structural frameworks: bibliographic; authority; and holdings.

BIBLIOGRAPHIC RECORDS

A bibliographic record essentially describes the work. Based upon the vendor, the number of descriptive elements of the record may vary from minimal data to intricately described data. The bibliographic structure uses a combination of fixed and variable length fields. Fixed fields contain excerpted information in predetermined length strings to allow ease in searching the datasets. Variable fields have no predetermined lengths, can contain extensive amounts of information, and are of variable length because the amount of information differs for each item. All information is entered into defined fields, designating the type of data, which is then further subdivided into discrete pieces. Not all data in the record are available to the public. Some of the data are used for general housekeeping operations for the database vendor.

The PubMed record format is borrowed from the MARC (Machine Readable Cataloging) format, which was developed by the United States Library of Congress in the 1960s. The current iteration of MARC is MARC 21, now an international standard, whose uniform data structure has been enhanced with the development of the Z39.50 standard for the electronic sharing of data and with the use of the XML (Extensible mark-up language) format. Unlike Hyper-Text Markup Lnguage (HTML), which was developed to display data on graphical web interfaces, XML was created to transport and store data. Unlike HTML, which uses pre-defined tags, XML allows the author to define his or her own tags and to create his or her own document structure. For example, the National Library of Medicine's PubMed database provides a searchable fields map to existing fields in a bibliographic record (see Figure 11.1),

In addition to these searchable fields, a bibliographic record also may contain non-searchable fields (e.g., the digital object identifier, doi; PubMed field: AID) and the dates when the item was received and accepted. Further, certain fields are repeatable fields, such as author fields and MeSH (Medical Subject Headings). Each author has his or her own name field entry, with the names formatted as to full name and/or to last name and initials. Multiple subject headings provide numerous access points that also allow the use of filters to improve relevance and specificity. The addition of the MeSH term "humans" to the English language field allows users to retrieve English-only articles with "humans" as the research population, as opposed to retrieving all articles in every language with animal and human studies (see Figure 11.2).

AUTHORITY RECORDS

In addition to the bibliographic record, authority records establish the semantic interoperability of controlled subject terminology and classification data. Authority control allows the user to find all items on a particular topic or by an author, regardless of the many term variations, synonymous terms, or languages that might be available in a database. Authority records achieve consistency among bibliographic records and provide a linking

Abstract/Index Tags [itag]	ISSN [issn]	Publication Status [status]
Acid Free	ISSN Type [is]	Publication Type [pt]
All Fields [all]	Item Type [item]	Publication Year [dp]
Author [au]	Journal [jo]	Publication End Year [eyr]
Broad Subject Term(s) [st]	Language [la]	Publication Start Year [syr]
Corporate/Conference Name [cn]	MeSH Major Topic [majr]	Publisher [publ]
Country of Publication [pl]	MeSH Subheadings [sh]	PubMed Central Holdings
Current Format Status [cfs]	MeSH Terms [mh]	Resource Type [res type]
Current Indexing Status	NLM Unique ID [nlmid]	Series [ser]
Current Subset	Olio [olio]	Title [ti]
Currently/Previously Indexed for MEDLINE	Other Number [other num]	Title Abbreviation [ta]
Filter [sb]	Other Term [ot]	URL [url]
Full Author Name [fau]	Personal Full Name as Subject [fps]	Version Indexed
Indexing Subset [xs]	Personal Name as Subject [ps]	Publication Status [status]
ISO Abbreviation [isoabbr]		

FIGURE 11.1 Field Descriptions and Tags in a PubMed Bibliographic Record.

Retrieved from *NLM* (2007). *NLM catalog help*, http://www.ncbi.nlm.nih.gov/books/NBK3799/#catalog. Overview.

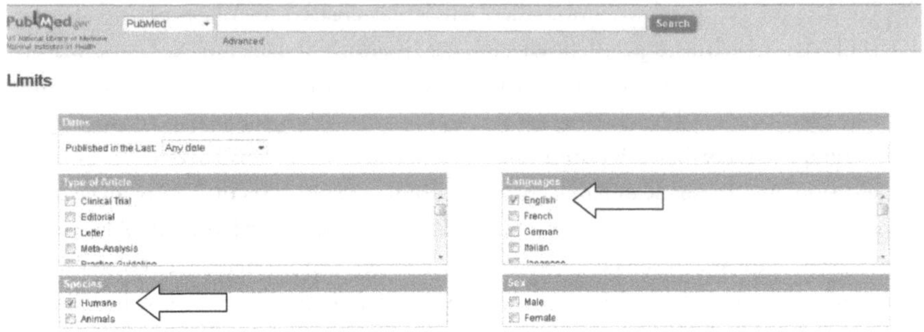

FIGURE 11.2 Screenshot of Limits Feature Using Species and Languages.
Retrieved from http://www.ncbi.nlm.nih.gov/pubmed/limits.

framework for related names and subjects. An authority record includes three basic components: (1) headings; (2) cross references; and (3) notes. The heading is the standardized "authoritative" form of a name, subject, or title that is used on bibliographic records. There are two types of cross references. The first type, a *see* reference, directs a user from a variant form of a name or subject to the authoritative form. The second type is a *see also* reference. The *see also* reference directs the user from one authoritative form to another authoritative form because they are related to one another. The references are carried on the record for the authoritative heading, and a well-designed system will allow these references to lead searchers to the correct heading. Notes contain general information about standardized headings or more specialized information, such as citations for a consulted source used to verify a form of name or a definition.

In PubMed, for example, authority records are created for subject, names (personal, corporate, meeting, and geographic), series and uniform titles, and name/title authority records. In the PubMed authority records, associated references and scope notes are also provided. Using NLM's LocatorPlus, the authority record for the phrase "mental disorders" shows "mental disorders" in the 150 field, which makes it a preferred term for use in PubMed. The next seven phrases (in the 450 fields) are *see* terms. *See* terms automatically map the user to the preferred term, which is "mental disorders." *See also* terms are found in the 550 field. A *see also* term is a related term that has a conceptual relationship with the term in the 150 field (Figure 11.3). The purpose of the *see also* terms is to allow the user to expand or narrow his or her search to additional concepts.

HOLDINGS

Holdings records generally contain information about whether an institution or vendor can provide access to bibliographic items, in what formats, which parts of a bibliographic item it holds, and where to find them. Holdings records are linked to the bibliographic record through the use of unique identifiers, which may be numeric or alphanumeric in format. In the case of digital records, in addition to the unique identifier linking the user to the bibliographic record, there will be another unique identifier, known as a digital object identifier (doi), which links the user to the authoritative version of the digital document.

150 __ |a Mental Disorders 450 __ |w nnna |a Behavior Disorders 450 __ |w nnna |a Diagnosis
450 __ |w nnna |a Behavior Disorders
450 __ |w nnna |a Diagnosis
450 __ |w nnna |a Diagnosis, Psychiatric
450 __ |w nnna |a Psychiatric Diagnosis
450 __ |w nnna |a Disorder, Mental
450 __ |w nnna |a Disorders, Behavior
450 __ |w nnna |a Disorders, Mental
450 __ |w nnna |a Mental Disorder
550 __ |a Mentally Ill Persons

Psychiatric illness or diseases manifested by breakdowns in the adaptational process expressed primarily as abnormalities of thought, feeling, and behavior producing either distress or impairment of function.

FIGURE 11.3 NLM LocatorPlus Authority Record for Term "Mental Disorders," National Library of Medicine.
NLM LocatorPlus. http://locatorplus.gov/.

Information-Seeking Behaviors

An international analysis of user needs determined that there are four generic information tasks which users perform when performing a search (IFLA Study Group on the Functional Requirements for Bibliographic Records, 1998). The first task is to find works that correspond to the user's stated search criteria. This allows the user to find all documents on a given subject, or a search for a work issued under a particular title. The second task is to identify the document, which is described in a record, that corresponds to the document sought by the user. This also allows the user to disambiguate, that is, to distinguish between two works that have the same title. For example, a user searches on the phrase "President's New Freedom Commission on Mental Health" with the intent to retrieve the Commission's final report. Twenty-five items are retrieved: the final report; 16 subcommittee reports; an executive summary of the Commission's final report; an interim report; three supplemental reports; a fact sheet; and a news release.

The third task is to select a work that is appropriate to the user's needs. In addition to subject analysis, critical data, in this case, provide information on the language of item or available formats (e.g., .pdf, .html, or .wav) that are compatible with the user's hardware and operating system. The final task is to obtain access to the work that is described, whether it is to download the item immediately, create an account for access, order the item through an online vendor, or to place a request through the website or through a library's interlibrary loan system (IFLA ..., 1998).

These principles are still the foundation of best practice, including the notion of specificity, the consideration of the user as the principal basis for subject-heading decisions, the practice of standardizing terminology, the use of cross-references to show preferred terms and hierarchical relationships, and solving the problem of the order of elements (Heron & Hanson, 2003). Not only do these practices organize the information in such a way that allows the user to eliminate irrelevancies, the focus on specifics reduces cognitive overload *and* saves the time of the user. For the access that web-based search engines may provide to digital materials, nothing comes close to the relevance and precision in a search that a well-designed catalog or database can provide.

SUBJECT ACCESS VERSUS KEYWORD SEARCHING

Researchers who are serious about retrieving the most targeted materials on a topic use subject access as opposed to keyword searching. Understanding the hierarchical structure of a thesaurus or controlled vocabulary allows the user to "see" clusters of concepts that share common characteristics as well as the natural language terms useful in the context in which the thesaurus will be used (Heron & Hanson, 2008). Let's take a very basic example. Depression, bipolar disorder, and obsessive-compulsive disorder all share the common characteristic of being a *mental illness*. They also share additional characteristics, such as treatment and diagnosis. These terms constitute the beginnings of a *mental disorders* facet. Sometimes the terms in a facet can be divided into subfacets by secondary characteristics. For example, within the *mental disorders* facet, there is a facet for *mood disorders*, which comprise depressive disorders, bipolar disorders, substance-induced mood disorders, alcohol-induced mood disorders, benzodiazepine-induced mood disorders, and interferon-alpha–induced mood disorders. Another facet would be created for obsessive-compulsive disorder, which is *anxiety disorders*. Yet another facet would be *personality disorders*. Facets and subfacets are then arranged as simple hierarchies of terms, from general to specific.

There are several benefits to using a faceted approach. First, users can see naming consistency, order, hierarchical relationships, relationships to other groups, and current or superseded terms. Second, a faceted approach is extensible, so it is easier to add new terms or establish new relationships among existing terms within the thesaurus. Third, a faceted approach reinforces an important concept in knowledge organization and management, that is, *cognitive miserliness*. Coined by social psychologists Fiske and Taylor (1991), the term *cognitive miser* describes an individual's interest in conserving energy and reducing cognitive load, that is, sifting through the mass of information that bombards us every day, ignoring anything unimportant to us, and retaining the information that is important. Clearly, it is much easier for a user to understand a set of hierarchically organized facets as a conceptual map (which shows the precise level and set of associations of a term) than to negotiate a long list of alphabetized terms or 450,000 hits (retrieved by a web search engine or a "one-search" metasearch).

To provide the most effective subject approaches to traditional and networked resources, vendors, librarians, and information specialists must account for the many different patron strategies and vendor models currently used in information retrieval. The Boolean model, which uses exact match across inclusive and exclusive groupings (AND, OR, NOT), tends to provide more precision in one's search. However, with the emphasis on natural language searching, other tools (such as ranking algorithms, vector, and probabilistic models) attempt to compensate for their loss of precision to a certain degree by methods of statistical ranking and computational linguistics (based on term occurrences, term frequency, word proximity, and term weighting).

Controlled vocabulary offers the benefits of consistency and accuracy with better recall through synonym control and term relationships and greater precision through homograph control. Although controlled vocabulary will not replace the apparent "ease" of keyword searching, it supplements keyword searching to enhance retrieval results. However, from an informatics perspective, the issues that emerged in the early days of online access still remain.

In 1999, Batty observed "There is a burden of effort in information storage and retrieval that may be shifted from shoulder to shoulder, from author, to indexer, to index language designer, to searcher, to user. It may even be shared in different proportions. But it will not go away." Ten years later, Colati et al. (2009) suggested, "Creating broadly accessible descriptive metadata is a way to maximize access by current users and attract new user communities through online access." The apparent "ease" of keyword searching is very attractive to the novice searcher, but places the cognitive responsibility on the researcher. Controlled vocabulary, created by trained indexers, offers the benefits of consistency and accuracy with better recall through synonym control and term relationships and greater precision through homograph control, simplifying the task of the researcher. Although controlled vocabulary will not replace keyword searching, it supplements keyword searching to enhance retrieval results. Certainly, information provision is moving to "user-focused" or "task-based" frameworks. Whether the focus is on the user or the task, new ways of conceptualizing information retrieval will allow a greater degree of personalization in information strategies and retrieval.

In addition, retrieval tools, such as Google, have changed users' expectations in accessing information. Unlike other Internet search engines, Google is similar to academic vendors because it uses database management as a core informational tool. Unlike Web 1.0, Web 2.0 brought to information retrieval a more user-centered design and new web applications (Bennett & Flach, 2011). In addition to the proliferation of Web 2.0 tools, there are additional issues to address in designing interfaces to increase user success in creating effective search strategies and increasing relevance in his or her recall of materials (the display of retrieved items). Functional interface design requires an understanding of the information system structure and the user. The use of server logs, for example, record user interactions with the interface, providing insights into user search behavior and efficiency of the search process. Other data-mining approaches use association rules, clustering, and classification to visualize the usability and functionality of interfaces for databases.

One of the more important changes in interface design is the incorporation of back-end thesauri and controlled vocabulary in the front-end display. Searches are more precise if controlled vocabularies are available in the database. For example, preferred headings and related terms are easily displayed as cues to the user for determining the relevance of the topics in an article and whether or not the item is worth reading. Augmenting controlled vocabularies with natural language (a.k.a. keyword) searching is almost *de rigueur* (i.e., standard) in today's more sophisticated search engines. The use of similarity cues, such as "Did you mean X," provide an easy transition for the user to subject analysis and terms.

From an informatics perspective, a natural evolution is the use of a "layered" interface, which provides options to operate at different levels of granularity. By incorporating these types of knowledge frameworks into the interface design, presentation of results is improved and query specifications are enhanced, resulting in more precision and relevance for users. One example is the use of simple and advanced search features. The simple search feature in PubMed, for example, allows the user to use natural language or keyword searching in a single field entry. The advanced search feature allows the user to build a search across 39 fields (using a drop-down box) and displays the index for ease of selection and insertion into the search builder feature. In addition, the advanced search option links to the limiting features available, including dates, type of article (e.g., clinical trial, meta-analysis, etc.), species, subsets (e.g., history of medicine, nursing, etc.), text options (full-text, free full-text, and/or abstracts), languages, gender, and ages (14 age groups). A third feature is the ability to go directly into MeSH and build a search directly from its controlled vocabulary, including the use of subheadings. In Figure 11.4, the search using mood disorders maps displays three terms: *mood disorders, seasonal affective disorder*, and *affective disorders, psychotic*.

Choosing *mood disorders*, the screen displays a definition, the year introduced, and subheadings, which are the search headings most likely to be associated with this term. For example, if the focus of one's search is on the rehabilitation of persons who have mood disorders, one can select the subheading "rehabilitation" and then automatically add the term and subheading to the search builder ["Mood Disorders/rehabilitation"[MeSH]] and search PubMed. One of the really nice features of PubMed is that the results automatically display lists if there are any review articles in the search retrieval. Once the above search is completed (with over 1,400 results), one can then go into "Limits" and "limit by language" [English] and by free full-text.

FEDERATED SEARCH ENGINES

Another important development in information retrieval is the use of federated search engines. A federated search engine searches across a wide range of heterogeneous resources

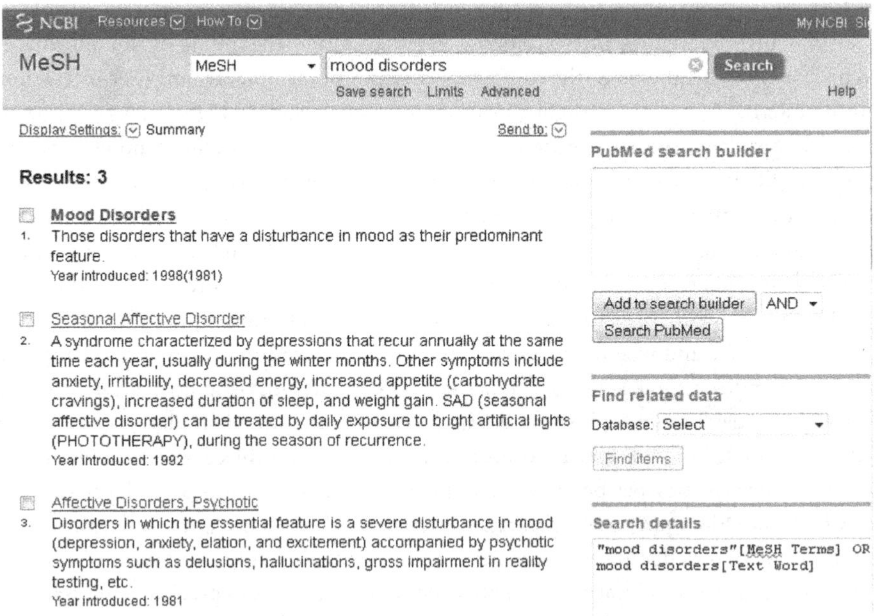

FIGURE 11.4 Results of MeSH Search on Mood Disorders (Screenshot).

(e.g., catalogs, reference databases, citation databases, subject gateways, and e-journals) that differ in the format of the information, the technologies used, and the types of materials contained in the resources. The user's query is broadcast to each resource, and results are returned to the user. There are several criteria to use when evaluating federated search engines: extent of metadata provided, and by whom; the intended scope (subject, geographical, language); and quality criteria and quality control.

Unlike the National Library of Medicine's PubMed database, which uses a controlled vocabulary and mapping, the U.S. Government Printing Office (GPO, 2011) has implemented Federal Depository Library Program (FDLP) Desktop, a federated search engine, to search across 54 federal databases, including reference databases, digital repositories, and subject-based web portals. Built upon Ex Libris's MetaLib product, descriptive information is provided for each item, which may include holdings information, classification, subject heading and keyword assignation, and summary information.

Current and Emerging Technologies

Major barriers to information access include time, resource reliability, trustworthiness and/or credibility of information, and "information and/or dataset overload." Dataset overload is particularly problematic due to the increasingly large number of datasets generated by surveys and other data collection tools using a variety of platforms, structural frameworks, and interfaces that make it much more difficult to integrate and analyze data. With the number of databases and search engines increasing at almost an exponential rate, it is important to step back and examine some of the current emerging technologies that enhance access and (hopefully) decrease barriers. As with the development of any technology application, there is also a standards group for web-based services and protocols.

The W3C (World Wide Web Consortium) is an international community that develops open standards to ensure the long-term growth of the web. Most W3C work revolves around the standardization of Web technologies, using an international consensus process similar to that of the International Organization for Standardization (ISO). In 2011, a W3C Web Services Package was formally approved as ISO/IEC standards by the ISO Joint Technical Committee JTC 1 (Information Technology) and the International Electrotechnical Commission (IEC). The core of the package utilizes the SOAP protocol.

SOAP 1.2 (formerly known as Simple Object Access Protocol), for example, bridges competing technologies and facilitates interoperability across services, objects, and servers. Considered a service-oriented architecture (see Figure 11.5), it defines the use of XML in the creation of a message, as well as the protocols used to send that message across the web (HTTP, *HyperText Transfer Protocol* and HTTPS, HTTP Secure). There are a number of advantages in using SOAP. Not only is it versatile enough to use across a variety of transport protocols, it is platform independent. Further, it is language independent, which makes it usable from an international perspective, and it is extensible.

SOAP consists of three parts: (1) an envelope that defines a framework for describing what is in a message and how to process it; (2) a set of encoding rules for expressing instances of application-defined data types; and (3) a convention for representing remote procedure calls and responses. The ISO/IET package specifically includes the SOAP

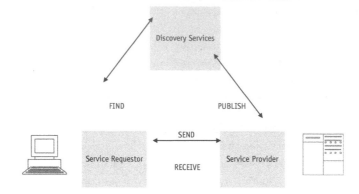

FIGURE 11.5 Service-Oriented Architecture.

Message Transmission Optimization Mechanism (SOAP MTOM), WS-Addressing 1.0 (addressing and correlation capabilities), and the WS Policy language 1.5. The WS Policy language provides a general purpose model and corresponding syntax to describe the policies of entities in a Web services-based system, using any Web Service Description (W3C, 2011).

A service-oriented architecture (SOA) also lends itself to gateway services, which act as entrances to another network. Gateway services handle data discovery functions, while OpenURL applications (e.g., SFX) provide context-sensitive linking services that assist users in either obtaining the actual material or expanding upon the data already discovered. Linking syntaxes utilize standard methods of identification or attributes (metadata) of the discovered object. The method creates a unique and persistent identifier, which links the query to the authoritative document. The digital object identifier (doi) is a key component in the OpenURL Framework for Context-Sensitive Services. The OpenURL became an ANSI/NISO standard (Z39.88–2004) in April 2005 (NISO, 2005). ANSI/ NISO Z39.88–2004 describes details of a publication (metadata) in a systematic way.

The metadata use standard descriptors, ISSN (International Standard Serial Number), volume, author last name, collection name, and so on, to create the query to describe the work and to deliver the requested item. Metadata, which may be derived from descriptive cataloging, comprise the administrative elements for resource management. The metadata allow context-sensitive linking through its link server, which determines which target(s) should be delivered to the user and the addresses (URLs) for those targets. Link servers contain the data in a single place on all the resources, print or electronic, that a university, vendor, or agency wants their users to be able to link.

Building upon the descriptive standards and the move to a context-sensitive query leads to the Semantic Web. The Semantic Web is a part of Web 3.0 development. According to the W3C (2011), the Semantic Web "provides a common framework that allows data to be shared and reused across application, enterprise, and community boundaries" (HTML, no pagination).

The Semantic Web would allow a user to start off in database A and then move through an unending set of databases (∞) that are connected together by context (i.e., being about the same thing). By encouraging the inclusion of semantic content in web pages, the

Semantic Web aims at converting the current web of unstructured documents into a "web of data." It builds on the W3C's Resource Description Framework (RDF).

The RDF data model is similar to classic conceptual modeling approaches, such as entity-relationships or class diagrams, both used extensively in library and information science. An entity is an object (e.g., a person, group, place, thing, or activity) that stores data. An entity relationship (ER) is the visual representation of all data stored in a system. It is a means of visualizing how the information a system produces is related. Many ER diagrams resemble flowcharts. Entities may be represented by rectangles, relationships may be represented by diamond shapes, and connecting lines connect an entity to a relationship. Attributes, also used in ER diagrams, are drawn as ovals and are connected by lines to a single entity or relationship (see Figure 11.6).

Based upon the idea of making statements about resources (in particular web resources) in the form of subject-predicate-object expressions, the RDF has a series of file formats for encoding data and interpretation mechanisms so that resources can be described in such a way that specific software can access and use the information. It is important to translate and code the data held in relational databases so they can be machine-processed and the semantics (context) properly made accessible. Controlled vocabulary and ontologies come into play as critical resources.

An ontology formally represents knowledge as a set of concepts (vocabulary and taxonomy) within a domain, and the relationships between those concepts, that is, the structural frameworks for organizing information. In the Semantic Web, Web Ontology Language (OWL) is a family of knowledge representation languages to create ontologies. For a more accessible example, we examined the Unified Medical Language System (UMLS) of the National Library of Medicine, which is a compendium of many controlled vocabularies in the biomedical sciences. The UMLS addresses the granularity and problems that can emerge with context-based searching:

> A concept is a meaning. A meaning can have many different names. A key goal of Metathesaurus construction is to understand the intended meaning of each name in each source vocabulary and to link all the names from all of the source vocabularies that mean the same thing (the synonyms). (NLM, 2009, p. 4)

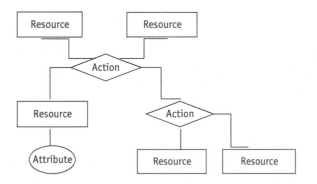

FIGURE 11.6 Entity-Relationship-Attribute Model.

With over 1 million medical concepts from more than 100 specialized vocabularies in the UMLS metathesaurus, synonymous terms are clustered into a concept, a preferred term is chosen, and a unique identifier (CUI) is assigned to the term (NLM, 2009). In addition to names, synonyms, terms, and codes, hierarchies and mappings are created (relationships), and attributes are defined. The CUI links the concept data across the files (NLM, 2009).

The UMLS is also a semantic network in its development of semantic types (135 categories) and semantic relationships (54) between categories (NLM, 2009). The Semantic Network serves as an authority for the semantic types assigned to concepts in the Metathesaurus. The Network uses both textual descriptions and hierarchical information to define its semantic types. The meaning of each term is defined "by its source, explicitly by definition or annotation; by context (its place in a hierarchy); by synonyms and other stated relationships between terms; and by its usage in description, classification, or indexing" (NLM, 2009, Chapter 5, p. 1). In Figure 11.7, we see the use of an "isa" link ("is a"), which is the primary link in the Semantic Network. This establishes the hierarchy of types within the Network and is used for deciding on the most specific semantic type available for assignment to a Metathesaurus concept. For example, starting at the bottom left of the figure, a *mental process* is an *organism function,* which is a *physiologic function,* which is a *biologic function.* Further, one could say that the functions of the organism, the organ, the cell, and at the molecular level may be related to the concept of mental process.

In addition, the UMLS also identifies a set of non-hierarchical relations between the types: "physically related to"; "spatially related to"; "temporally related to"; "functionally related to"; and "conceptually related to." In Figure 11.8, we see a very small example of the Semantic Network, illustrating either the hierarchical or associative relations that exist between semantic types.

With a natural language search as the default search strategy by many users, the UMLS SPECIALIST Lexicon was developed to provide the lexical information needed for the SPECIALIST Natural Language Processing System (NLP). Intended to be a general

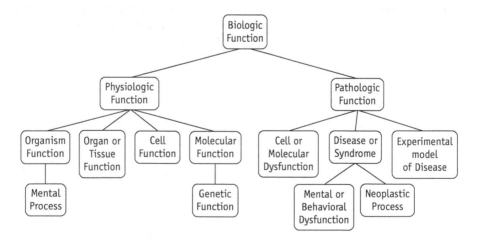

FIGURE 11.7 A Portion of the UMLS Semantic Network: "Biologic Function" Hierarchy.

From NLM (2009). Chapter 5 "Semantic network" in *UMLS Reference Manual.* Retrieved http://www.ncbi. nlm.nih.gov/books/NBK9679/#ch05.I51_Overview.

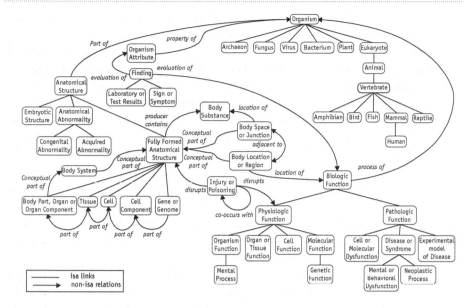

FIGURE 11.8 A Portion of the UMLS Semantic Network: Relations.
From NLM (2009). Chapter 5 "Semantic network" in *UMLS Reference Manual.* Retrieved http://www.ncbi.
nlm.nih.gov/books/NBK9679/#ch05.I51_Overview.

English lexicon with biomedical terms, SPECIALIST NLP coverage includes both commonly occurring English words and biomedical vocabulary. Each lexicon entry records the "syntactic category, inflectional variation (e.g., singular and plural for nouns, the conjugations of verbs, the positive, comparative, and superlative for adjectives and adverbs), and allowable complementation patterns (i.e., the objects and other arguments that verbs, nouns, and adjectives can take)" (McCray, Srinivasan, & Browne, 1994, p. 235). This allows the normalization of terms when users search syntactic, morphological, and orthographic information needed by the SPECIALIST NLP System. For example, if the normalized term is "eye patch," then the term "eye-patch" maps to "patches, Eye" and "Eye Patch" (McCray, Srinivasan, & Browne, 1994, p. 236).

In addition, the MetaMap Transfer (MMTx), one of the Lexical Tools in the UMLS, is specifically designed to map arbitrary terms to concepts in the Metathesaurus, or, equivalently, to discover Metathesaurus concepts within free text.

The use of the semantic web is increasing in health services research and practice. The W3C Semantic Web Health Care and Life Sciences Interest Group (HCLSIG) were interested in developing tools for researchers to navigate and annotate potentially relevant literature in neuroscience (Ruttenberg, et al., 2007). The HCLSIG created an application to allow researchers to collect, annotate, and share their observations on study methodologies and hypotheses. Another area was the application of natural language processing to scientific texts to encode entities and relationships within the texts. The result was SWAN (Semantic Web Applications in Neuromedicine; http://swan.mindinformatics.org/), which currently focuses on the research on Alzheimer's disease and other neurodegenerative diseases, with a series of specialized ontologies: relationships; scientific discourse; collections; provenance; authoring and versioning (iterations, drafts, e.g., who wrote what version when); and FOAF (friend of a friend), describing and connecting social websites and the people they describe (Ruttenberg, et al., 2007).

Shotton (2009) writes how the Semantic Web may enhance the use of scholarly journal articles through the publication of data and metadata. He defines "semantic publishing" as "anything that enhances the meaning of a published journal article, facilitates its automated discovery, enables its linking to semantically related articles, provides access to data within the article in actionable form, or facilitates integration of data between papers" (Shotton, 2009, p. 86). More importantly, semantic publishing provides a way for computers to understand the structure and the meaning of the published information. For example, the inclusion of appropriate metadata, from established thesauri or ontologies, may increase the "findability" of a resource and enable its retrieval with a higher level of precision and relevance in one search. Many publishers, such as PLoS (Public Library of Science), have made their articles downloadable in both .pdf and XML formats. The Centers for Disease Control and Prevention provide access to statistical tables in an .xls format as well as the capacity to generate dynamic charts and tables.

Another interesting use of the Semantic Web is CiTO (*Ci*tation *T*yping *O*ntology). CiTO, written in the Web Ontology Language OWL, describes the nature of reference citations in scientific research articles and other scholarly works (Shotton, 2010). It examines a number of relationships between citing publication and cited publication, including the in-text and global citation frequencies of each cited work and the nature of the cited work itself (e.g., publication and peer review status). Authors can use any of the 20 possible relationship fields to annotate their articles for the web, including cites to, is cited by, agrees with, disagrees with, disputes, includes excerpt from X, includes quotation from Y, is cited as authority by, is cited as data source by, among others. CiTO's metadata framework is strongly influenced by FRBR (IFLA, 1998) and includes the SWAN Scientific Discourse Relationships Ontology, although there are subtle discrepancies in the targets and definitions of relationships (Shotton, 2010). This type of tool may change how scholarly works are accessed and understood, especially in academia.

Implications for Mental Health Informatics

Information retrieval appears deceptively simple; however, that is a false perception. Since language and cognitive processing are involved in effective information retrieval, automated search functions are extremely difficult to automate. Not only are there scalability problems, but user needs vary from one subject domain to another. Therefore, optimal indexing and retrieval mechanisms vary substantially from field to field. To organize information, a variety of standards are used to describe data, including structural frameworks, cataloging rules and interpretations, class schedules, and subject access.

As we move into the next decade, persons interested in mental health informatics should think of the opportunities provided in electronic collection management. Not only are there exciting developments in managing access to and creating metadata, we urge active participation in standards or systems development.

Clearly, there is much to offer and to learn in the development of intelligent tools for integrated access across heterogeneous resources. Bringing Semantic Web technologies, for example, into health care toolkits to address interoperability increases beneficial collaboration, improved patient care, and enhanced clinical research outcomes.

References

Batty, D. (1998). WWW: Wealth, weariness or waste: Controlled vocabulary and thesauri in support of online information access. *D-Lib Magazine, November*, http://www.dlib.org/dlib/november98-11batty.html.

Bennett, K. B., & Flach, J. (2011). *Display and interface design: Subtle science, exact art.* Boca Raton; London: CRC Press

Colati, J. B., Dean, R. & Maull, K. (2009). Describing digital objects: A tale of compromise. *Cataloging & Classification Quarterly, 47*(3), 326–369.

Cutter, C. A. (1904). *Rules for a dictionary catalog,* 4th ed. Washington, DC: Government Printing Office.

Fiske, Susan T., & Taylor, Shelley E. (1991). *Social cognition,* 2nd ed. New York: McGraw-Hill.

Greenberg, S. A. (2009). How citation distortions create unfounded authority: Analysis of a citation network. *BMJ, 339*, b2680. doi:10.1136/bmj.b2680.

Heron, S. J., & Hanson, A. (2008). Describing geospatial information. In J. Abresch, A, Hanson, S. J. Heron, & P. Reehling (Eds.), *Integrating geographic information systems into library services: A guide for academic libraries* (pp. 82–113). Hershey, PA: IGI Global.

Heron, S. J, & Hanson, A. (2003). From subject gateways to portals: The role of metadata in accessing international research. In N. Callaos (Ed.), *Conference proceedings of the SCI 2003: The 7th world multiconference on systemics, cybernetics, and informatics* (pp. 529–533). Orlando, FL: International Institute of Informatics and Systemics.

IFLA Study Group on the Functional Requirements for Bibliographic Records. (1998). *Functional Requirements for Bibliographic Records, Final Report* (UBCIM Publications, New Series; v. 19). München: K. G. Saur. Retrieved from http://www.ifla.org/VII/s13/frbr/frbr.pdf.

McCray, A. T., Srinivasan, S., & Browne, A. C. (1994). Lexical methods for managing variation in biomedical terminologies. *Proceedings of the 18th Annual Symposium on Computer Applications in Medical Care* (pp. 235–239). Bethesda, MD: NLM. Retrieved from http://www.ncbi.nlm.nih.gov/pmc/articles/PMC2247735/?tool=pubmed

National Library of Medicine. (2009). Metathesaurus—UMLS® Reference Manual. Bethesda, MD: NLM. Retrieved from http://www.ncbi.nlm.nih.gov/books/NBK9684/pdf/ch02.pdf.

NISO. (2005). *Z39.88–2004, The OpenURL Framework for context-sensitive services.* Retrieved from http://www.niso.org/standards/z239-88-2004.

President's New Freedom Commission on Mental Health. (2003). *Achieving the promise: Transforming mental health care in America. Final Report* (DHHS Pub. No. SMA-03-3832). Rockville, MD: President's New Freedom Commission on Mental Health. Retrieved 19 May, 2009, from http://web.archive.org/web/20101106222826/http://www.mental-healthcommission.gov/reports/Finalreport/toc.html.

Ruttenberg, A., Clark, T., Bug, W., Samwald, M., Bodenreider, O., Chen, H., …, & Cheung, K. H. (2007). Advancing translational research with the Semantic Web. *BMC Bioinformatics, 9*(8 Suppl 3), S2. doi: 10.1186/1471-2105-8-S3-S2.

Shotton, D. (2010). CiTO, the Citation Typing Ontology. *Journal of Biomedical Semantics, 1*(Suppl 1), S6. doi: 10.1186/2041-1480-1-S1-S6.

Shotton, D. (2009). Semantic publishing: The coming revolution in scientific journal publishing. *Learned Publishing, 22*, 85–94. http://dx.doi.org/10.1087/2009202.

Svenonius, E. (2000). The intellectual foundation of information organization. *Digital libraries and electronic publishing.* Cambridge, MA: MIT Press.

Tillett, B. (2003). *What is FRBR? A conceptual model for the bibliographic universe.* Washington, DC: Library of Congress, Cataloging Distribution Service.

U.S. Department of Health and Human Services. (1991). *Healthy people 2000: National health promotion and disease prevention objectives.* Washington, DC: U.S. Government Printing Office.

U.S. Department of Health and Human Services. (2000). *Healthy people 2010, With understanding and improving health and objectives for improving health* (2 vols.), 2nd ed. Washington, DC: U.S. Government Printing Office.

U.S. Department of Health and Human Services, Office of the Surgeon General. (1999). *Mental health: A report of the Surgeon General.* Rockville, MD: Dept. of Health and Human Services, U.S. Public Health Service.

U.S. Government Printing Office. (GPO, 2011). *Accessing federal information using MetaLib's federated search.* Retrieved from http://www.fdlp.gov/collections/building-collections/822-metalib.

WC3 (2011, November). *W3C Semantic Web Activity.* Retrieved from http://www.w3.org/2010/08/ws-pas.html.

W3C (2011). *W3C web services package PAS explanatory report.* Retrieved from http://www.w3.org/2010/08/ws-pas.html.

Our choices add up; each one influences others, and cumulatively a series of
delightful short-term choices can leave us much worse off in the long run.

DANIEL AKST, 2011

12 Selected Mental Health Informatics Databases

Any discussion of information sources must start with a disclaimer. Information-seeking,
finding, and retrieval require complex cognitive and behavioral processes. As shown in
previous chapters, there are a variety of entities, including government, academic, professional, consumer, and advocacy groups, which publish (or simply disseminate) numerous types of information. Each entity has its preferred distribution or communication
channels, formats, and schedules. It would require an encyclopedia to address all of the
authoritative resources available to savvy (re)searchers. This chapter addresses selected
open access and proprietary resources for persons interested in mental health informatics
databases.

Determining databases pertinent to persons working in mental health informatics can be daunting. Persons working with mental health informatics include clinicians,
administrators, program specialists, computer programmers, systems administrators, and
state and regional coordinators. From the perspectives of library and information science, mental health services research, and public health perspectives, there are important
elements to consider in the selection of databases. These include back-end development to
enhance precision, relevance, and recall in one's retrieval and serendipity, so that the user
may find novel and innovative information on the cusp of being known. In the databases
that appear in the balance of this chapter, *lagniappes* (i.e., unexpected benefits) will be identified, including multiple avenues to create search strategies, clearly defined vocabulary(ies),
current awareness alerts, and personalization features.

Computer and Information Science: CiteSeer^X

CiteSeer^X is a digital library for the scientific literature that focuses primarily on the literature on computer and information science. Created in 1997, CiteSeer^X has been a leader in harnessing new web technologies and standards. For example, CiteSeer^X uses autonomous citation indexing (ACI) to create a citation index, which allows the user to track who has cited whom and what. Other features include reference linking, allowing the user to cross-link articles when reviewing an article's bibliography, full-text indexing with support for full Boolean, phrase, and proximity searching, and a "related documents" feature utilizing citation- and word-based measures. CiteSeer^X provides extensive metadata on all indexed articles and is compliant with the Open Archives Initiative Protocol for Metadata Harvesting, a standard proposed by the Open Archive Initiative to facilitate content dissemination.

In addition, CiteSeer^X harvests research papers from the web using a focused (topical) web crawler, using prediction algorithms, and reinforcement learning (Liu, Milios, & Korba, 2008). One of its newer features is MyCiteSeer^X, a personalized content portal that allows the user to create personalized search settings and collections, establish syndication feeds when the site or specific content is updated, and take advantage of social bookmarking and network facilities. MyCiteSeer^X uses data mining algorithms and recommendation in the creation of a personal portal. Another interesting component of CiteSeer^X is the ability to track institutional data.

Since CiteSeer^X allows full Boolean, phrase, and proximity searching across its simple search, and advanced search features, it is fairly easy to construct and retrieve relevant items according to the level of specificity built into the search strategy. In addition, CiteSeer allows the user to expand his or her search to include the citations. Starting with a natural language search on the phrase "mental health informatics" (using the simple search feature and no citation searching), over 20,000 items were retrieved. With citation searching included, almost 30,000 items were retrieved. Taking advantage of Boolean and phrase searching "mental health AND informatics," almost 200 items were retrieved. On the first page of ten, topics included the use of nursing informatics to improve outcomes and quality of care, using health informatics in autism. Clearly, a more relevant search was achieved by taking advantage of Boolean and phrase searching.

The record display also offers the user additional opportunities for serendipity and assessment (Figure 12.1). Users can view the summary (abstract), the active bibliography, co-citation, clustered documents, and version history.

In the Summary view, the Citations listed under the Abstract provide links to other works by Oberleitner et al. cited in CiteSeer^X in Figure 12.1. Co-citation displays any related documents that cited articles in the current article's bibliography. Clustered documents and iterations show how many versions of a document are held in CiteSeer^X. Iterations, or versions of a manuscript, need to be differentiated as to the final, authoritative version to ensure that data or findings are not misreported. In the upper right quadrant of the screen, one can opt to save the item to a list, add it to his or her collection, correct errors, and request an update when there are any changes to the record. In the lower right quadrant of the screen, the doi for the record is displayed, as is the citation in BibTeX, a reference management software (Fenn, 2006), and a number of social bookmarking tools (CiteULike, Connotea, BibSonomy, delicious, Digg, and reddit).

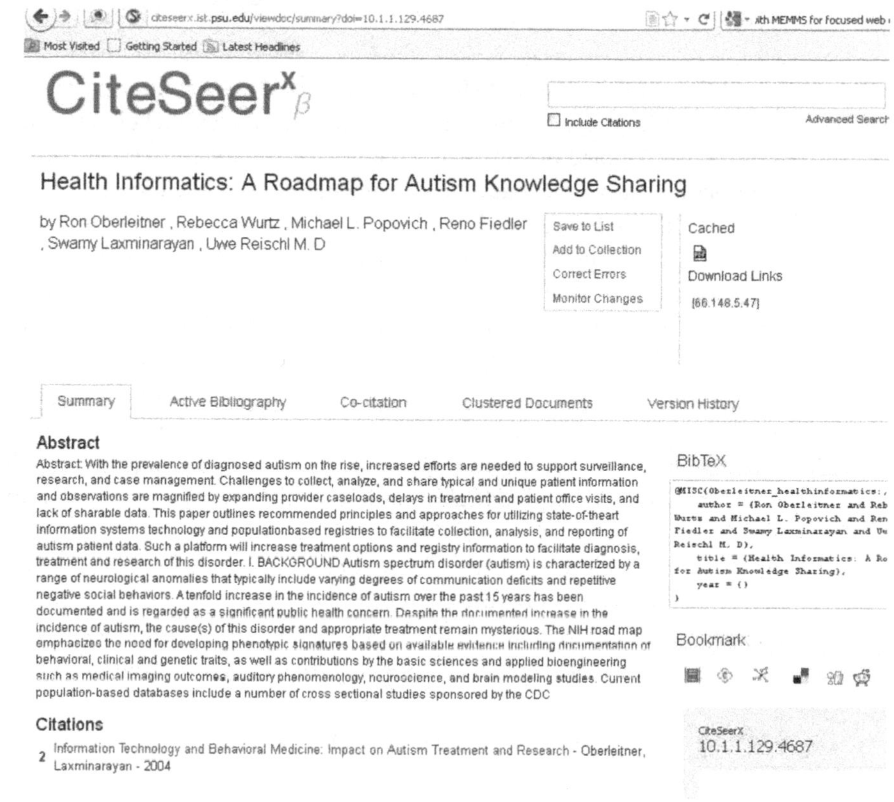

FIGURE 12.1 Screenshot of Record in CiteSeer^X.
Retrieved http://citeseerx.ist.psu.edu/viewdoc/summary?doi=10.1.1.129.4687. Used with permission.

Statistics: Federal Data

The national health information infrastructure was defined as "not just technologies but, more importantly, values, practices, relationships, laws, standards, systems, and applications that support all facets of individual health, health care, and public health" (National Committee on Vital and Health Statistics, 2002, p. 1). When examining statistics in mental health services research and policy, one faces a number of obstacles, the most important being there is no central repository of current data on the utilization of mental health services, the epidemiology of mental disorders, or linkages to all the areas of state and federal governments which must collect this data. One of the best federal gateways to national data was the Department of Health and Human Services (DHHS) Gateway to Data and Statistics. The site used standard terminology to normalize the vocabulary across the different agencies, had numerous interactive applications and tools, and provided meta-tags for geographically referenced materials. Unfortunately, this site was terminated by the Department. In its place, DHHS provides a Directory of Health and Human Services Data Resources, which is a selective listing by agency of the published and aggregated statistics each (agency) has available. Each listing includes the following information on the available datasets: description, limitations, status, and access. In addition, there are a number of public use websites, such as the Centers for Disease Control WISQARS (Web-based Injury Statistics Query and Reporting System) which provides fatal and non-fatal injury data as well as violent death data. WISQARS now provides additional interactive tools. These include a cost of injury report if the patient was treated at a hospital or emergency room department and a mapping module that allows users to produce customized, color-coded maps depicting injury-related death rates throughout the United States.

The Census Bureau site also has new geomapping tools that allow the user to "drill down to the street level" on a query and to see the associated data sets attached to the address. For example, one can see if it is available in the Public Use Microdata Area, Census Tract, Metro Statistical Area/Micro Statistical Area dataset, Congressional and legislative districts, or Urban or rural designation. Clicking on the dataset, the system returns the tables matching the larger geographical location. Clicking on the Census Tract data set, the user can see housing data: occupied and vacant housing rates; year the housing was built; and the number rented or owned. However, the children data reverts to the larger metropolitan area. Health data, broadly defined as health not just mental health, focuses on health insurance.

Mental health data is difficult to easily find. There is no federal database which one can query and determine incidence and disorder clusters. Even *Mental Health United States*, a biennial federal report, does not have current data on mental disorders. In the 2010 report, for example, the most current data available is 2009 and data sets may have relatively old data, as in the case of prevalence (2002) or data on the shortage of mental health professionals (2006). State, county, and city data is even more unavailable.

Federal Legislation: FDsys and THOMAS

Tracking the authoritative version of a federal document can be difficult. The best places to do so are FDsys, the new digital library system of the U.S. Government Printing Office (104th–112th Congress; 1995 to date) or the Library of Congress THOMAS site for federal legislative information (100th–112th Congress; 1995 to date).

Using a content management system, FDsys is the preservation repository of official publications from all three branches of the federal government. Its purpose is to ensure content integrity and authenticity of government documents. To do so, FDsys has a system design document (SDD) describing the system architecture (consistency check, continuity of access, continuity of operations, custom application, and file processor) and the publishing protocol (repository, search API, search configuration, and site map). There is also a data management document (DMD), which contains detailed data processing information for each type of the publication collection managed by the system. Metadata is provided using XML. In addition, FDsys allows the use of advanced Boolean and field operators to construct complex searches, filters to narrow results, and downloads in multiple formats, including the Metadata Object Description Scheme (MODS) and Preservation Metadata Implementation Strategy (PREMIS) data dictionary.

FDsys allows the user to browse by Congressional committee, date, or collection. The Congressional committee section is first subdivided by Senate and House, then by type of committee (joint, standing, select, special, and other), caucuses, Congressional commissions, and Congressional panels. The date option ranges from the last 24 hours to the earliest publication contained in the system. For example, on a particular day, 43 documents had been added to FDsys within the previous 24 hours. Of the 43, the most relevant was the addition of the amended H.R. 3559 (IH), the Insurance Data Protection Act, which restricts the sharing of any non-publicly available data by insurance companies. There are approximately 50 collections in the FDsys, including the U.S. budget, the Code of Federal Regulations, presidential documents (1993 to date), the *Congressional Record*, and public and private laws (104th–112th Congress; 1995 to date).

A search using "mental health informatics" resulted in 714 retrievals (Figure 12.2). In the left-hand column, there are a number of filters available to narrow the search: collection; publication date; government author; organization; person (listed within the report); place published; and additional keywords that may be of value in refining future search strategies. These options are generated by the metadata created by FDsys for each item. In the inset black-banded box in Figure 12.2, the search has been narrowed using a filter of Public and Private Laws and then refined using the additional terms of outcomes and assessments, resulting in three bills that address outcomes and assessments in mental health informatics.

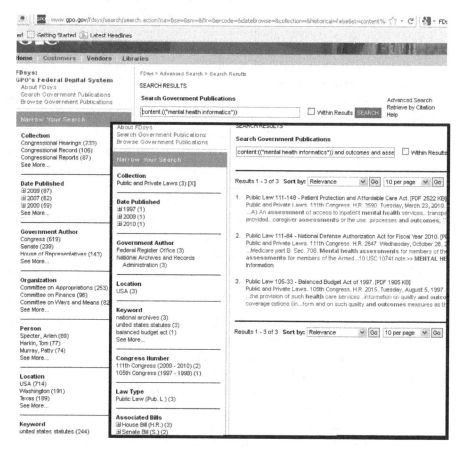

FIGURE 12.2 Screenshots of FDsys Illustrating Filter Options.
Retrieved from http://www.gpo.gov/fdsys./

Public and Private Laws are also known as "slip laws." A slip law is an official publication of the law that is admissible evidence in all courts and tribunals in the United States. Public laws affect the nation. Public Law 104–191, the Health Information Portability and Accountability Act (HIPAA), radically changed the way in which health information is utilized across the United States. Private laws affect individuals or groups, such as a petition to change immigration status or for compensation for emergency work conducted after a major disaster. FDsys retrieves the .pdf of the document, a .txt document, and a page with the metadata for the Act. Not only are there data on the category of the document, the collection in which it was located, and the date it was approved, but the bill number of the originally sponsored bill is listed, as are the House and Senate reports on the bill, the legislative history, the United States Code (USC) citations, and the statutes at large citations.

Statutes at large (a.k.a. "session laws") are compiled from the slip laws enacted during every session of Congress. It represents the chronological arrangement of the laws in the exact order in which they have been enacted. Public laws are incorporated into the United States Code every six years. Until the public law is incorporated into the United States Code (USC), a supplement to the USC is published every year to document the present status of laws. Each amendment of the law (over the six years) is incorporated in the supplement until the authoritative USC volume is published. This is critical information if one is tracking changes in federal legislation to determine if previous legislation is affected by the newly passed law. We would question including a citation for Public Law 104–191 in an academic or research paper if the base URL was www.ohappydays.com. Although it may look like the right document, the user must decide if it is worth taking a chance if it is not the current version, if it has been altered deliberately, or if it is a corrupted file. Always err on the side of caution. If there is a federal authoritative site, locate it and use it.

In 1995, during the start of the 104th Congress, the Library of Congress launched THOMAS. Congress then instructed the Library of Congress to make federal legislative information freely available to the public. Similar to FDsys, THOMAS contains Congressional documents, the *Congressional Record*, schedules and calendars, committee information and reports, presidential nominations, and treaties (see Figure 12.3). THOMAS also uses a number of Web 3.0 tools, such as Real Simple Syndication (RSS), and a variety of social media, such as Twitter, Digg, Reddit, Facebook, Stumbleupon, Diigo, Technorati, Delicious, MySpace, Yahoo, and Google. In addition, there is also a personalization feature, myLOC. The social media and myLOC are available from Share/Save icon on the upper right hand side of the screen.

However, unlike FDsys, not all of the information in THOMAS is full-text. For the full-text, THOMAS advises users to search FDsys. THOMAS is the keeper of legislative activity. A search in the bill text of the 112th Congress (limited to enrolled bills) on the phrase "mental health informatics" indicates that there were zero bills on the phrase exactly as entered (think "mental+health+ informatics" in machine language), zero bills that contained all the search words near each other in any order, zero bills that contained all the search words but not near each other. However, there were 15 bills that contained one or more of the search words. If the search is revised to "mental health AND informatics," the same zero sum for articles that have all the words now reveals 84 bills that have one or more of the search words. Before reviewing those 84 items, performing a final search for just the term "informatics" retrieves no bills for that session. Hence, searching on the bill

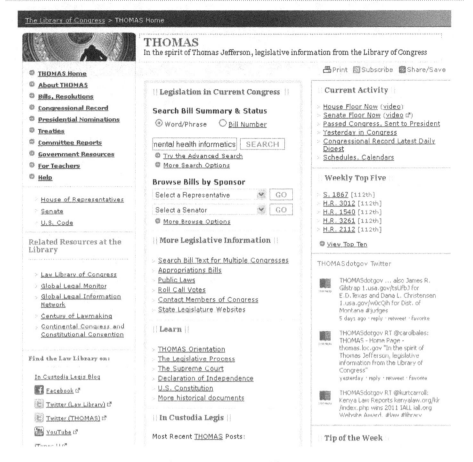

FIGURE 12.3 THOMAS Interface (http://thomas.loc.gov).

number and/or the most unique word makes for the most efficient search. However, by simply selecting the option "search multiple Congresses," the search retrieved seven bills that contained all three of the words but not near each other. The display lists the seven with all the words, followed by over 1,300 documents that contained one or more of the search words (see in Figure 12.4).

The myLOC personalization feature offers the opportunity to bookmark items in the Library of Congress. For example, in THOMAS, on the bill summary and status of H.R. 1101, the Medicare Telemedicine and Medical Informatics Demonstration Act of 1997, the user can click on the "Share/Save" feature on the right-hand side of the page, select "myLOC" as the option, and the item is tagged and saved to myLOC. The user can then create a folder entitled "informatics legislation" and continue to build a collection folder on the topic. When reviewing the folder, the link takes the user back to the page where he or she can access the legislative text, read the list of co-sponsors, review the CRS summary, the titles of the bill, and the committees that reviewed it, as well as major Congressional actions, all Congressional actions, and all Congressional actions with amendments. There are also links to *Congressional Record* pages, votes, and reports.

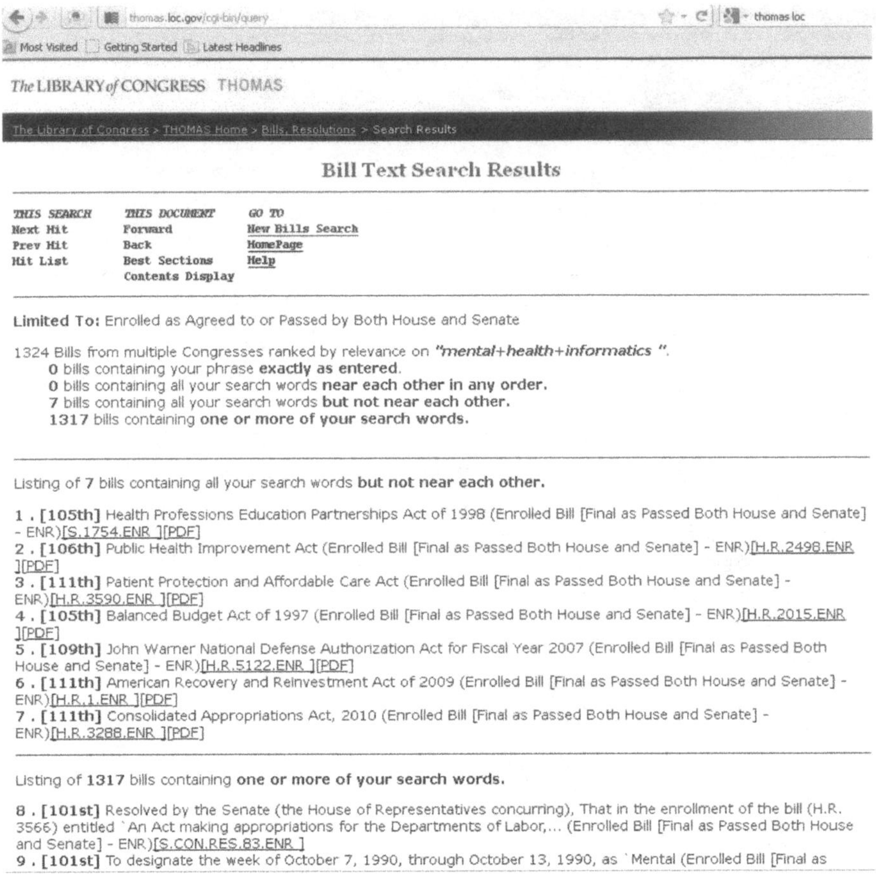
thomas.loc.gov/cgi-bin/query

Most Visited Getting Started Latest Headlines

The LIBRARY of CONGRESS THOMAS

The Library of Congress > THOMAS Home > Bills, Resolutions > Search Results

Bill Text Search Results

THIS SEARCH	THIS DOCUMENT	GO TO
Next Hit	Forward	New Bills Search
Prev Hit	Back	HomePage
Hit List	Best Sections	Help
	Contents Display	

Limited To: Enrolled as Agreed to or Passed by Both House and Senate

1324 Bills from multiple Congresses ranked by relevance on *"mental+health+informatics "*.
0 bills containing your phrase **exactly as entered.**
0 bills containing all your search words **near each other in any order.**
7 bills containing all your search words **but not near each other.**
1317 bills containing **one or more of your search words.**

Listing of **7** bills containing all your search words **but not near each other.**

1 . **[105th]** Health Professions Education Partnerships Act of 1998 (Enrolled Bill [Final as Passed Both House and Senate] - ENR)[S.1754.ENR][PDF]
2 . **[106th]** Public Health Improvement Act (Enrolled Bill [Final as Passed Both House and Senate] - ENR)[H.R.2498.ENR][PDF]
3 . **[111th]** Patient Protection and Affordable Care Act (Enrolled Bill [Final as Passed Both House and Senate] - ENR)[H.R.3590.ENR][PDF]
4 . **[105th]** Balanced Budget Act of 1997 (Enrolled Bill [Final as Passed Both House and Senate] - ENR)[H.R.2015.ENR][PDF]
5 . **[109th]** John Warner National Defense Authorization Act for Fiscal Year 2007 (Enrolled Bill [Final as Passed Both House and Senate] - ENR)[H.R.5122.ENR][PDF]
6 . **[111th]** American Recovery and Reinvestment Act of 2009 (Enrolled Bill [Final as Passed Both House and Senate] - ENR)[H.R.1.ENR][PDF]
7 . **[111th]** Consolidated Appropriations Act, 2010 (Enrolled Bill [Final as Passed Both House and Senate] - ENR)[H.R.3288.ENR][PDF]

Listing of **1317** bills containing **one or more of your search words.**

8 . **[101st]** Resolved by the Senate (the House of Representatives concurring), That in the enrollment of the bill (H.R. 3566) entitled `An Act making appropriations for the Departments of Labor,... (Enrolled Bill [Final as Passed Both House and Senate] - ENR)[S.CON.RES.83.ENR]
9 . **[101st]** To designate the week of October 7, 1990, through October 13, 1990, as `Mental (Enrolled Bill [Final as

FIGURE 12.4 Search Results in THOMAS (http://thomas.loc.gov).

When searching all of the Library of Congress, the search engine provides similar displays, with a number of filters, including available online, all items, original format, online format, publication date, sites and collections, contributor, and subject. In this case, the Library of Congress uses the Library of Congress Subject Headings (LCSH), which is the system utilized by many academic and research libraries. For example, starting with a broad search using the term "informatics," there are 184 items available online, with a total of 1,707 items overall, all in numerous formats. The search can be narrowed from the choice of the Subject list "Telemedicine" and refined further with a second subject heading "Congressional Reporting Requirements." By adding value through the use of additional subject metadata, Library of Congress catalogers reduce search time significantly.

Mental Health Services Research and Informatics: National Library of Medicine (NLM)

The National Library of Medicine (NLM) provides a number of resources and tools for individuals working in mental health services research and informatics. Bibliographic resources of particular interest to mental health informatics include MEDLINE/PubMed, which contains journal citations from 1950 to the present; the NLM catalogue of monographs, serials, and media; and the NLM Bookshelf, the UMLS® Metathesaurus, Meeting Abstracts, and Health Services Research Projects in Progress (HSRProj).

Searches can be conducted using Boolean, proximity, MeSH, field tags, and natural language from the Gateway search engine. It links to the specific search and retrieval mechanisms in MEDLINE/PubMed (advanced query parser, Related Articles, and LinkOut functions) and in the NLM Catalog (Related Records function). Users have the option to set preferences, such as which elements of a record to see in the display of results. As described in Chapter 11, a number of fields are searchable. The default search for the NLM Gateway is the subject search; if it cannot find the term, then it defaults to mapping for the natural language term or phrase. A summary of results is presented in three broad categories: (1) bibliographic resources; (2) consumer health resources; and (3) other information resources. The user can access an individual collection's results directly through its link on the summary. Most of these databases allow one to export a search into citation management software (including ProCite, EndNotes, and RefWorks).

Two of the resources, HSRProj and HSTAT (Health Services Technology Assessment Texts series), provide access to historical information on projects and health technology assessments. The HSRProj, for example, contains descriptions of research in progress funded by federal and private grants and contracts before results are available in a published form. The HSRProj record contains the title of the research, the names and contact information of the principal investigator(s), the names of performing and sponsoring agencies, beginning and ending year(s) of the project, state and country, status, and an abstract. In the structured abstract, there is information about study design and methodology, demographic characteristics of the study group, number of subjects in the study population, population base of the study sample, and source of the project data. All records have supplemental metadata with Medical Subject Headings (MeSH®). Additional metadata is supplied from the National Institutes of Health's CRISP (Computer Retrieval of Information on Scientific Projects) keywords. Users can also refine "on the fly" by selecting keywords, project status, investigator, and performing and supporting organizations. This is an excellent focused source for health services research. For a larger review of federal health funding, the NIH RePORTER (RePORT Expenditures & Results) allows users to search a repository of all NIH-funded research projects and to access publications and patents resulting from NIH funding.

The HSTAT series is a full-text resource on health information designed to support health care decision making. HSTAT includes evidence reports, technology assessments, prevention guidelines and protocols. It also includes consensus conference reports, treatment improvement protocols, and reports of the Surgeon General. Each item opens with basic bibliographic information (author, title, series number, date and place of publication, report number, and copyright notice). Next is a structured abstract, which is followed by the table of contents. The record ends with the name of the sponsoring agency, and the contract number. Both archived and current texts are available. Many are available as .pdfs. All are available in HTML. In some cases, the NLM record is the only access to the item.

Another health services resource available at NLM is the Health Services/Sciences Research Resources (HSRR). Supported by the National Information Center on Health Services Research and Health Care Technology at NLM, HSRR is a searchable database on data resources (research data sets, instruments/indices and software) used in health services research, the behavioral and social sciences, and public health. Data sets are considered a file or group of files associated with one part of a study, such as a single data file or a series of data files with a machine-readable codebook. Instruments/indices contain research instruments, which includes the operational definitions of all measures related to the research and questionnaires, which only contain the questions and answers with no supporting documentation. HSRR supports phrase searching using quotation marks ("."), Boolean operators, nested search constructions, and field searching.

Items first display by record type: research data sets; instruments/indices; and software; then alphabetically by title. The core bibliographic record contains at a minimum eight fields: (1) title URL; (2) record type; (3) source; (4) source URL; (5) purpose; (6) description; (7) keywords; and (8) date revised. However, the individual record by type of resource may be far more extensive (see Table 12.1). In addition, the records also contain pre-defined query searches for the items to PubMed, and the URLs of providers for additional information or access to the resources. Again, through the use of an extensible bibliographic record, there is a variety and depth to the information available on items with HRSS.

There are several interesting features in the NLM interfaces that take advantage of newer technologies. The broad search feature in the NLM Gateway does support phrase searching (using quotation marks) and Boolean. One can select "highlight output," which then highlights the text/phrase that was searched. As with other online databases, one can browse and select, then download selections at one time. Options for download include save to file or display for printing, format selection (text or HTML), and level of detail (brief or complete). In HSRR, output options include formats (brief, complete, or tagged) and output (text, file, or e-mail). The tagged format provides an importable format into many of the citation management programs. In HSRProj, users can email or export as HTML, text, or XML.

Further, one can elect to use a number of Web 2.0 and 3.0 tools, including application programming interfaces (APIs); mobile applications and widgets; utilities, tools, and executable files; as well as communication tools, such as RSS. Two APIs of interest to database builders are the Unified Medical Language System (UMLS) API and the RxTerms API, both of which allow users to download functions for retrieving terms from the respective

TABLE 12.1

Fields Available in HRSS Record Format

Title	Price Information	Population
Title Acronym	Survey Type	Geographic Region
Topic Subset	Method/Technique	Unit of Analysis
Source	Special Software	Validity
Source URL	Sample Design	Variables
Purpose	Sample Size	References
Description	Interval	Keywords
Data Format	Year of Availability	Date Revised
Special Software	Media	Contacts
Restrictions	MEDLINE Search Strategy	Vendors

www.nlm.nih.gov/nichsr/hsrr_search/.

databases. From a web perspective, an API is typically a defined hypertext transfer protocol (HTTP) request and response message, usually written in XML or JavaScript Object Notation (JSON) format. An API takes advantage of controlled vocabulary (syntax and elements of a specific language), as in the case of chemical databases, or it can integrate several programming languages to overlay data from one application to another. One common example is a restaurant API that overlays its information over a map application to show proximity and distance. In addition, an API can program for behaviors that push or pop information to the user, such as RSS (real simple syndication) feeds.

NLM mobile apps and widgets include AIDSInfo, Medline Plus Mobile, and PubMed Mobile, as well as number of disaster apps for first responders and families. ReUnite is a mobile app for use to help reunify families after a disaster. Available in English, French, and Spanish from iTunes, it provides a format to upload missing person information, a photo of the person, metadata tagging, geo-location, and notes using both text and voice. In addition to numerous utilities, tools, and executables (62 at last count), NLM also provides several tools of interest to information providers and consumers. First, there is LinkOut, which allows third parties to link directly from PubMed and other NLM databases to full-text publications, other databases, consumer health information, and research tools. For example, many health science libraries create links to their full-text journals through an authenticated user gateway. MedlinePlus Connect joins electronic health record systems to health information contained in Medline, which can be used as clinical guidelines or for decision making. PubMed Clinical Queries is a targeted subset of PubMed, with a focus on clinicians and health services researchers. Clinical Queries limits by clinical study category, filters for systematic reviews, and medical genetics. Several other tools, including Taxonomy Browser and Common Tree, address taxonomies, which are central in building controlled vocabulary and semantic mapping. From a consumer perspective, there are several tools, such as MyMedicationList, which allows users to manage medication lists and make records readily available. NIHSeniorHealth provides easily accessible information related to improving and maintaining senior health.

Communication tools include specialized portals, such as AIDSInfo, Disaster Information, Health Services Research Information Central, MedlinePlus, and a number of social media tools. Users can follow specialized areas on Twitter, including AIDs, NCBI updates, Medlineplus, caregivers, global health, disaster medicine, and public health, refugee health, and women's health. Users can be a fan of NLM specialty areas on Facebook, as well as exhibitions and programs. Finally, there are a number of RSS feeds, podcasts, and webcasts in which users can participate, such as topical areas of UMLS and PubMed. RSS feeds range from new resources to clinical updates, updates on the UMLS, clinical morbidity and mortality alerts, and new resources and services. NLM podcasts allow users to keep current with NLM materials; users can participate in interactive webcasts, such as topical areas of UMLS and PubMed. Although seen as "old" technology, NLM offers a number of e-mail lists that may be announcement-only or interactive.

The Cochrane Collaboration: Cochrane Reviews

Systematic reviews are considered important resources when researching interventions. First, a systematic review is a rigorous, not anecdotal, evaluation of a topic. A review clearly explains its method of analysis, including inclusion and exclusion criteria, with very complete documentation as to how the review was conducted. Using a simple search interface (one search box), users can search the Cochrane Summaries using phrase, Boolean, and nested searching. A search on the string "mental health" and "controlled trials" AND "interventions" retrieved over forty records. There are several filters displayed on the search screen: new and/or updated; health topics, which break out additional clinical areas, such as complementary and alternative medicine; and the number of articles in the area. The display also lists available podcasts and the number of PEARLS ("Practical Evidence About Real Life Situations"), which offer guidance and advice for real-time decision making. Each summary page displays a plain language summary, the formal abstract, a link to the podcast, and related topics. The Cochrane Summaries also use "ShareThis" to allow users to sign on to over 30 social media (e.g., Facebook, Twitter, LinkedIn, Google, Yahoo) as well as other applications, including CiteULike and Connotea, both free online reference management software programs.

The Cochrane Summaries (http://www.cochrane.org/reviews/) provides free online access to summaries. If the user is working from an authenticated site or interface, he or she will be able to link in to the Cochrane Library, a proprietary resource hosted by Wiley Online Library. On the Wiley interface, users have access to a number of tools, including a My Profile account, export citations to citation management software, related records ("More articles like this"), and share across a variety of social media (CiteULike, Connotea, delicious, Mendeley, Twitter, Digg, Facebook, Diigo, Google Reader, and StumbleUpon). Another feature is the iteration view, where users can see earlier and later versions of the systematic review. Finally, users may also look at other Cochrane resources, including clinical trials, methods studies, health technology assessments, and economic evaluations (the British National Health Service economic evaluation database). Subscriptions to the *Cochrane* suite of databases are often available at universities that have medical schools or schools/colleges of public health.

The National Academies Press

The National Academies Press (NAP) is considered an authoritative source for materials addressing critical issues in science, technology, and health policy published by the National Academy of Sciences, the National Academy of Engineering, the Institute of Medicine, and the National Research Council. The NAP reports are freely available online for reading, and provide executive summaries of the reports. A number of the reports are available for free download; reports that are not downloadable are available for purchase. Unlike Google Books where portions of text may be missing, NAP monographs are full text and searchable with a simple text search engine.

There are a number of features on the NAP site. Users can browse across broad topic (subject) areas, such as behavioral and social sciences or engineering and technology. The search feature uses a simple construct enclosed within double quotes, e.g., "mental health" or simple Boolean, such as "mental health" AND "informatics." The search is across the full-texts, so the more specificity in the search reduces the number of less relevant returns.

Results can be ordered alphabetical by title or by year of publication. Users may search within the book using phrases ("within double quotes") or using single words. Certain words are not searchable, such as possessives or "stop words." The "show in context" feature takes users right to the page where the word or phrase is located, rather than having to skim or read the entire chapter.

In addition, the NAP site provides two digital discovery tools, the Web Search Builder and the Reference Finder. The Web Search builder allows one to use the book's keywords to explore within the book, across the NAP collection, or across the web. By selecting a chapter from a book, Web Search Builder generates paired searches and a list of keywords, which can be selected to further refine searches using a paired search (see Figure 12.5). Using the "Why Health Technology Doesn't Work" chapter from *Frontiers of Engineering: Reports on Leading-Edge Engineering from the 2009 Symposium*, Web Search Builder generated paired combinatorial searches using "medical informatics," "informatics associations," and "health data" ("medical informatics" AND "informatics associations," "medical informatics" AND "health data," and "informatics associations" AND "health data"), which generated almost 100 unique search terms. Selecting the phrases "automated translation" and "health data" as the paired search with the search parameter of the Google Scholar retrieved approximately 30 entries, Yahoo! and Bing retrieved approximately 60 results, Google Web retrieved over 1,200 entries, Google Books resulted in a 404, and National Academies Press retrieved over 4,700 entries.

Title	Price Information	Population
Title Acronym	Survey Type	Geographic Region
Topic Subset	Method/Technique	Unit of Analysis
Source	Special Software	Validity
Source URL	Sample Design	Variables
Purpose	Sample Size	References
Description	Interval	Keywords
Data Format	Year of Availability	Date Revised
Special Software	Media	Contacts
Restrictions	MEDLINE Search Strategy	Vendors

FIGURE 12.5 National Academies Press Web Search Builder.

Reference Finder is a "find more like this text" search tool. Working from an existing text, users can paste in up to eight pages of text, and Reference Finder will search the NAP site for relevant reports or search the web across Google, Yahoo, MSN, and press sites. Similar to Web Search Builder, Reference Finder extracts a series of keywords from the provided text, puts them into the NAP search engine, then aggregates and displays the NAP texts that seem most appropriate. Since Reference Finder builds searches based upon keywords in the text, it is good for serendipitous finds. However, both Web Search Builder and Reference Finder lack the precision of a controlled vocabulary. On the other hand, it does use algorithmic key weighting, which examines word and phrase frequency, term placement, co-occurrence with other terms/phrases in building searches for Web Search Builder and Reference Finder. For very targeted keywords and phrases, both offer a quick review of available resources. However, these types of analytical tools require expert use to increase precision and relevance in one's search.

In addition to these digital discovery tools, NAP uses a number of Web 2.0 and 3.0 technologies. Users may subscribe to its *Newsletter* on a topic of interest, view short biweekly podcasts, or sign up for RSS feeds (14 readers are supported) for ongoing updates on content and new releases, or log on as an authorized user to access .pdfs of reports. NAP provides a number of tools to share URLs of the reports and a widget that can be posted on other websites to allow users to pull an authoritative version from the NAP site. NAP's "Share" icon leads the user to over 330 social media sites, to tweet the site, recommend it on Facebook, or publicly recommend on Google+.

Agency for Health Care Research and Quality (AHRQ)

The AHRQ provides access to a number of software and clinical tools for use with its databases as well as other administrative data sets. For example, the AHRQ quality indicators use inpatient hospital data to examine prevention, inpatient quality of care, patient safety, and pediatric quality of care. Of particular interest is the clinical classifications software (CSS) suite, developed for the ICD-9-CM and the subsets for mental health and substance abuse, comorbidity, and chronic cases; the ICD-10, and the services and procedures suite (Current Procedural Terminology codes and Healthcare Common Procedure Coding System codes). The CSS classify the codes into clinically meaningful categories, which can then be used for aggregate statistical reporting.

Another tool is My Own Network AHRQ (MONAHRQ), a desktop software tool that quickly generates an interactive health care reporting website by health organizations. MONAHRQ summarizes hospital and area-level data on the quality of care, health care utilization, preventable hospitalizations, and rates of conditions and procedures utilizing hospital discharge data, inpatient measures from CMS Hospital Compare, and/or HCAHPS survey measures (AHRQ, 2011).

AHRQ is also responsible for the United States Health Information Knowledgebase (USHIK), which supports the metadata registry project for HL7. The USHIK focuses on the data elements used in the transactions, medical data code sets, and transaction users (providers, health plans, sponsors, and pharmacy) covered in HIPAA legislation. Medical code data sets include the ICD-9-CM, National Drug Codes, Code on Dental Procedures and Nomenclature, Health Care Financing Administration Common Procedure Coding System, and Current Procedural Terminology, 4th edition.

The role of USHIK is to move the national health record infrastructure to uniform query and interface standards using standards developed by national organizations, including the Accredited Standards Committee X12 Subcommittee N-Insurance (X12N), the American Dental Association, the American Society for Testing and Materials Committee E31 on Healthcare Informatics (ASTM E31), Health Industry Business Communications Council (HIBCC), Health Level Seven (HL7), the Medical Device Communications Industry Group (IEEE 1073), and the National Council for Prescription Drug Programs (NCPDP). Other participants include the Centers for Disease Control and Prevention, the Department of Defense Health Affairs, National Cancer Institute, National Committee on Vital and Health Statistics, the Government Computer-based Patient Record Project, and the Health Care Financing Administration.

The purpose of the registry is to have a central repository describing data characteristics and attributes, support data sharing across systems and organizations for common units of data, and to create crosswalks and definitions for a common understanding of how data is named, defined, represented, and identified to ensure interoperability across disparate data

TABLE 12.2

ANSI/ADA 1000: Standards Clinical Data Architecture for the Structure and Content of an Electronic Health Record

Individual	Patient Health	Health Services	Care Delivery
Individual Identification	Patient Health Facts	Health Services	Healthcare Event
Individual characteristics	Patient Specimen	Health Services Outcomes	Health Service Resources
POPULATION	Patient Object	Health Services Objects	Health Material
Population	Patient Health Condition Diagnosis	CLINICAL RESEARCH	Health Material Item
Population characteristics	Patient Service Plan	Clinical Investigation	SUPPORTING
POPULATION HEALTH	Patient Treatment Plan	Clinical Investigation Protocol	Codes & Nomenclature
Population Health Facts	Patient Health Service	Clinical Investigation Trials	Organization
Population Health Condition Diagnosis		Clinical Investigation Analysis	Location Communication

Retrieved from http://ushik.ahrq.gov/model_ADA.html?Referer=Models.

TABLE 12.3

USHIK Information

Data Elements	Views
Value Domains	Information Models
Constraints	Organizations
Functional Groups	Data Agreements
Conceptual Domains	Collections
Contexts	Initiative
Vocabularies	Organizations
Representational Classes	

Retrieved from http://ushik.ahrq.gov/.

systems. For example, Table 12.2 illustrates the broad clusters of data elements required by the ANSI/ADA 1000: Standards Clinical Data Architecture for the Structure and Content of an Electric Health Record.

Currently in version 2.4.8.2, USHIK also utilizes information models to visually display information in a graphical representation, allowing users to drill down via a variety of sub-views and hierarchical relationships. Information models currently in use include X12N: Insurance, Clinical Care Classification (CCC) System; Consolidated Health Informatics (CHI); Federal Health Information Exchange (FHIE); Healthcare Information Technology Standards Panel (HITSP); the Continuity Assessment Record Evaluation (CARE); MHS Functional Area Model—DATA (FAM-D); National Committee on Vital and Health Statistics (NCVHS); NCPDP and NCPDP-SCRIPT; the National Health Information Model of Australia (NHIM); the Health Care Service Data Reporting Guide (HCSDRG); and the Small Scale Harmonization Project (SSHP). Table 12.3 shows the information available through USHIK.

Measuring Quality of Care: The Quality Data Set (QDS) Framework

Measuring quality of care is an intrinsic outcome with the implementation of the EHR and the national health information infrastructure. In the 1990s, the National Committee for Quality Assurance (NCQA) expanded the Healthcare Effectiveness Data and Information Set (HEDIS) to accommodate additional measures and domains of care for the managed care accreditation process (Grimaldi, 1997). With over 60 standards across 40 conditions and areas of care, many of the HEDIS measures can be calculated from claims data. However, there are several measures that require clinical information not available in claims data (Tang et al., 2007). A similar effort was undertaken by the Joint Commission on Accreditation of Healthcare Organizations (JCAHO) when it released ORYX, which attempted to incorporate objective measurement of care processes into the hospital accreditation process (Braun, Koss, & Loeb, 1999). Several years later, JCAHO established core measures in four clinical areas, which were used in its accreditation process (Getting started, 2002). The Centers for Medicaid and Medicare Services (CMS) expanded JCAHO's four core areas into eight domains of care for its quality improvement initiatives. After the implementation of the Medicare Modernization Act of 2003, CMS implemented the Physician Quality Reporting Initiative (PQRI), which supports 153 process and outcome measures in an array of clinical specialty areas (Danberg et al., 2009).

However, developing outcome measures to address quality of care is very complicated, especially when examining data that needs to be in a record (inputted by someone) for the data to be extracted for reports, assessment, and evaluation. The use of multiple reviewers, as well as the lack of familiarity with and problems with data abstraction tools, can lead to an inevitable variability in data, testing the boundaries of inter-rater reliability (Cassidy et al., 2002). Therefore, data collection methods, including evaluations of inter-rater reliability, crosswalks, and vocabulary across domains of care, need to be standardized and mapped to enable assessment of apples to apples, not apples to oranges.

Drawing upon the Institute of Medicine's (IOM) *Crossing the Quality Chasm* series and, in particular, its *Priority Areas for National Action* (Adams & Corrigan, 2003), the National Quality Forum (NQF) Health Information Technology Expert Panel (HITEP) was tasked to "define how HIT can evolve to effectively support performance measurement" (NQF, 2008, p. vi). Seven key recommendations were made, including the use of a coded interdisciplinary clinical problem list mapped to billing codes that could be used across care settings, an easily accessible and understandable data dictionary mapping HITEP data types and corresponding HISSP-recommended code sets, disambiguation between medication side effects and medication allergies to create standardized codes for each, and standardized codes for summary impressions of diagnostic test results. In addition, HITEP was asked to reassess, evaluate, and endorse quality measures as part of a continuous quality improvement process, and to work with other quality and information technology stakeholders to define additional quality measures that could be integrated or drawn from the EHR. A final recommendation dealt with new ways of presenting EHR medication data to address patient adherence to and compliance with medication treatment plans.

A year later, HITEP addressed the issue that clinical information needed for quality assessment was not adequately captured in EHRs. It drafted a quality data set (QDS) to leverage clinical longitudinal quality assessment from a patient-centric perspective across a variety of sources, including electronic health records (EHRs), personal health records (PHRs), registries, and health information exchanges (HIEs) (NQF, 2009). Future quality measure development will use the priorities and goals of the NQF National Priorities Partnership (28 national organizations) as a guide.

Implications for Mental Health Informatics

The National Health Information Infrastructure (NHII) provides the conceptual framework and the tools by which the United States will create an integrated, streamlined data collection system. Online and print resources are critical to understanding the complexity of creating such an infrastructure so that all stakeholders have a place at the table. Too often, informatics is seen as simply the "techie" side of health and mental health care. However, persons working in mental health informatics, as primary, secondary, or tertiary users of data, need to have more complete knowledge of the many factors that affect mental health services research and practice, especially when informatics is considered a key component of everyday work, from information seeking to retrieval to implementation.

This chapter addressed a select number of the many open access and proprietary databases used by individuals interested in mental health informatics. The next chapter will take a more global perspective in mental health informatics.

References

Adams, K., & Corrigan, J. M. (2003). *Priority areas for national action: Transforming health care quality.* Washington, DC: National Academies Press. Retrieved from http://www.nap.edu/catalog.php?record_id=10593.

Agency for Healthcare Research and Quality. (2011, September 8). *MONAHRQ Host User Guide, version 2.0.1.* Retrieved from http://monahrq.ahrq.gov/MONAHRQv201HostUserGuide.pdf.

Akst, D. (2011). *We have met the enemy: Self-control in an age of excess.* New York: Penguin Press.

Braun, B. I., Koss, R. G., & Loeb, J. M. (1999). Integrating performance measure data into the Joint Commission accreditation process. *Evaluation & the Health Professions, 22*(3), 283–297. doi: 10.1177/016327879902200301.

Cassidy, L. D., Marsh, G. M., Holleran, M. K., & Ruhl, L. S. (2002). Methodology to improve data quality from chart review in the managed care setting. *American Journal of Managed Care, 8*(9), 787–793.

Danberg, C. L., Sorbero, M. E., Hussey, P. S., Lovejoy, S., Liu, H., & Mehrotra, A. (2009). *Exploring episode-based approaches for medicare performance measurement, accountability and payment: Final report* (WR-653-ASPE). Washington, DC: U.S. Department of Health and Human Services. Retrieved from http://aspe.hhs.gov/health/reports/09/mcperform/report.shtml.

Fenn, J. (2006). Managing citations and your bibliography with BibTeX. *The PracTeX Journal, 4,* 1–19.

(2002). Getting started with core measures. *Joint Commission Perspectives, 22*(5), 7–8.

Grimaldi, P. L. (1997). New HEDIS means more information about HMOs. *Journal of Health Care Financing, 23*(4), 40–50.

Liu, H., Milios, E., & Korba, L. (2008). Exploiting multiple features with MEMMS for focused web crawling. In *Proceeding NLDB '08 Proceedings of the 13th international conference on natural language and information systems: Applications of natural language to information systems.* Berlin, Heidelberg: Springer-Verlag. doi: 10.1007/978-3-540-69858-6_11.

National Committee on Vital and Health Statistics. (2001). *Information for health: A strategy for building the national health information infrastructure.* Washington, DC: Author. Retrieved from http://ncvhs.hhs.gov/nhiilayo.pdf.

National Quality Forum. (2009, November). *Health information technology automation of quality measurement: Quality data set and data flow.* Washington, DC: Author. Retrieved from http://www.qualityforum.org/WorkArea/linkit.aspx?LinkIdentifier=id&ItemID=57067.

National Quality Forum. (2008). *Recommended common data types and prioritized performance measures for electronic healthcare information systems.* Washington, DC: Author.

Retrieved from http://www.qualityforum.org/WorkArea/linkit.aspx?LinkIdentifier =id&ItemID=22019.

Tang, P. C., Ralston, M., Arrigotti, M. F., Qureshi, L., & Graham, J. (2007). Comparison of methodologies for calculating quality measures based on administrative data versus clinical data from an electronic health record system: Implications for performance measures. *Journal of the American Medical Informatics Association, 14*(1), 10–15. doi: 10.1197/jamia. M2198.

Part 4 Globalization and the Future

Why should we promote international collaboration in Telemedicine and health telematics? The economic and social benefits of telemedicine and health telematics in health care delivery are certainly more of regional and national importance. However, the rapid sharing of knowledge and expertise in areas of sciences and human needs now bypass geographical and political barriers.

—LaCroix et al., 2002

13 Globalization of Information

The previous chapters have focused on mental health informatics from a United States perspective. In this chapter, we want to expand our perspective to a more global approach to informatics. In this chapter, we will examine the international aspects of telemental health, including the creation of measures and standards, issues in tracking health care services, and reforms in developing and emerging nations, and we conclude with a section on implications for mental health informatics.

Global Aspects of Telemental Health

Approximately half of the telemedicine studies come from the United States. This means there is a wide range of research, from small-scale studies to large-scale implementations, examined from global perspectives that are relevant to implementation of a national health information infrastructure in the United States. However, any review of global health initiatives must account for differences in health care systems and technological infrastructure that may affect successful adoption and implementation of technology within health and mental health care. Nevertheless, as the United States continues reforms in its health care systems, a review of global infrastructures and system practices may be useful for health systems reform.

One early initiative was the G-8 Global Healthcare Applications Subproject-4 (G-8 GHAP-SP-4) (LaCroix et al., 2002). The G-8 nations are part of an economic summit group, comprising representatives from Canada, France, Germany, Italy, Japan, the United Kingdom, United States, and Russia. Between 1998 and 1999, five thematic forums were held, with over 650 invited participants from 16 countries. Each forum addressed a key issue, including clinical and technical quality and standards, evaluation and cost effectiveness of telemedicine, impact of telemedicine on health care management, interoperability of telemedicine and telehealth systems, and medico-legal aspects of national and international applications. In addition, a number of professional organizations participated, including the World Health Organization, the U.S. National Library of Medicine, the Canadian Institute of Health Information, the National Aeronautics and Space Administration, the Institute of Medicine, the National Academies of Science, the International Medical Informatics Association, and academic centers from the G-8 countries.

A series of 21 recommendations (five sub-sets) were prepared by the national representatives of the G-8 GHAP SP-4 to present to policy makers, political leaders, and health care managers (see Table 13.1). The first subset of recommendations addressed standards, network reliability, security, and applications concerning a number of primary issues. First, there was the need to adopt and harmonize all standards as much as possible with the recommendations of the International Standard Organization working groups. Second, a process model for each discipline involved in health care should be developed, with technical needs defined in terms of quality of service (QoS), security, and application interoperability that can be understood by the clinical user. This recommendation moves technology from the rarified stratum of the technical area to a more everyday understanding of the clinical and professional staff. In other words, it makes this information part of the common workflow process. The remaining two recommendations stressed the need for infrastructure to be compatible, interoperable, and evolutionary, with current and emergent technologies and access to bandwidth appropriate to the application in use.

The second subset of recommendations addressed the role of national governments in the role of technology in health care. The second set focused on organizational issues. By recognizing the health and economic benefits of telehealth, national governments should make a strategic argument for telehealth to improve its nation's health. They should create and promote working models and cultivate partnerships between industry and health. In particular, national governments should address issues of licensures, credentialing, and health care provider reimbursement at both national and international levels. Finally, national governments should play a leadership role in building consensus and creating health care systems that integrate telehealth.

The third subset of recommendations addressed how national governments should support telehealth from a humanistic perspective. National governments should provide financial support for the telehealth training and education for health professionals and students, as well as financial incentives for established professionals to adopt and implement telehealth in their practices. There should be funding for evaluation of telehealth systems from a combined humanistic and systems perspective. In addition, governments should ensure that there is technical assistance available for telehealth users, as well as for those who wish to implement systems. Finally, a key component is the development of multilingual health information and services delivery in telehealth.

The fourth subset of recommendations was concerned with evaluation of telehealth, particularly how it related to improved health outcomes, identification and treatment of population needs, reliability of services, and cost-effectiveness and cost-efficacy when compared to other interventions. A major element of evaluation was the assessment of telehealth as it related to government policies and programs, as well as to other measures

TABLE 13.1

Summary of G8SP-4 Working Group Recommendations

Standards, Network Reliability, Security & Applications	Organizational Issues: Role of National Governments	Human Factors	Evaluation	Medico-Legal Aspects
Adopt and harmonize with ISO	Recognize health and economic benefits	Support training and education	Assess outcomes, population needs, reliability, & cost-effectiveness	Legal framework & international infrastructure
Discipline-based process model understandable to clinical user	Working models; Industry/health sector partnerships	Provide incentives to adopt and use telehealth systems	Assess the systemic aspects & interactions with government frameworks	Informed consent; ethical use of information, privacy & confidentiality
Compatible, interoperable, and adaptable	Licensures, credentialing, reimbursement	Fund & evaluate key human factors and systems	Measure impact on acceptability, workforce & professional competence	International ethical & medico-legal guidelines
Access to bandwidth	Consensus building	Provide access to technical expertise; Support multilingual system development	Develop practice documentation, dissemination of EBP & management	Telemedicine activity occurs at the site of the consultant

Adapted from http://mi.medu-tokai.ac.jp/g7sp4/final.htm.

of service delivery and system outcomes. Workforce distribution and competency of the telehealth workforce should be measured for their impacts on population health. Finally, evaluation incorporates best practices regarding documentation of protocols, practice, and management to improve health outcomes and dissemination of best practices.

The last subset of recommendations related to medico-legal concerns, which spanned government responsibility, patient responsibility, and professional responsibility. Governments should maintain an open dialogue at the international level to ensure that there is an appropriate legal framework for telehealth practice, legislation, and regulation. Patient privacy, confidentiality, and informed consent are critical issues for the ethical and legal use of patient information. Professional and patient organizations should work together to clearly understand and disseminate patient rights regarding privacy, confidentiality, and consent procedures. Another joint patient-professional responsibility addressed licensing. The remote site of the consultant is the "practice" site. Therefore, patients should abide by the rules of the remote "practice" site as if they were at the local site where they would be physically present. Finally, there was strong consensus for an internationally representative group to develop an global ethical, medical, and legal framework for the practice of telehealth.

In addition, the G-8 sub-project-4 conducted the IMPACT (International Multipoint Project of Advanced Communication in Telemedicine) feasibility study, which conducted multipoint telemedicine exchanges between academic centers of the participating G-8 and other countries, with a focus on emergency medicine.

In 2000, the United Nations (UN, 2000) officially adopted Resolution 55/2, the *United Nations Millennium Declaration*, which addressed peace, security, disarmament; development and poverty eradication; environmental sustainability; human rights, democracy, and good governance; protecting vulnerable populations; and meeting the special needs of Africa. In 2011, these goals were reaffirmed, with an emphasis on eradicating poverty and hunger, establishing universal education, improving maternal and child health, creating gender equity, combating AIDS, increasing environmental sustainability, and improving global partnerships. The *Millennium Declaration* also emphasized the use of technology to achieve these goals, as well as the importance of international cooperation.

In 2003 and 2005, the UN hosted the World Summit on the Information Society. At the 2003 summit, a *Declaration of Principles* and a *Plan of Action* were adopted. The *Declaration of Principles* defined a common vision and key principles of the information society. Capacity building, access to information, the role of governments, information communication technology (ICT), infrastructure, ethical concerns, maintaining cultural and linguistic diversity and identity, and international cooperation were stressed (World Summit, 2003 December 13).

A *Plan of Action* identified a number of objectives, goals, and targets (World Summit, 2003 December 12). A major goal was connectivity for all communities, including government offices, health and educational facilities, scientific and research centers, public libraries, cultural centers, museums, post offices, and archives. Similar to the 1998–1999 G-8 summit forums, the role of the national governments was addressed in promoting and implementing ICTs to aid in infrastructure development and sustainability, to increase access, and to build capacity. E-health was specifically addressed, emphasizing collaborative efforts between governments and other stakeholders, the development of international standards for the exchange of health data, and the strengthening of ICT initiatives for medical and humanitarian assistance in disasters and emergencies. In addition, a number of public health concerns were identified, including surveillance of communicable diseases and the strengthening of public health research and prevention efforts (World Summit, 2003 December 12).

In 2007, Crisp (2007) reiterated the need for developed nations, specifically the United Kingdom, to assist in the improvement of health in developing countries. He suggested that developing countries should "take the lead and own the solutions" for improved health outcomes and care, working in tandem with international, national, and local partnerships based on mutual respect. He also suggested that the United Kingdom and other industrialized countries assist in the training, education, and employment of health workers in developing countries on a more massive scale. Finally, he urged greater use of communication, information, and biomedical technologies, working from a best practices or evidence-based practice approach (Crisp, 2007). However, telehealth initiatives in developing countries raise very difficult questions regarding sustainability, resource use, and access to health care.

In 2011, the G-8 endorsed the Deauville Accountability Report, which reiterated the G-8's commitments to health and food security as well as supporting Internet initiatives that address health and education, privacy and confidentiality concerns, intellectual property, multi-stakeholder governance, cyber-security, and protection from crime.

Measuring Impacts of Health

Measuring the impacts of health is complex, especially considering the burden of diseases on individuals, populations, and nations. However, there are additional factors that make measuring health difficult. Although the relationship between disability and disease resulted in the development of the DALYS, there are other less obvious risk factors related to disease. From an epidemiological perspective, these include factors with long latency periods such as cancer, or factors that have nonspecific outcomes, meaning that they could be manifestations of many other illnesses. Further, complex (multifactorial) diseases, which are determined ultimately by a number of genetic and environmental factors, are difficult to determine at the population level. These disease clusters are defined as "an unusual aggregation, real or perceived, of health events that are grouped together in time and space and that is reported to a public health department" (CDC 1990, HTML). To establish an environmentally related disease cluster, first there must be verification of a disease or adverse health outcomes (surveillance). Next, one must determine the geographical region that is affected and the period during which the disease occurs (surveillance). It is not enough to determine the environmental exposure. It is critical to clearly establish a connection between the hazard and the disease and/or the adverse health outcome. Finally, the disease cluster or adverse health outcomes are confirmed through statistical tests.

Constructing summary measures can be difficult, especially when trying to identify the relative magnitude of diseases, injuries, *and* risk factors. Sanders (1964) suggested that the end-product of health care, that is, increasing the productive disability-free years from a given cohort, should be measured across identified issues in community health. This is particularly important, as communities that have adequate health care have a higher prevalence of chronic morbidity, since persons with chronic conditions live longer due to medical advances. However, realistically, an index of community health must select and summarize measures that can be obtained either from the government or from local, state, regional, or national surveys. Sullivan (1966) argues that such an index should "attempt to reduce the assessment of health activities to a rational and empirical formula" (p. 1). Therefore, to construct an index of health, researchers must select the concepts to be measured (such as mortality and morbidity), specify operational definitions for these concepts, determine the measures to be used, and develop a method of combining them into a single index.

X causes Y—a simple statement. However, the notion of causal attribution to disease is not so simple. In epidemiology, categorical attribution and counterfactual analysis are commonly used methods to attribute morbidity, mortality, and risk. In categorical attribution, using a defined set of rules, an event is attributed to a single cause. These rules become harder to interpret when the event exhibits comorbidity or multi-causality. Counterfactual analysis creates an ideal "what if" scenario and then compares current levels of a summary measure with the ideal. For example, if person X did not have a substance abuse problem, would he or she have contracted HIV/AIDS? Counterfactual analysis must take into account both direct and indirect consequences. Needle sharing is a direct consequence of transmission. Unsafe sexual activity that occurs to an individual who is under the influence of alcohol or drugs is an indirect consequence. Mathers et al. (2001) explain that health gap measures use categorical attribution to attribute morbidity and mortality due to disease and injury to "an exhaustive and mutually exclusive set of disease and injury categories" (p. 7), while counterfactual analysis attributes "the burden of disease to health determinants and risk factors" (p. 7).

In 1990, the WHO conducted a global burden of disease (GBD) study using a different type of metric. Traditionally, health impact assessment in public health measures health liabilities using a measure of mortality, years of life lost (YLL). In this global study, the mortality measure (YLL) was combined with a measure of years of life lived with a disability (YLD). The disability-adjusted life years (DALYS) metric provides a way to see the impacts of years of life lost in terms mortality and morbidity (Murray & Lopez, 1996). One DALY is equal to one year of life lost. Using a summary measure of population health, such as the DALY, allows health researchers to compare different diseases and disability through a standard methodology using a standard disease classification tool, the *International Classification of Diseases* (ICD). Although there are a number of other measures, the DALY is most easily applied across cultures and is used by the WHO to measure health gaps by comparing the difference to the actual situation compared to an ideal situation.

The results of the 1990 GBD were published as a four-volume set in 1996. Volume 1, *The Global Burden of Disease* (Murray & Lopez, 1996), gave the rationale to incorporate social, physical, and mental disabilities in health assessments. By using the DALY, they determined that depression was the fourth leading cause of disease burden in 1990 and extrapolated that it would be the single leading cause of disease burden by 2020. In addition, it predicted that HIV would be comparable to tuberculosis in its burden of disease. The successive volumes examined global health statistics, health dimensions of sex and reproduction, and the epidemiology of infectious diseases.

In 2000, the WHO conducted another Global Burden of Disease study, which updated estimates of incidence, health state prevalence, severity and duration, and mortality for over 130 major causes, for 112 member states. In the 2004 update, mental disorders and alcohol use disorders were among the 20 leading causes of disability worldwide. However, less than 25% of persons affected by mental disorders had access to treatment (WHO, 2008). Further, 45% of the adult disease burden in low- and middle-income countries globally was attributable to noncommunicable disease, based primarily upon population aging and changes in the distribution of risk factors (WHO, 2008).

In addition to the Global Burden of Disease studies, the WHO also conducted a number of other surveys, such as the World Health Survey (WHS) and the Global Observatory on eHealth (GOe) Survey (2005). The WHS was conducted across 70 countries during 2000–2002 to create a baseline for comparative studies on health status, outcomes, and evaluative methods from a health systems infrastructure perspective (WHO, 2002). Questionnaires were created for households and individuals, as well as for high-income and low-income countries. A number of interesting studies have emerged from the initiative and the data, ranging from methodological issues in the development of health surveys in developing countries (Timaeus et al., 1988) to an examination of war deaths using sibling history from the WHS (Obermeyer, Murray, & Gakidou, 2008).

The Global Observatory on eHealth (GOe) Survey was established in 2005 to provide member states with information and assistance on effective policies and practices in eHealth. It was the first worldwide assessment on eHealth by the WHO and utilized three priorities jointly identified by the World Summit on the Information Society and WHO. The first priority was to create, describe, and analyze eHealth profiles from a country, region, and international perspective. The second priority focused on key action areas, specifically identifying and evaluating which measures support the development of eHealth. The final priority was to establish standards for eHealth tools and services for the WHO member states. All 192 member states were invited to participate in the survey. Survey questions were grouped around the following:

1. Enabling environment;
2. Infrastructure;
3. Content;
4. Cultural and linguistic diversity, and cultural identity;
5. Capacity (including human resources knowledge and skills);
6. National centres for eHealth; and
7. eHealth systems and services (WHO, 2006).

The first three questions addressed policies and strategies to support eHealth, access to ICTs, and access to information and knowledge. A second survey was planned as a follow-up to the first survey, with fewer respondents, but with a more detailed questionnaire to enable a more robust analysis.

In 2010, the World Health Organization (WHO) suggested a more comprehensive approach to the socioeconomic impact of telehealth, particularly in terms of benefits to social care systems, infrastructure costs, and other services (Stroetmann et al., 2010). Since the WHO defines health as a state of physical, mental, and social well-being, it is important to view health as a "more continuous and holistic service provided both in response to evident need and to avoid unanticipated acute responses and phases of costly treatment" (Stroetmann et al., 2010, p. 3). To move toward this perspective, an integrated approach to care, with the appropriate health information and technology infrastructure, is critical.

However, there are key gaps in the evidence base for telehealth. Studies differ widely in design, complexity of interventions, populations (often a small n), allocations of resources, change management, and service integration. Further, many studies do not address longitudinal impacts or scalability. Debates over the evidence for telehealth urge more rigorous empirical studies. Although the randomized clinical trial is the gold standard, there is an increased call to engage in naturalistic evaluations of health care technologies under routine conditions and the impact of additional investment in telehealth services on health and social care systems. For example, increased investment in telehealth care infrastructure to support continuity of care across sectors may actually decrease costs in the social services sector.

Economic analyses and dynamic impact modeling may provide the long-view perspective critical to understanding impacts over time, place, and populations, such as identifying barriers to care that are as yet unknown and/or determining the costs and consequences of decisions. These types of analyses may show telehealth solutions that are cost-effective or have cumulative net benefits in one country (type of health system or governance) that may not be seen as such in other countries with different infrastructures and resources. Qualitative studies as well as mixed methods studies, such as information on the impacts on provider-patient experience or the provider-network experience, will provide substantiation for adoption, implementation, and sustainability of evidence-based practices.

Governance issues, for example, may be particularly difficult to discern. Governance refers to the codification, administration, and regulation of the performance of services across service sectors. These rules and regulations may affect the ability of telehealth to integrate effectively across service sectors, organizational silos, and/or national systems. Telepsychiatry, for example, may be effective in providing services to a person with schizophrenia with functional limitations; however, it may not "work" to coordinate supported housing or assisted transportation services in the community. Governance issues also affect how the public and private sectors provide, reimburse, and distribute financing for health care (Cronquist Christensen & Remler, 2007). As expected, there are considerable differences across countries regarding liability, reimbursement, and credentialing for telehealth services, and even more when trying to measure the impact of ICTs to a national level.

Measuring Impacts of ICTs

As part of the 2000 UN Millennium Declaration, member nations committed themselves to Millennium Development Goals (MDGs). Each of the MDGs has a series of targets with benchmarks to measure progress over time. Goal 8, "Develop a global partnership for development," has eight targets (UN, 2008). Target 8F is "to make available the benefits of new technologies, especially information and communications" (UN, 2008). Its three metrics are (1) the number of telephone lines per 100 of the population; (2) the number of cellular subscribers per 100 of the population: and (3) the number of Internet users

TABLE 13.2

Overview of ITU Questionnaires

Name of Questionnaire	Short World Telecommunication/ ICT Indicators (WTI) questionnaire	Long World Telecommunication/ ICT Indicators (WTI) questionnaire	Tariff Indicators Questionnaire	Questionnaire on ICT Access and Use by Households and Individuals
Addressed to	Government agency in charge of telecommunications/ ICT (Ministry, regulatory authority)	Government agency in charge of telecommunications/ ICT (Ministry, regulatory authority)	Government agency in charge of telecommunications/ ICT (Ministry, regulatory authority)	National Statistical Offices
Format	Online	Online	Online	Excel
Periodicity	Annually	Annually	Annually	Annually
Collection period	March	June/July	September	March/April
Number of indicators	Approximately 10	Approximately 70	Approximately 35	12 core indicators + classificatory variables
Data published	June and November/ December	November/December	November/December	June; November/December

Adapted from International Telecommunication Union. (2011). Overview of ITU questionnaires. Retrieved from http://www.itu.int/ITU-D/ict/datacollection/.

per 100 of the population (UN, 2008). By 2010, over 80 countries around the world had adopted or planned to adopt a national broadband strategy (International Telecommunication Union, 2011). Further, over 40 countries include broadband in their universal service definitions, and a number of them consider access to broadband a legal right.

Measuring this target is the purview of the International Telecommunication Union (ITU), an agency of the United Nations. The role of the ITU is to identify and define the statistics to be measured and then produce official statistics on ICT implementation and use for the international community. To do so, it collects three key sets of data. The first set of data details existing infrastructure. The second set of data enumerates tariffs associated with ICTs. The last set of data indicates access and use of ICTs by individuals and households.

Just as international standards are developed, a standard vocabulary lists the definitions of things to measure, so that apples are compared to apples. In addition, there are standards to describe how one derives measures mathematically and how a series of measures are combined to produce a larger measure. For example, a fixed telephone line (112) is "an active* line connecting the subscriber's terminal equipment to the public switched telephone network (PSTN) and which has a dedicated port in the telephone exchange equipment" (ITU, 2010, p. 1). An active* line is defined as a line that has beenactive during the past three months. To determine the number of fixed telephone lines, one must count the active number of analog fixed telephone lines (112a) plus ISDN channels (28c) plus fixed wireless (WLL) plus public payphones (1112) plus VoIP subscriptions (112IP) [112 = 112a + 28c + 1112 + 112IP] (ITU, 2010, p. 1). Definitions, indicators, and measures for telecommunication/ICT infrastructure and access and for tariff data are in the ITU's *Indicators Handbook* (2010). Indicators on access to and use of ICTs by households and individuals are in the *Core ICT indicators*. Table 13.2 lists the four surveys conducted by ITU to compile the necessary data to determine national progress toward the MDGs.

Additional Issues in Global Telemental Health

Broadband not only supports the development of cutting-edge approaches to health care, broadband-enabled telemedicine services also shift the health care paradigm by real-time patient monitoring, increased disease surveillance, disease prevention, and in-home care. Further, private and public sector partnerships encourage the use of telehealth innovations, pushing governments to invest in next-generation networks to realize the full range of broadband-enabled telemedicine tools and services (Davidson & Santorelli, 2009). For example, there are a number of international organizations and nonprofit nongovernmental organizations (NGO) that are using a variety of ICTs, networking locally and nationally, to improve health (Wooten, Patil, Scott, andf Ho, 2009). One example is the International Society for Telemedicine and e-Health (ISfTeH). and GNU Solidario. A nonprofit NGO established in Switzerland, ISfTeH has a broad membership base, including individuals, corporations, institutions and organizations, professional societies, regional and national councils, and government agencies. It provides technical assistance centers and staff to facilitate the dissemination of telehealth initiatives in developing nations.

A second example is GNU Solidario, another nonprofit NGO, also works in the areas of health and education with free software. A recent initiative was GNU Health training, offered through the United Nations University. The health information software used and deployed by the United Nations University, GNU Health is available through the GNU general public license as a health and hospital system. Designed as a multiplatform system, it works across operating systems, database management systems, and enterprise resource planning systems. GNU Health is currently used in a number of countries and is hosted on the European Commission portal and the Portal do Software Público Brasileiro (SPB).

Digital technologies have had three primary impacts on telemedicine: (1) efficient and fast transmission of large amounts of data over long distances; (2) the sending, receiving, managing, and storing of data; and (3) cost savings due to the adoption and implementation of these technologies. Telehealth has significantly increased the outreach of mental health services, prevention, and health promotion across difficult-to-reach populations, such as individuals living in rural and frontier areas, persons with chronic long-term disabilities, seniors aging "in place," and survivors of disasters, using a variety of technologies.

Outreach in Rural and Frontier Areas

There are a number of issues in the provision of services in rural and frontier areas. From a global perspective, there is little consensus as to the definition of a village or even if the term *village* is used as a term of measurement. National definitions of what constitutes a village, town, city, or metropolitan area vary significantly, depending upon what type of definitions and data are used. Generally, data are expressed in overall quantities, in per population ratios, or per household ratios (ITU, 2008).

Since most national statistical systems provide data at the province or state level, administrative definitions created by local governing boards contain the population defined as "urban" (UN, 1974). Everything outside the "urban" boundary is classed as "rural." This may be under- or overestimated, depending upon how often unincorporated areas become incorporated into an urban area. Another issue in using administrative data is that the level of administrative oversight may not extend to a village level. For example, in Malawi, the level of administrative oversight stops several steps above the village level (ITU, 2008). In some countries, a different type of criterion defines "urban": the size and type of economic activity. In other countries, the level of existing infrastructure (roads, utilities, etc.) may be the defining factor. There is also a geographic definition based upon an internationally recommended definition of "localities" (i.e., densely settled population clusters) (UN, 1974).

There are 15 different definitions of *rural* in the United States (Coburn et al., 2007). Even the differences between using the Census Bureau definition of *rural* and that of the Office of Management and Budget (the two most commonly used definitions) result in very different sets of places defined as rural (Coburn et al., 2007).

Since rural definitions are used to identify rural populations, settings, and/or health care providers, consequences from a poorly constructed definition can adversely affect policy to improve health and population outcomes for rural and frontier areas. Hence, caution is essential in making cross-country comparisons. However, for the purposes of this chapter, we are using the definition of rural from the WHO (2009): *rural areas* are considered to be those areas that are not urban in nature. An *urban agglomeration* refers to the de facto population contained within the contours of a contiguous territory inhabited at urban density levels without regard to administrative boundaries. (UN, 2009, p. 6). With this definition in mind, the following section examines the use of ICT in the provision of health and mental health services.

AUSTRALIA: WEB-BASED MENTAL HEALTH DECISION SUPPORT

In 2006, the Australian government implemented the Better Access to Mental Health Care (BAMHC) program. The BAMHC program provides general practitioners (GPs) additional support in the provision of mental health services using online decision support tools and a service directory using a website (Ollerenshaw, 2009). In the Ballarat and District Division of General Practice (BDDGP), 107 GPs and 6 GP registries cover 7,300 square kilometers and over 120,000 patients. After the launch of the website, the annual review of its usage showed 50% of site visitors came directly from the BDDGP website. Almost 25% of visitors used the service directory, and an additional 14% went directly to the decision support tool. The results suggest repeat visits by GPs, which may indicate research on mental health referrals and supports.

SOUTH AFRICA: HEALTH PROMOTION OVER COMMUNITY RADIO

Telehealth may involve a variety of media. For example, in many rural or underdeveloped areas, there may be little access to broadband applications by the general population. However, other telecommunications technologies, such as radio, may be the primary source of community and health information. The South African Medical Research Council (MRC) conducted a pilot project on the use of health information among community radio stations in South Africa. Snyders, van Wyk, and van Zyl (2010) examined the use of community radio to determine the frequency of health information broadcast to the community relevant information, where community radio stations found health information, and what types of audio products were most needed by the community. Working cooperatively with the stations and their staff, the MRC was able to create targeted content to address health concerns to the community and provide audio content to the radio stations through a user friendly website on health information.

MHEALTH: ADOPTION ACROSS WHO MEMBER NATIONS

Another innovation in health care is the use of mobile and wireless technologies (mobile health). According to the International Telecommunication Union (2011), there are now over 5 billion wireless subscribers; over 70% of them reside in low- and middle-income countries. Further, commercial wireless signals cover over 85% of the world's population (ITU, 2011). Mobile health (mHealth) services and processes are most easily incorporated into areas with existing telephone networks, such as health and mental health call centers, toll-free numbers, and emergency services. However, in less developed countries, the use of mHealth for surveillance, health promotion, and decision support systems is more limited.

The Global Observatory for eHealth (GOe, 2011) defines mHealth or mobile health as "medical and public health practice supported by mobile devices" (p. 6). Mobile devices range from mobile phones, patient monitoring devices, personal digital assistants (PDAs), and other wireless devices to network services and applications, including voice and short messaging service (SMS), general packet radio service (GPRS), third and fourth generation mobile telecommunications (3G and 4G systems), global positioning system (GPS), and Bluetooth technology.

Eighty-three percent of WHO Member States have implemented between one to four mHealth initiatives (low-income countries, 77%, $n = 22$; high-income countries, 87%, $n = 29$)). Health call centers, telephone help lines, and emergency and/or disaster toll-free telephone services are the most common mHealth initiatives (GOe, 2011, p. 19). Health call centers and telephone help lines account for 60% of mHealth use in most Member States, except in Africa (40%). Health issues, such as HIV/AIDS, H1N1, reproductive health/family planning, pandemics, and drug abuse (p. 19) are among the most common health issues.

Where There Is No Connectivity

There are many areas of the world where there is no connectivity to the Internet. This makes it particularly difficult for medical and community health practitioners to remain current in best practices or to have access to the literature. Early initiatives used microform, CD-ROMs, and DVDs. However, for those areas, which have little or no electricity, the WHO created the Blue Trunk Library (BTL) project (Mouhouelo, Okessi, & Kabore, 2006). Each BTL contains over 100 books on medicine and public health. The blue trunk, in which materials are packed, also doubles as a bookcase. The bulk of the materials are practical manuals. Topics are addressed at several practitioner levels, including physicians, nurses, nurses' aides, and community health workers.

As of December 2010, 84 countries have received approximately 2,100 BTLs (WHO, 2011). In addition, health districts in the sub-Saharan countries have received over 850 BTLs. However, there are requests to expand the BTL project to nursing schools and NGOs.

PERSONS WITH CHRONIC LONG-TERM DISABILITIES AND AGING "IN PLACE"

Chronic illnesses contribute to mental decline and loss of mobility, requiring additional care outside the home. Further, the world overall is aging. At the world level, the number of older persons is expected to exceed the number of children for the first time by the year 2045 (United Nations, 2009). Two U.S. studies estimate the adoption of policies that reduce barriers and accelerate implementation of broadband-based health resources could result in the reduction in health care expenditures by a net of $197 billion (in constant 2008 dollars) and save over $920 billion in health care costs for seniors and people with disabilities (Litan, 2008; Litan, 2005).

Chronic illnesses and an aging population influence numerous factors, such as family composition and living arrangements, migration trends, epidemiology, and the need for health care services. Higher prevalence of chronic illnesses, for example, leads to treatment expansion, as the numbers of persons affected by disease increase due to the progression of disease(s) and aggressive detection and treatment of disease (Howard, Thorpe, & Busch, 2010). Further, as the incidence of chronic diseases increase, changes in medical practice and reductions in mortality rates result in persons living longer with a reduced quality of life. Of the 57 million deaths that occurred in 2008, the WHO reported non-communicable diseases were responsible for 63% of those deaths, in particular, cancers, chronic respiratory disease, cardiovascular diseases, and diabetes (Alwan et al., 2011). Further, preventable risk factors were identified as elevated blood pressure (13% of deaths globally), tobacco use (9%), elevated blood glucose (6%), physical inactivity (6%), and overweight and obesity (5%) (Alwan et al., 2011). Concurrent with these physical illnesses, persons may also experience mental illnesses, such as depression or substance use disorders.

Older persons living alone are at greater risk of experiencing social isolation and economic deprivation. For example, the proportion of Japanese who live in multi-generational households has fallen from almost 50% in 1985 to 20% in 2006 (United Nations, 2009). In Africa, especially with the HIV/AIDS epidemic, older adults are responsible for their grandchildren and extended family whose parents have succumbed to AIDS (United Nations, 2009). With the death of their adult children, these elderly individuals are unable to receive the level of family support that normally occurs in their societies. This increases the possibility of intergenerational poverty and deprivation.

Telehealth contributes to maintaining independence for the elderly and for persons with chronic illnesses. As care for the elderly and persons with chronic illnesses shifts from family members to the formal health sector (home health care, nursing homes, and hospitals), home care is most feasible only when individuals are capable of living independently. The European Commission (2010) published a *Digital Agenda for Europe*, which focuses on how information and communications technologies will assist in creating positive social challenges, such as improving how energy is used, enhancing health services and public services, supporting e-governance, and collaboration across the European Union and other nations. One of its emphases is on the ability of individuals, especially seniors, to "age in place."

The International Society for Gerontechnology (IST), a standing committee of the International Association of Gerontology and Geriatrics and a member of the Ambient Assisted Living Forum, has as its mission the design of "technology and environment for independent living and social participation of older persons in good health, comfort and safety" (IST, 2011). Hosted by Technische Universiteit Eindhoven (TUe) in the Netherlands, IST envisions an inclusive society where all members (aging, disabled, or healthy) live, thrive, and age in optimal environments. Thus, planning for an aging society must start before that society has aged. By incorporating the best of design and technology to create livable, sustainable environments, there are enhanced health and environmental outcomes for society. Addressing issues of telesurveillance to improve diagnosis and monitoring of persons with dementia, for example, allows persons with dementia or other cognitive or developmental disorders to remain at home longer and in a protected environment (Kearns et al., 2011). The use of gaming in increasing movement (e.g., Wii) for elders can also be used for persons with traumatic brain injury, spinal cord injuries, amputees, and neuromuscular disorders, as well as to encourage movement in persons of all ages, reducing obesity and obesity-related diseases (Aarhus et al., 2011). In addition, such research also allows us to be better prepared to handle the injuries and trauma suffered by survivors of disasters.

SURVIVORS OF DISASTERS

Disasters contribute to increased morbidity and mortality with significant economic impacts worldwide. Consider that the psychological, physical, and social sequelae of disasters are evident years after the initiating event. Problems with socioeconomic and infrastructure issues before a disaster are exacerbated following a disaster. Further, many medical and public health technologies are underutilized due to the lack of inclusion in local, regional, and national preparedness planning, and training activities as well as planning for effective network infrastructure and connectivity costs. Determining risk and implementing risk management requires a number of steps, ranging from prospective risk management (before the disaster) to compensatory risk management (mitigating existing vulnerabilities) (United Nations Development Programme, 2004). The MDG has as one of its stated goals in target 8 (developing a global partnership for development) to reduce the effects of natural and manmade disasters (UN, 2008).

The use of ICTs for disaster response is not new. In 1986, Japan determined that it was feasible to send medical information using its domestic communication satellite with a 30/20 GHz simple communication system with one-telephone-equivalent channel (Otsu et al., 1986). In 1988 and 1989, there was a joint telemedicine "spacebridge" between Armenian, U.S., and Russian medical centers and teams to assist in triaging and treatment of medical problems following the December earthquake in Armenia and the June 1989 gas explosion near Ufa. Of the 209 interactive patient consultations (across 20 specialty areas), 185 patients received altered diagnoses (54), new diagnostic studies (70), new diagnostic processes (47), and modified treatment plans (47) (Houtchens et al., 1993).

In 1989, the global community launched the International Decade for Natural Disaster Reduction (United Nations General Assembly, 1989) in order to increase awareness of the importance of disaster reduction. During this time, several important initiatives emerged, including the Yokohama strategy and plan for action (United Nations World Conference on Natural Disaster Reduction, 1994). The Yokohama strategy emphasized the importance of a culture of prevention, vulnerability reduction, and the use of existing and new technologies to reduce the impact of disasters. Activities were devised at the community and national levels, regional and sub-regional levels, and at international levels through the use of formal bilateral and multilateral agreements.

In 1997, then Vice President Albert Gore requested the formation of a Disaster Information Task Force (DITF) to determine the feasibility of creating a global disaster information network. The DITF working groups originally focused by function (users, providers, and disseminators), by disaster types (severe weather, geologic, fires, and man-made), and by disaster phases (pre- and post-). The findings identified by the DITF resulted in a consensus document for the Global Disaster Information Network (GDIN, 1997), now part of the International Charter "Space and Major Disasters," an international agreement among space agencies to support data and information relief in the event of major disasters.

In 1999, the International Strategy for Disaster Reduction (UNISDR) was created. Part of the United Nations, the ISDR follows the Geneva Mandate on Disaster Reduction (1999) as its founding document (General Assembly Resolution GA 54/219). In 2001, the UNISDR expanded its mandate to become the coordinator for disaster reduction activities of the United Nations system and its regional organizations and activities (GA resolution

56/195). Its "International Strategy for Disaster Reduction" revolves around three major concepts: (1) natural hazards; (2) vulnerability; and (3) risk (Inter-agency Task Force on Disaster Reduction, 2001). At this time, the ISDR accepted its mandates from two UN General Assembly resolutions: to cooperate at an international level to reduce the impact of El Niño (54/220); and to strengthen Early Warning capacity for disaster management (54/219) (Inter-agency Task Force on Disaster Reduction, 2001). At the 2005 World Conference on Disaster Reduction, the Yokohama Strategy was reevaluated in light of a decade's worth of work and technology innovations. The Hyogo Framework for Action 2005–2015 was adopted. Its five priorities (United Nations International Strategy for Disaster Reduction, 2005, p. 15) included:

1. Ensure that disaster risk reduction is a national and a local priority with a strong institutional basis for implementation ;
2. Identify, assess, and monitor disaster risks and enhance early warning;
3. Use knowledge, innovation and education to build a culture of safety and resilience at all levels;
4. Reduce the underlying risk factors; and
5. Strengthen disaster preparedness for effective response at all levels.

The Hyogo Framework emphasized the establishment of national platforms for disaster reduction encompassing public, private, and civil participation from all agencies and organizations within a country. It recommended a number of information-seeking actions, including the dissemination of risk maps, identification of vulnerable areas/infrastructures, development of indicator systems and scales to rank disaster risk and vulnerabilities, and the collection and analysis of disaster occurrences, impacts, and losses. It also urged compilation and standardization of regional disaster risks, impacts, and losses; as well as the use, application, and affordability of recent information, communication, and space-based technologies/services to support disaster risk reduction and risk prediction. These requests for information require generic, realistic, and measurable indicators that can collect essential data across emerging, developing, and developed nations.

However, there are a number of conceptual and methodological challenges in measuring disaster loss. For example, what occurrences can be attributed directly to a disaster, and what can be indirectly attributed to a disaster? Direct costs are attributed to physical damages (industries, crops, inventories, etc.), economic infrastructures (roads, utilities, etc.), and social infrastructures (housing, schools, churches, etc.). Indirect costs describe disruption to goods and provision of services and the consequences from the increased incidence of morbidity and mortality. In addition, there are secondary effects, which result from short- and long-term impacts on the socioeconomics of a locality, a population, and a nation. These range from redistribution of local and national monies post-disaster to the costs of relocation and/or migration of populations, industries, and workforces. However, the major obstacle to describing and analyzing the impact of a disaster is the lack of reliable data and information that must be collected from numerous individuals, agencies, and organizations over time in order to determine a disaster's full scope. Further, the data must be able to be framed into a people-centered approach, so that collective action and knowledge can be generated to minimize risk and vulnerability of a population.

One such example is the development of early warning systems. Considering the devastation that occurred in 2004 with the tsunami in the Indian Ocean, Cyclone Nargis in Myanmar in 2008, and more recently with the earthquakes in 2010 and 2011 in Haïti and Japan, it is critical to understand that early warning is not only a technology but also "an understanding of risk and a link between producers and consumers of warning information, with the ultimate goal of triggering action to prevent or mitigate a disaster" (International Federation of Red Cross and Red Crescent Societies, 2009, p. 17). Figure 13.1 illustrates the four elements of early warning and response systems. Of these, we will look at the issues surrounding dissemination.

In addition to satellite-based telecommunications sub-systems and the data-collection services of meteorological satellites, dissemination may rely on both technological and non-technological solutions among numerous agencies and first responders before warnings are broadcast to the general population. Technologies may include satellite radio, cellular phones, and traditional broadcast media. However, in many poorer communities, electricity to power broadcast media may be limited or nonexistent. In this case, wind-up or solar-powered radios can deploy over AM, FM, and shortwave frequencies. The International Federation of Red Cross and Red Crescent Societies (2009) describe the case of the Maldives, which comprises 200 populated islands in a 1,200-island chain. Over 90% of the unpopulated islands have been converted to tourist resorts, which may account for approximately 20% of the islands' populations during the tourist season. There is extensive cell phone use by tourists and the Maldivians. After the 2004 tsunami, cell broadcasts over

RISK KNOWLEDGE

Systematically collect data & undertake risk assessment

Identify hazards & vulnerabilities

Review patterns and trends

Identify availability of/access to risk maps & data

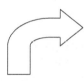

RESPONSE CAPABILITY

Build national & community response capabilities

Currency of response plans

Response systems testing

Local capacities and knowledge

Public preparedness

TECHNICAL MONITORING & WARNING

SERVICE

Develop local & global hazard monitoring / early warning services

Select appropriate parameters

Best practices for forecasting

Feasibility, accuracy, & timely

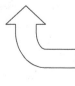

DISSEMINATION AND COMMUNICATION

Communicate risk information and early warnings

Do warnings reach all of those at risk?

Are the risks and the warnings well understood?

Is the warning information clear and usable?

FIGURE 13.1 Elements of Early Warning and Response Systems.
Adapted from UNISDR (n.d.) http://www.unisdr.org/ppew/whats-ew/basics-ew.html.

mobile phones were considered for emergency warning systems (International Federation of Red Cross and Red Crescent Societies, 2009).

Cell broadcast is the ability to "push" (send) a single text or binary message for distribution to multiple mobile phones within a "cell" area (Udu-gama, 2009). Cell broadcasts are considered a "one-to-many" mode of communication, unlike SMS, which is a one-to-one mode; cell broadcasts are not queued and do not require individual phone numbers. There is less opportunity for bandwidth congestion and loss of service. Cell broadcasts are effective on 2G and 3G networks. In addition, cell broadcasts can be repeated within 2-second to 32-minute intervals, and multi-language broadcasts can be broadcast to multiple channels simultaneously. Finally, cell broadcasts are more secure transmissions (encryption and decryption) and can be generated by an official government agency or office (Udu-gama, 2009). However, there are limitations to cell broadcast systems. A cell broadcast system is not meant to be a stand-alone network. Further, if cell tower infrastructure is disrupted, cellular communications cease; in extremely remote or formidable terrain, or if there is a lack of telecommunications carriers, the effectiveness of cell broadcast systems is limited (Udu-gama, 2009).

Implications for Mental Health Informatics

There are a number of reasons to promote international collaboration in telemedicine and telehealth. Obvious reasons are the socioeconomic benefits in improving and enhancing the delivery of health and mental health care. Further, the sharing of expertise now exceeds geographical and political barriers. More industrialized nations have a responsibility to test and develop new technologies that can improve health care and health outcomes in less industrialized countries. From a larger perspective, all nations have rural and frontier areas in desperate need of access to care, and all nations are susceptible to natural and manmade disasters, which can obliterate a nation's sense of security and access to health care.

As discussed in this chapter, measuring the impact of ICTs and health is confounded by many factors. Something as simple as defining a rural population or counting at a village level or agreeing upon a definition for POTS (plain old telephone services) becomes infinitely more complex when viewing administrative levels and governance issues within a nation, much less across nations. Unclear definitions can result in different outcomes from those originally intended for specified target areas and populations. An indicator that is unavailable in country X limits the ability to determine progress toward benchmarks. Finally, there may be dire consequences to populations when policy is not grounded in reliable data created from a shared understanding of terms.

At an international level, the two most commonly used classifications of country groupings are those of the WHO and the World Bank. Although each country classification schema have strengths and constraints, it is difficult, if not impossible, to crosswalk data collected or to compare analyses at a local or national level, or health and socioeconomic impacts. For example, the WHO country grouping crosswalks to WHO's strategic analysis, planning, and operational actions, based upon the GOe data. However, other agencies outside the WHO framework may have difficulty interpreting or applying the GOe data to their own data. The World Bank (2012) income grouping is a simple four-level scale based on gross national income (GNI) per capita (high, upper-middle, lower-middle, and low income). Clearly defined within an economic framework, it allows easy comparison across countries and WHO regions. However, it is constrained by the lack of indicators addressing other sociodemographics of a population (e.g., health and age).

Economic evaluations of telemedicine, at an international level, also raise particular challenges for evaluators. If a telemedicine system has multiple uses and joint costs across agencies, partnerships, or nations, it may be difficult to apportion the costs of service X to agency Y. Further, a telemedicine system developed for one use may expand to include other services, requiring additional resources and capacity. Finally, obsolescence in technology happens exponentially. Changes in technologies may require a new way of evaluating costs and consequences of delivering specific services.

Cost-effectiveness analysis is the most common method used for health issues and helps to assess whether the expected health benefits are worth the investment. However, governance issues affect both public and private regulation, licensing, credentialing, and reimbursement. Decisions regarding the use of telemedicine will need to consider not just the costs of eHealth but if the health benefits are worth the cost. Economic evaluations also should factor in the costs of monitoring and evaluating telehealth services.

Finally, the WHO definition of underserved areas covers geographical areas where persons live in poverty, areas that have limited access to health services and providers, rural or remote areas, regions in conflict or post-conflict, and refugee camps (WHO, 2009, p. 6). When examining global telehealth applications, it is critical to have inter-jurisdictional, national, and regional cooperation and involvement of the user community in identifying linguistic and cultural requirements to ensure appropriate and timely distribution of and access to health and early warning information. Low technology is as important, if not more so, when looking at improving and securing global health. Public trust in its local, national, regional, and international governments and nongovernmental organizations is essential. Health and disaster information and services must be reliable, timely, current, and deliverable. Finally, interoperability as to standards, definitions, classifications, and technologies must be seen as standard operating procedure in the development of new or updated technologies.

References

Aarhus, R., Grönvall, E., Larsen, S.B., & Wollsen, S. (2011). Turning training into play: Embodied gaming, seniors, physical training and motivation. *Gerontechnology; 10*(2), 110–120. doi:10.4017/gt.2011.10.2.005.00

Alwan, A., Armstrong, T., Cowan, M., & Riley, L. (2011). *Noncommunicable diseases country profiles 2011*. Geneva: World Health Organization. Retrieved from http://whqlibdoc.who.int/publications/2011/9789241502283_Eng.pdf.

Centers for Disease Control. (1990). Guidelines for investigating clusters of health events. *MMWR: Recommendations and Reports, 39*(RR-11):1–23. Retrieved from http://www.cdc.gov/mmwr/preview/mmwrhtml/00001797.htm.

Coburn, A. F., MacKinney, A. C., McBride, T. D., Mueller, K. J., Slifkin, R. T., & Wakefield, M. K. (2007). Choosing rural definitions: Implications for health policy. *Rural Policy Research Institute Health Panel, Issue Brief #2*, 1–8. Retrieved from http://www.rupri.org/Forms/RuralDefinitionsBrief.pdf.

Crisp, N. (2007). *Global health partnerships. The UK contribution to health in developing countries.* London: COI, 2007. Retrieved from http:// http://www.dh.gov.uk/en/ Publicationsandstatistics/Publications/PublicationsPolicyAndGuidance/DH_065374.

Cronquist Christensen, M., & Remler, D. (2007). Information and communications technology in chronic disease care: What are the implications for payment? *Medical Care Research & Review, 64*(2), 123–147.

Davidson, C, M., & Santorelli, M. J. (2009). The impact of broadband on telemedicine: A report to the U.S. Chamber of Commerce. Washington, DC: U.S. Chamber of Commerce, Environment, Technology & Regulatory Affairs. Retrieved from http://www. uschamber.com/sites/default/files/about/0904Broadband_and_Telemedicine.pdf.

European Commission. (2010). Pillar VII: ICT for social challenges. In *Digital agenda for Europe.* Retrieved from http://ec.europa.eu/information_society/newsroom/cf/pillar. cfm?pillar_id=49.

G8 (2011, May). *Deauville G8 declaration: renewed commitment for freedom and democracy.* Retrieved from http://www.worldvision.org/resources.nsf/main/press-G8-experts/$file/ Deauville_Declaration.pdf.

Global Disaster Information Network. (1997). Harnessing information and technology for disaster management. Retrieved from http://www.westerndisastercenter.org/ DOCUMENTS/DITF_Report.pdf.

Global Observatory for eHealth. (2005). *Global eHealth Survey 2005.* Geneva: WHO. Retrieved from http://www.who.int/entity/kms/initiatives/Global_EHealth_survey_ FINAL.doc.

Global Observatory for eHealth. (2011). mHealth: *New horizons for health through mobile technologies: Based on the findings of the second global survey on eHealth* (Global Observatory for eHealth series, Volume 3). Retrieved from http://www.who.int/goe/publi- cations/goe_mhealth_web.pdf.

Houtchens, B. A., Clemmer, T. P., Holloway, H. C., Kiselev, A. A., Logan, J. S., Merrell, R. C., Nicogossian, A. E., … & Siegel, J.H. (1993). Telemedicine and international disaster response. Medical consultation to Armenia and Russia via a telemedicine spacebridge. *Prehospital & Disaster Medicine, 8*(1), 57–66.

Howard, D. H., Thorpe, K. E., & Busch, S. H. (2010). Understanding recent increases in chronic disease treatment rates: more disease or more detection? *Health Economics, Policy, & Law, 5*(4),411–435.

Inter-Agency Task Force on Disaster Reduction. (2001). *Framework for action: For the imple- mentation of the International Strategy for Disaster Reduction (ISDR).* New York: United Nations. Retrieved from http://www.eird.org/fulltext/marco-accion/ framework-english.pdf.

International Federation of Red Cross and Red Crescent Societies. (2009). *World Disasters Report 2009: Focus on early warning, early action.* Geneva: The Federation. Retrieved from http://www.ifrc.org/Global/Publications/disasters/WDR/WDR2009-full.pdf.

International Society for Gerontechnology (2012). Society home. Retrieved from http://www. gerontechnology.info/index.php/journal/pages/view/isghome.

International Telecommunication Union. (2011). Increased competition has helped bring ICT access to billions. *ITU snapshot* (5). Geneva: ITU. Retrieved from http://www.itu.int/net/ pressoffice/stats/2011/01/index.aspx.

International Telecommunication Union. (2008). *ITU measuring information and communication technology availability in villages and rural areas.* Geneva: ITU. Retrieved from http://www.itu.int/ITU-D/ict/material/Measuring%20ICT_web.pdf.

International Telecommunication Union. (2010, March). *Definitions of world telecommunication/ICT indicators, March 2010.* Geneva: ITU. Retrieved from http://www.itu.int/ITUD/ict/material/TelecomICT_Indicators_Definition_March2010_for_web.pdf.

Kearns, W. D., Fozard, C. H., Nams, V. O., & Craighead, J. D. (2011). Wireless telesurveillance system for detecting dementia. *Gerontechnology; 10(2),* 90–102. doi:10.4017/gt.2011.10.2.004.00.

LaCroix, A., Lareng, L., Padekan, D., Nerlich, M., Bracale, M., Ogushi, O.... & McDonald, I. (2002). *International concerted action on collaboration in telemedicine: Final report and recommendations of the G8 Global Healthcare Applications Project 4.* Retrieved http://mi.med.u-tokai.ac.jp/g7sp4/final.htm.

Litan, R. E. (2005). *Great expectations: Potential economic benefits to the nation from accelerated broadband deployment to older Americans and Americans with disabilities.* New Millennium Research Council. Retrieved from http://www.newmillenniumresearch.org/archive/Litan_FINAL_120805.pdf.

Litan, R. E. (2008). *Vital signs via broadband: Remote health monitoring transmit savings, enhances lives.* Retrieved from http://www.corp.att.com/healthcare/docs/litan.pdf.

Mathers, C., Vos, T., Lopez, A., Salomon, J., & Ezzati, M. (2001). *National burden of disease studies: a practical guide, edition 2.0.* Geneva: World Health Organization, Global Program on Evidence for Health Policy. Retrieved from http://www.who.int/healthinfo/nationalburdenofdiseasemanual.pdf.

Mouhouelo, P., Okessi, A., & Kabore, M.-P. (2006). Where there is no Internet: Delivering health information via the Blue Trunk Libraries. *PLoS Med 3*(3), e77. doi:10.1371/journal.pmed.0030077. http://www.plosmedicine.org/article/info:doi/10.1371/journal.pmed.0030077

Murray, C. J., & Lopez, A. D. (1996). *The global burden of disease: A comprehensive assessment of mortality and disability from diseases, injuries, and risk factors in 1990 and projected to 2020.* Cambridge, MA: Harvard University Press.

Obermeyer, Z., Murray, C. J., & Gakidou, E. (2008). Fifty years of violent war deaths from Vietnam to Bosnia: Analysis of data from the world health survey programme. *BMJ, 336*(7659), 1482–1486. doi: 10.1136/bmj.a137.

Ollerenshaw, A. (2009). Internet tool box for rural GPs to access mental health services information. *Rural & Remote Health, 9*(2), 1094. Retrieved from http://www.rrh.org.au/articles/subviewnew.asp?ArticleID=1094.

Otsu, Y., Choh, T., Yamazaki, I., Kosaka, K., Iguchi, M., & Nakajima, I. (1986). Experiments on the quick-relief medical communications via the Japan's domestic communication satellite CS-2 for the case of disasters and emergencies. *Acta Astronautica; 13*(6–7), 459–466.

Partnership on Measuring ICT for Development. (2010). *Core ICT indicators 2010.* Geneva: ITU. Retrieved from http://www.itu.int/dms_pub/itu-d/opb/ind/D-IND-ICT_CORE-2010-PDF-E.pdf.

Sanders, B. S. (1964). Measuring community health levels. *American Journal of Public Health, 54,* 1063–1070.

Snyders, J., van Wyk, E., & van Zyl, H. (2010). Investigating health information needs of community radio stations and applying the World Wide Web to disseminate audio products. *Studies in Health Technology and Informatics, 160*(Pt. 1), 514–517. doi: 10.3233/978-1-60750-588-4-514.

Stroetmann, K. A., Kubitschke, L., Robinson, S., Stroetmann, V., Cullen, K., & McDaid, D. (2010). *How can telehealth help in the provision of integrated care?* (Policy brief #13). Copenhagen: WHO Regional Office for Europe. Retrieved from http://www.euro.who. int/en/what-we-do/data-and-evidence/health-evidence-network-hen/publications/2010/ how-can-telehealth-help-in-the-provision-of-integrated-care.

Sullivan, D. F. (1966). *Conceptual problems in developing an index of health* (Public Health Service Publication, no. 100). Washington, DC: U.S. Government Printing Office.

Timaeus, I., Harpham, T., Price, M., & Gilson, L. (1988). Health surveys in developing countries: the objectives and design of an international programme. *Social Science & Medicine, 27*(4), 359–368.

Udu-gama, N. (2009). *Mobile cell broadcasting for commercial use and public warning in the Maldives.* Colombo, Sri Lanka: LIRNEasia. Retrieved from http://lirneasia.net/ wp-content/uploads/2009/07/CB_Maldives_FINAL_2009_041.pdf.

United Nations. (1974). *Methods for projections of urban and rural population: Manual 8* (United Nations publication, Sales No. E.74.XIII.3). New York: UN. Retrieved from http://www.un.org/esa/population/techcoop/PopProj/manual8/chapter1.pdf.

United Nations. (2008). *Millennium development goals indicators.* Retrieved from http:// mdgs.un.org/unsd/mdg/Host.aspx?Content=Indicators/OfficialList.htm.

United Nations. (2009). *World population ageing 2009* (ESA/P/WP/212). United Nations Department of Economic and Social Affairs Population Division. Retrieved from http:// www.un.org/esa/population/publications/WPA2009/WPA2009_WorkingPaper.pdf.

United Nations Development Programme. (2004). *Reducing disaster risk: A challenge for development: A global report.* New York: UN. Retrieved from http://www.adaptation- learning.net/research/2-united-nations-development-programme-undp-1004-reducing-dis aster-risk-challenge-developme.

United Nations General Assembly. (1989). A/Res/44/236 International Decade for Natural Disaster Reduction. Retrieved from http://www.un.org/documents/ga/res/44/a44r236.htm.

United Nations General Assembly. (2000). *55/2 United Nations millennium declaration.* Retrieved from http://www.un.org/millennium/declaration/ares552e.htm.

United Nations International Strategy for Disaster Reduction. (2005). *Hyogo framework for action 2005–2015: Building the resilience of nations and communities to disasters.* Kobe: ISDR. Retrieved from http://www.unisdr.org/2005/wcdr/intergover/official-doc/L-docs/ Hyogo-framework-for-action-english.pdf.

United Nations World Conference on Natural Disaster Reduction. (1994). *Yokohama Strategy and plan of action for a safer world: Guidelines for natural disaster prevention, prepared- ness and mitigation.* Yokohama: United Nations World Conference on Natural Disaster Reduction. Retrieved from http://nidm.gov.in/amcdrr/yokohama.pdf.

Wooten, R., Patil, N. G., Scott, R. E., Ho, K. (2009). *Telehealth in the developing world.* London: Royal Society of Medicine Press Ltd. Retrieved from http://web.idrc.ca/ openebooks/396-6/.

World Bank. (2012). *How we classify countries.* Retrieved from http://data.worldbank.org/ about/country-classifications.

World Health Organization. (2002). *World health survey instruments and related documents.* Geneva: WHO. Retrieved from http://www.who.int/healthinfo/survey/instruments/en/ index.html.

World Health Organization. (2006). *E-health tools & services: Needs of member states.* Geneva: WHO. Retrieved from http://www.who.int/kms/initiatives/tools_and_services_ final.pdf

World Health Organization. (2008). *The global burden of disease: 2004 update.* Geneva: WHO. Retrieved from http://www.who.int/healthinfo/global_burden_disease/2004_ report_update/en/index.html.

World Health Organization. (2009). *Increasing access to health workers in remote and rural areas through improved retention: Background paper for the first expert meeting to develop evidence-based recommendations to increase access to health workers in remote and rural areas through improved retention.* Geneva: WHO. Retrieved from http://www.who.int/hrh/ migration/background_paper.pdf.

World Health Organization. (2010). *Telemedicine: Opportunities and developments in Member States: Report on the second global survey on eHealth 2009.* Geneva: WHO. Retrieved from http://www.who.int/goe/publications/goe_telemedicine_2010.pdf.

World Health Organization. (2011). *Blue trunk libraries.* Retrieved from http://www.who.int/ ghl/mobile_libraries/bluetrunk/en/index.html.

World Summit on the Information Society. (2003, December 12). *A plan of action* (Document WSIS-03/GENEVA/DOC/5-E). Geneva: The Summit. Retrieved from http://www.itu. int/wsis/docs/geneva/official/poa.html.

World Summit on the Information Society. (2003, December 13). *Declaration of principles: Building the information society: a global challenge in the new millennium* (Document WSIS-03/GENEVA/DOC/4-E). Geneva: The Summit. Retrieved from http://www.itu. int/wsis/docs/geneva/official/dop.html.

Policy analysis must create problems that decision-makers are able to handle with the variables under their control and in the time available ... by specifying a desired relationship between manipulable means and obtainable objectives.

AARON WILDAVSKY, 1979, 16

14 Policy and Practice

So far, the previous chapters have focused on the intersection between mental health services research, education, and practice with mental health informatics, examining local, state, national, and global perspectives. This chapter will present emergent trends, upcoming legislation, and new ways of conceptualizing the intersection of mental health services research, practice, and informatics, and will conclude with implications for the field, keeping in mind the challenges faced by public sector health and mental health providers, educators, and researchers.

Issues and Concerns

By the middle of the twenty-first century, health care will consume one-quarter of the country's gross domestic product as per capita health care spending grows more rapidly than per capita GDP:

> CBO [Congressional Budget Offie] projects that, without changes in law, total spending on health care will rise from 16 percent of GDP in 2007 to 25 percent in 2025 and 49 percent in 2082. Federal spending on Medicare (net of beneficiaries' premiums) and Medicaid would rise from 4 percent of GDP in 2007 to 7 percent in 2025 and 19 percent in 2082. (Orszag, 2008, p. 1)

What accounts for this exponential increase in health care cost? Two factors frequently discussed in this text included an increase in the costs per beneficiary in private and public health insurance programs, and the increase in chronic illnesses. However, the CBO has suggested that the emergence, adoption, and implementation of new health technologies and services by the U.S. health and mental health care system may be a more significant factor, as the cost of these technologies are passed on to the consumer, for example, in the cost per beneficiary of a health plan, or passed on in the cost of care in a hospital or residential setting (Orszag, 2008).

IMPACT OF LEGISLATION

Without a doubt, legislation affects service delivery, care and treatment, distribution of resources, allocation of staff, and funding streams. By investing in HIT systems, it is estimated that typical hospitals will generate savings of some $25,000 to $44,000 per bed per year, and $30 billion to $40 billion annually when looking at the hospital industry nationally (Laflamme, Pietraszek, Rajadhyax, 2010). If we extrapolate this savings into the larger health and mental health provider networks, from individuals to large group practices, as well as community-based, public, and private providers, we are looking at significant changes in health care delivery, optimizing the use of labor, reducing the number of adverse drug events and duplicative tests, and instituting a more efficient management of revenue (Levin & Hanson, 2011).

The Patient Protection and Affordable Care Act of 2010 (ACA) contains many provisions intended to increase access to and to lower the cost of health care. To do so, the ACA has adopted public health measures built upon health promotion and disease prevention. This emphasis on population health mandates insurance companies to cover programs that focus on the public health model of identifying and minimizing risk, such as regular examinations, appropriate screening tests, wellness programs, and free vaccinations. In addition, the ACA has extended portions of the Health Information Technology for Economic and Clinical Health (HITECH) Act. The "meaningful use" rule stops short of requiring changes in health care outcomes to be aligned with the fiscal incentives offered by the HITECH Act. Although providers must report quality data to show successful implementation, broad systemic changes would take more time before the "meaningful use" rule would show any significant changes in specific quality of care and patient outcomes. Think of it this way: the "meaningful use" rule becomes the guideline to achieve the ACA's strategic goal of improving the nation's health.

Although the "meaningful use" regulation originally required health care professionals, providers, and hospitals to incorporate systems that effectively use the electronic health record, the latest extensions in the ACA address payment reform, particularly in accountable care organizations and Medicare. These changes are significant to the provision of health care and the use of health care information technology (HIT). Earlier chapters discussed the issues involved in creating an electronic health record, with a brief look at reimbursement and standardization. Consider the following example. Mr. I. M. Apatient is seen by four different provider organizations over the course of a year. At each facility, he is given a different medical patient number. Tracking Mr. Apatient across multiple numbers can lead to unintentional errors. It makes sense from an HIT perspective to create a single master patient index to more easily track instances and reimbursement of care for Mr. Apatient.

However, data is still problematic when examining the wide variations in quality of care, outcomes, and health care practice. Behavioral health data are complex. Each behavioral health agency, organization, and delivery system has separate health information systems consisting of legacy and new databases that contain diverse formatting structures that may or may not be crosswalked to each other. Further, data collection and reporting requirements vary widely. Each entity has its preferred distribution or communication channels, its preferred formats, and its preferred schedules. Every time state agencies are reorganized, they create or inherit highly decentralized information management, infrastructure, technology, and operations (Hanson & Levin, 2010). Further, health and mental health data are combinations of numerous city, county, state, regional, national, regulatory, administrative, oversight, and financial data sets. These data, required by each state or federal agency, are then reported to other state and federal agencies that have oversight for Medicaid, Medicare, and other public entitlement programs (Hanson & Levin, 2010). These cumulated data are then used in program and patient outcomes evaluations, including comparative effectiveness research (CER).

CER was legislated in P.L. 111-5, the American Recovery and Reinvestment Act (ARRA, 2009). Over $1.1 billion has been allocated to support research on CER in two areas. The first area supports research to compare clinical outcomes, effectiveness, and appropriateness of services and procedures used to prevent, diagnose, or treat diseases. The second area encourages "the development and use of clinical registries, clinical data networks, and other forms of electronic health data to generate or obtain outcomes data" (ARRA, 2009). Further, CER has minimum threshold criteria that must be met, including decreasing the prevalence and burden of disease, treatment and utilization costs, variability in patient outcomes, and increasing patient benefit.

Implementing clinical decision-making tools into an MIS (management information system) or EHR (electronic health report) system increases the ability of practitioners to locate new diagnostic tools, and evidence-based practices will increase patient and practice outcomes. Surveillance data, a critical component of public health and mental health practice, plays an important role in health promotion, disease management, and disease prevention. Clinical trial data, combined with surveillance data, may create more effective disease registries, in which research on patient histories may determine the best clinical and health education practices at the individual and population health levels. However, the creation of new databases and analytic tools will need to bear in mind the federal requirements for and expected outcomes of health information technology.

MEASURING OUTCOMES DATA

According to the World Health Organization, mental illnesses account for more collective disability burden in developed countries than any other group of illnesses, including cancer and heart disease. The effects of mental illnesses on a person's ability to effectively function on a daily basis and the link between mental and physical health (chronic disease) generate disability. To determine the level of disability in a population requires evaluation. But what data are used? How are data codified? What does this mean from national and global perspectives?

In the United States, mental health measures are included in a number of established health surveillance surveys, such as the Centers for Disease Control and Prevention's

(CDC) National Health Interview Survey (NHIS), the National Health and Nutrition Examination Survey (NHANES), and the Behavioral Risk Factor Surveillance System (BRFSS). Surveillance surveys also capture the cost of care in a general population or with a focus on a specific identified public health issue, such as the Agency for Healthcare Research and Quality's Medical Expenditure Panel Survey, the Substance Abuse and Mental Health Services Administration's (SAMHSA's) National Survey on Drug Use and Health (NSDUH), and in the National Science Foundation's Panel Study of Income Dynamics.

In addition to these surveys, there are also national epidemiologic mental health data. The best known national epidemiologic surveys were the Epidemiologic Catchment Area Study (Regier et al., 1993), the National Comorbidity Survey (Kessler et al., 1994), the National Comorbidity Survey Replication (NCS-R) (Kessler & Merikangas, 2004), and the Collaborative Psychiatric Epidemiology Surveys (CPES) (Heeringa et al, 2004). The CPES integrated three surveys (the NCS-R, the National Survey of American Life, and the National Latino and Asian American Study) to provide national-level data on cultural and ethnic influences on mental and substance use disorders, utilization of mental health services, and chronic medical conditions. Not only have these data sets established benchmarks for rates of specific lifetime and previous 12-month mental disorders, they have also been used to document the prevalence of mental illnesses for the Surgeon General's reports and used as baseline data sources for measuring objectives in *Healthy People*.

There are new ways of using numeric and spatial data. Sayani (2012) describes a GIS application that provides graphical depictions of medically underserved areas; underserved populations; regions with a shortage of primary care, mental health, and dental health professionals; as well as the location of federally qualified health centers and hospitals, local health departments, and facilities with a shortage of health professionals. From a mental health informatics perspective, a number of questions emerge, including questions surrounding data source; data authenticity; data currency; the quality of data; uses of GIS data in program and outcomes assessment; and evaluation of GIS services, resources, and applications.

However, one of the more pressing questions deals with the use of personal health information in publicly available data sites and interactive maps and how such use complies with the Health Insurance Portability and Accountability Act (HIPAA). HIPAA requires the redaction of federally defined patient protected health and personal information to ensure confidentiality and privacy. This is particularly pertinent to small rural or neighborhood-level data, where populations are far more constrained as to the incidence of disease. Since different approaches will be needed to ensure confidentiality, this is an opportunity for new applications in informatics to create new blinded, cross-referencing, and de-identifying applications. However, new program applications would need approval by the appropriate local, state, and national agency review board(s), depending upon the scope of the data and its use. Interoperability, portability, and standard classifications and definitions, at national and international levels, would also need to be addressed.

Similar to U.S. health information systems, which rely upon a range of population-based and health facility–based data sources, global health is measured through the use of census, household surveys, vital registration systems, public health surveillance, administrative data, health services data, and health system monitoring data, also derived from local, state, regional, and national sources. The World Health Organization, for example, is focusing on a common monitoring and evaluation framework to strengthen health systems.

Health systems have been described in terms of six core components or "building blocks": (1) service delivery; (2) health workforce; (3) health information systems; (4) access to essential medicines; (5) financing; and (6) leadership/governance (WHO, 2010, p. vi). The WHO suggests that there are five components to a monitoring and evaluation framework. Three of these address associated progress and performance reviews, which evaluate all major disease programs and health system activities, and documentation of institutional capacity. In addition, the WHO emphasizes public access and synthesis of all health data sources to monitor performance and harmonization of indicators and measurement strategies across its partners in this initiative. These five components will provide critical information on the WHO's overall goals and strategies to improve population health.

From outcomes and informatics perspectives, there remain several challenges, particularly in the reconciliation of disparate systems and the discrepancies within and across systems to create a reliable and functional performance system. Consider the range of data used in the United States to determine the state of mental health services, performance, and outcomes. To be a partner using the WHO's monitoring and evaluation framework requires the United States to crosswalk its data across the WHO framework for health systems performance assessment (2000); the World Bank control knobs framework (Roberts et al., 2008); and the WHO building blocks framework (2007). In addition, the performance of national statistics offices may be measured by other international organizations, such as the United Nations (1994; Hoffmann, 1999) and the International Monetary Fund (DeVries, 1998; IMF, 2003).

Therefore, from an informatics perspective, data quality assurance is critical, especially when conducting comparative analyses across a diverse range of health care systems and practices. Generally, data quality assurance distinguishes assessment criteria for data outputs from those criteria that address the quality of institutional frameworks (the latter, of course, is a prerequisite for the generation of reliable data). Some quality frameworks will be used to assess national health data, while others will assess data at the international level. So, again, there will be added complexity in data collection, management, sharing, and analyses that must be addressed when assessing public health and mental health outcomes at national and global levels. Thus, for each metric or framework created, standards in definitions, classification, indicators, data sources, reporting formats, and data collection are critical to ensure objectivity and comparability over time and across localities, states, regions, and countries.

EVIDENCE-BASED POLICY MAKING

Another issue of great interest is the moving of evidence-based research to practice and to policy. There are two major advantages to evidence-based policy making: transparency and accountability. Understanding how a decision is made requires information about the process of decision making by policy makers, as well as an understanding of the criteria they use in their process. Further, to see the construction and representation of stakeholders in a specific decision-making event, it is critical to make sense of how an issue is "problematized," how information is analyzed, and how the information is integrated to determine best practices. Since policy processes go through different stages, from agenda setting to formulation to implementation, evidence therefore has the potential to influence the policy making process at each stage. However, different evidence and different mechanisms may be required at each of the policy stages.

Shaxson (2005) argues that we need evidence for a number of reasons: understanding the policy environment; appraising and assessing different policy options; showing clear lines of argument and evidence between future goals and the current situation; determining what is needed to meet strategic goals or intermediate objectives; influencing others to help achieve and implement policy; and effectively communicating the quality (breadth and depth) of the evidence to substantiate policy decisions.

However, the knowledge base for evidence-based policy making is consists of scientific, professional, political, institutional, and stakeholder knowledge. Scientific knowledge is generated by systematic research conducted by academic and research institutions. Professional knowledge of practitioners and professionals provides both explicit and tacit knowledge of the implementation and effectiveness of programs and policies in their settings, as in what works under what conditions. Institutional sources of expertise provide us with the knowledge of the role and function of these heterogeneous systems in the implementation and assessment of a policy decision. Stakeholder knowledge, in this case, defined narrowly to address the needs of the service users and their caregivers, provides the perspective and experiences of the patients in a service delivery system. All of these sources of knowledge generate an enormous amount of quantitative and qualitative data, including but not limited to statistics, observational studies, systematic reviews, meta-analyses; and experimental, longitudinal, and comparative studies; as well as expert opinions and descriptive studies. But what is good data for policy making?

From an evidence perspective, good data is effective data. It allows policy makers to show the parameters ("what, why, when, and how") of their decision, as well as the possible effects of one decision over another. In addition, more sophisticated quantitative and qualitative methodologies are being developed to provide different types of data that were impossible to determine previously. Hence, evidence-based policy making requires the existence and availability of reliable evidence at different stages in the public policy-making process. Scott suggests, "Evidence-based policy-making means that, wherever possible, public policy decisions should be informed by careful analysis using sound and transparent data" (Scott, 2005, p. 1). Scott further defines evidence-based policy making as "the systematic and rigorous use of statistics" to bring an issue to the attention of policy makers, to inform policy choices and program design to address the issue, to forecast future impacts of addressing or ignoring the issue, to monitor policy implementation, and to evaluate policy impact (2005, p. 1).

Greenhalgh and Russell (2009) suggest that there are a number of challenges to evidence-based policy making and the design of policy alternatives. First, scalability is problematic for complex issues. Although there may be a common objective, such as improving the overall quality of a nation's health, there are numerous sub-objectives that must be identified and examined, and alternatives generated. Second, all policy objectives have a value, and all alternatives must be ranked to meet the needs of the stakeholders who will be affected by the new policy. Coordination of objectives often requires ranking incompatible values. Third, data may be ambiguous, irreconcilable, or deficient. Fourth, the framing of the problem may be poorly done or the underlying assumptions of the research question(s) are driven by another agenda other than effectively solving the problem.

Fifth, evidence may not be applicable to the local situation or context. For example, the success of evidence-based practices in developing countries is difficult to compare with developed countries. Finally, by the time a decision has been reached, the projected policy outcome may have changed due to a modification in objectives or to an unforeseen disaster event, such as a tsunami. Hence, there are opportunities for new methodologies in the field of informatics.

One such methodology for implementing evidence-driven program and policy design in the policy-making process may be computational modeling. DeSouza and Lin (2011) argue that computational modeling simulates various environments, interventions, and the processes in which certain outcomes emerge from the possible decisions available to policy makers. This allows policy makers to observe both the intended and unintended consequences of policy alternatives. The first step is to construct a conceptual model. DeSouza and Lin (2011) identify four steps to establishing a conceptual model:

1. Identify key constructs and processes;
2. Translate them into model variables and mechanisms;
3. Set up model inputs and outputs based on specific policy problems; and
4. Specify assumptions that bound the inputs and outputs (DeSouza & Lin, 2011, p. 12).

By following these steps and creating a conceptual model, policy makers will have a better perception of the policy problem, its constituent components that need to be addressed, and its potential solutions.

Fox (2005) reminds us of the importance of other rigorous methodologies in policy making, such as systematic reviews. Like computational modeling, the cost of performing a systematic review of the literature ranges from $50,000 to $250,000 or higher (Fox, 2005). However, systematic reviews provide evidence as to the efficacy and effectiveness of many types of interventions, procedures, and treatments. For example, the Centers for Medicare and Medicaid Services began commissioning systematic reviews in 1999 as a step in making national coverage decisions. In 2000, the State of Oregon began collaborating with the Oregon Evidence-Based Practice Center to produce systematic reviews of drug classes to gather the best possible evidence for implementing its preferred drug list (PDL) (Oregon Health & Science University, 2012). That marked the beginning of the Drug Effectiveness Review Project (DERP), which has grown to a consortium of 15 states and 2 nonprofit organizations (Fox, 2005).

The DERP establishes priorities for evaluating drug classes through systematic reviews. The evaluations are conducted at one of the 13 Evidence-Based Practice Centers established by the Agency for Healthcare Research and Quality. Health practitioners and the general public are encouraged to comment during the review process. All completed and updated reviews are available on a website hosted by the Center for Evidence-Based Policy of the Oregon Health and Science University, which manages the project on behalf of the consortium (Oregon Health & Science University, 2012).

The use of the DERP reviews by policy makers has expanded, informing decisions about public employees' coverage and workers' compensation coverage (Fox, 2005). Further, the DERP reviews are written using probabilistic language, which clearly delineates what is certain knowledge and what is reasoned judgment, and the reviews do not make recommendations for policy. Hence, each review can lead to different coverage decisions.

There has been interest expressed in expanding the types of evidence to include observational and qualitative studies (Mundy & Stein, 2008), as well as health impact assessments and economic evaluations (Fielding & Briss, 2006). With more quantitative analyses created for use in policy making, there is a vital need to make statistics understandable and to have a clear foundation on what statistics can and cannot tell us. As discussed earlier, users of data may be primary, secondary or tertiary users, working with raw data, graphically interpreted data, or narrative data. Numerical and/or statistical literacy will be critical for persons working in mental health services research, practice, or informatics, as will be the ability to create effective syntheses of numeric, statistical, spatial, and narrative data. We also see the integration of qualitative and quantitative data to place decision making into local and/or situational contexts—a critical and salient opportunity for mental health informatics.

Implications for Mental Health Informatics

This chapter has reiterated several points that we feel are important: the potential impact of informatics on legislation, measurement of outcomes, and evidence-based practice. While we are leery of forecasting what is down the road since things change so quickly (in state and federal legislation, technology, communication, and organizations), we choose to provide a "short-term" perspective rather than a "long-term" perspective. Thus, we are certain about one aspect: mental health informatics must meet the needs of evolving health and mental health care systems, exchanging data, orchestrating the coordination of care across settings, improving clinical decision making, and improving the quality of life of persons with physical and mental illnesses in at-risk populations throughout the United States. It will be interesting to see how the field evolves to meet these challenges.

References

American Recovery and Reinvestment Act of 2009, Pub. L. 111-5, 111th Congress, §1401.

DeSouza, K. C., & Lin, Y. (2011). Towards evidence-driven policy design: Complex adaptive systems and computational modeling. *The Innovation Journal: The Public Sector Innovation Journal, 16*(1), Article 7. Retrieved from http://www.innovation.cc/scholarly-style/desouza_lin_policy_informatics_v16i1a7.pdf.

De Vries, W. (1998). *How are we doing? Performance indicators for national statistical systems.* Washington, DC: International Monetary Fund.

Fielding, J. E., & Briss, P. A. (2006). Promoting evidence-based public health policy: Can we have better evidence and more action? *Health Affairs, 25*(4), 969–978. doi: 10.1377/hlthaff.25.4.969.

Fox, D. M. (2005). Evidence of evidence-based health policy: The politics of systematic reviews in coverage decisions. *Health Affairs, 24*(1), 114–122. doi: 10.1377/hlthaff.24.1.114.

Greenhalgh, T., & Russell, J. (2009). Evidence-based policymaking: A critique. *Perspectives in Biology & Medicine, 52*(2), 304–318. doi: 10.1353/pbm.0.0085.

Hanson, A., & Levin, B. L. (2010). The complexity of mental health services research data. In B. L. Levin, K. D. Hennessy, & J. Petrila (Eds.). *Mental health services: A public health perspective* (3rd ed.). New York: Oxford Unviersity Press.

Heeringa, S. G., Wagner, J., Torres, M., Duan, N., Adams, T., & Berglund, P. (2004). Sample designs and sampling methods for the Collaborative Psychiatric Epidemiology Studies (CPES). *International Journal of Methods in Psychiatric Research, 13*(4), 221–240.

Hoffmann, E. (1999). *Standard statistical classification: Basic principles.* New York: United Nations Statistical Division, Bureau of Statistics.

International Monetary Fund. (2003). *Data quality assessment framework (DQAF) for national accounts statistics.* Washington, DC: International Monetary Fund. Retrieved from http://dsbb.imf.org/images/pdfs/dqrs_nag.pdf (see also http://dsbb.imf.org/vgn/images/pdfs/dqrs_Genframework.pdf).

Kessler, R. C., McGonagle, K. A., Zhao, S., Nelson, C. B., Hughes, M., Eshleman, S., Wittchen, H. U., & Kendler, K. S. (1994). Lifetime and 12-month prevalence of DSM-III-R psychiatric disorders in the United States: Results from the National Comorbidity Survey. *Archives of General Psychiatry, 51*(1), 8–19.

Kessler, R. C., & Merikangas, K. R. (2004). The National Comorbidity Survey Replication (NCS-R): Background and aims. *International Journal of Methods in Psychiatric Research, 13*(2), 60–68.

Laflamme, F. M., Pietraszek, W. E., & Rajadhyax, N. V. (2010). Reforming hospitals with IT investment. *McKinsey on Business Technology, 20,* 27–33.

Levin, B. L., & Hanson, A. (2011). Mental health informatics. In N. Cummings & W. T. O'Donohue (Eds.), *Understanding the behavioral healthcare crisis: The promise of integrated care and diagnostic reform* (pp. 59–82). New York: Routledge.

Mundy, K. M., & Stein, K. F. (2008). Meta-analysis as a basis for evidence-based practice: The question is, why not? *Evidence-Based Practice in Psychiatric and Mental Health Nursing 14*(4), 326–328.

Oregon Health & Science University. (2012). *Drug Effectiveness Review Project (DERP).* Retrieved from www.ohsu.edu/drugeffectiveness.

Orszag, P. R. (2008). *Growth in health care costs* (CBO Testimony). Washington, DC: The Congressional Budget Office. Retrieved from http://www.cbo.gov/ftpdocs/89xx/doc8948/01-31-HealthTestimony.pdf.

Regier, D. A., Farmer, M. E., Rae, D. S., Myers, J. K., Kramer, M., Robins, L. N., George, L. K., Karno, M, & Locke, B. Z. (1993). One-month prevalence of mental disorders in the United States and sociodemographic characteristics: The Epidemiologic Catchment Area study. *Acta Psychiatrica Scandanavica, 88*(1), 35–47.

Roberts, M. J., Hsiao, W., Berman, P., & Reich, M. R. (2008). *Getting health reform right: A guide to improving performance and equity.* New York: Oxford University Press.

Sayani, S. (2012). Geomapping health-related data. *Science Translational Medicine, 4*(119), 119mr4. doi: 10.1126/scitranslmed.3003383.

Scott, C. (2005). *Measuring up to the measurement problem: The role of statistics in evidence based policy-making.* Paris 21. Retrieved from http://www.paris21.org/sites/default/files/MUMPS-full.pdf.

Shaxson, L. (2005). Is your evidence robust enough? Questions for policy makers and practitioners. *Evidence and Policy: A Journal of Research, Debate and Practice, 1*(1), 101–111.

United Nations. (1994). *Fundamental principles of official statistics*. New York: United Nations. Retrieved from http://unstats.un.org/unsd/dnss/gp/fundprinciples.aspx.

Wildavsky, A. (1979). *Speaking truth to power: The art and craft of policy analysis*. Boston, MA: Little Brown.

World Health Organization. (2007). *Everybody's business: Strengthening health systems to improve health outcomes: WHO's framework for action*. Geneva: WHO. Retrieved from http://www.who.int/healthsystems/strategy/everybodys_business.pdf.

World Health Organization. (2010). *Monitoring the building blocks of health systems: A handbook of indicators and their measurement strategies*. Geneva: WHO. Retrieved from http://www.who.int/healthinfo/systems/monitoring/en/index.html.

World Health Organization. (2000). *World health report 2000: Health systems: Improving performance*. Geneva: WHO. Retrieved from http://www.who.int/whr/2000/en/.

Index